OXFORD
UNIVERSITY PRESS

SOUTHERN AFRICA

Oxford University Press Southern Africa (Pty) Ltd

Vasco Boulevard, Goodwood, Cape Town, Republic of South Africa
P O Box 12119, N1 City, 7463, Cape Town, Republic of South Africa

Oxford University Press Southern Africa (Pty) Ltd is a subsidiary of Oxford University Press,
Great Clarendon Street, Oxford OX2 6DP.

The Press, a department of the University of Oxford, furthers the University's objective of
excellence in research, scholarship, and education by publishing worldwide in

Oxford New York

Auckland Cape Town Dar es Salaam Hong Kong Karachi
Kuala Lumpur Madrid Melbourne Mexico City Nairobi
New Delhi Shanghai Taipei Toronto

With offices in

Argentina Austria Brazil Chile Czech Republic France Greece
Guatemala Hungary Italy Japan Poland Portugal Singapore South Korea
Switzerland Turkey Ukraine Vietnam

Oxford is a registered trade mark of Oxford University Press
in the UK and in certain other countries

Published in South Africa
by Oxford University Press Southern Africa (Pty) Ltd, Cape Town

Handbook of Family Medicine
Third edition published 2011
ISBN 978 0 19 599817 7

The moral rights of the author have been asserted
Database right Oxford University Press Southern Africa (Pty) Ltd (maker)

First edition published 2000
Second edition published 2006
Third edition published 2011
Third impression 2012

Publishing manager: Alida Terblanche
Commissioning editor: Marisa Montemarano
Development editor: Lisa Andrews
Project manager: Janine Loedolff
Designer: Judith Cross
Cover design: Oswald Kurten
Medical proofreader: Dr Bridget Farham
Indexer: Jeanne Cope

Set in 8 pt on 10 pt Utopia and 7 pt on 9 pt Myriad Pro by Elbert Visser
Cover reproduction by C2 Digital
Printed and bound by ABC Press, Kinghall Avenue, Epping Industria 2, Cape Town
118685

Abridged table of contents

iv

Contents

Contributors

Prof Julia Blitz
Division of Family Medicine
and Primary Care
University of Stellenbosch

Dr Graham Bresick
Division of Family Medicine
School of Public Health and
Family Medicine
University of Cape Town

Prof Nzapfurundi Chabikuli
Family Health International,
Nigeria
And Hon Lecturer, Department
of Family Medicine
University of Pretoria

Dr Maria Christodoulou
Division of Family Medicine
and Primary Care
University of Stellenbosch

Prof Ian Couper
Division of Rural Health
Department of Family
Medicine
University of the Witwatersrand

Prof Marietjie de Villiers
Deputy Dean of Education
Faculty of Health Sciences
University of Stellenbosch

Prof Sam Fehrsen
Former Head of Department of
Family Medicine, MEDUNSA
Hon Lecturer, Department of
Family Medicine
University of Pretoria

Dr Indiran Govender
Department of Family
Medicine
Nelson R Mandela School of
Medicine
University of KwaZulu-Natal

Prof Jannie Hugo
Department of Family
Medicine
University of Pretoria

Prof Bob Mash
Division of Family Medicine
and Primary Care
Department of
Interdisciplinary Health
Sciences
Stellenbosch University

Prof Khaya Mfenyana
Executive Dean
Faculty of Health Sciences
Walter Sisulu University

Dr Keymanthri Moodley
Bioethics Unit: Tygerberg
Division
Faculty of Health Sciences
University of Stellenbosch

Prof Soornarain S (Cyril) Naidoo
Department of Family
Medicine
Nelson R Mandela School of
Medicine
University of KwaZulu-Natal

Prof Gboyega A. Ogunbanjo
Department of Family
Medicine and Primary Health
Care
Medunsa Campus
University of Limpopo

Dr Michael Pather
Division of Family Medicine
and Primary Care
Department of
Interdisciplinary Health
Sciences
University of Stellenbosch

Prof Steve Reid
  Primary Health Care
  Directorate
  University of Cape Town

Dr Bev Schweitzer
  Division of Family Medicine
  School of Public Health and
  Family Medicine
  University of Cape Town

Chapters 7 and 8

Prof Hanneke Brits
  Department of Family
  Medicine
  University of the Free State
Prof Jimmy Chandia
  Department of Family
  Medicine
  Walter Sisulu University
Dr Indiran Govender
  Department of Family
  Medicine
  Nelson R Mandela School of
  Medicine
  University of Kwa-Zulu Natal
Dr Romona Govender
  Department of Family
  Medicine,
  Nelson R Mandela School of
  Medicine
  University of KwaZulu-Natal
Dr Liz Gwyther
  Division of Family Medicine
  School of Public Health and
  Primary Health Care
  University of Cape Town
Dr Louis Jenkins
  Division of Family Medicine
  and Primary Care
  Department of
  Interdisciplinary Health
  Sciences
  Stellenbosch University

Prof Bob Mash
  Division of Family Medicine
  and Primary Care
  Department of
  Interdisciplinary Health
  Sciences
  Stellenbosch University
Dr Mosedi Namane
  Division of Family Medicine
  School of Public Health and
  Family Medicine
  University of Cape Town
Dr John Ndimande
  Department of Family
  Medicine and Primary Health
  Care
  Medunsa Campus
  University of Limpopo
Dr Don O'Mahoney
  Department of Family
  Medicine
  Walter Sisulu University
Dr N Ranjith
  Division of Cardiology
  Department of Medicine
  Nelson R Mandela School of
  Medicine
  University of KwaZulu-Natal

Dr Zandy Rosochacki
Division of Family Medicine
and Primary Care
Department of
Interdisciplinary Health
Sciences
Stellenbosch University
Dr Andrew Ross
Department of Family
Medicine
Nelson R Mandela School of
Medicine
University of KwaZulu-Natal
Dr Helen Sammons
Centre for Rehabilitation
Studies
Stellenbosch University
Dr Bev Schweitzer
Division of Family Medicine
School of Public Health and
Family Medicine
University of Cape Town

Dr Claire van Deventer
Department of Family
Medicine
University of Witwatersrand
Dr Werner Viljoen
Division of Family Medicine
and Primary Care
Department of
Interdisciplinary Health
Sciences
Stellenbosch University
Dr Parimalarani Yogiswaren
Department of Family
Medicine
Walter Sisulu University

Disclaimer

While every effort has been made to check drug dosages in this handbook, it is still possible that errors have been overlooked. Dosages continue to be revised and new side effects recognized. Oxford University Press makes no representation, express or implied, that the drug dosages in this book are correct. For these reasons, the reader is strongly urged to consult the *South African Medicines Formulary* or the drug manufacturer's printed instructions before administering any of the drugs recommended in this clinical handbook. The authors and the publishers do not accept responsibility or legal liability for any errors in the text or for the misuse or misapplication of material in this work.

The authors and the publishers gratefully acknowledge permission to reproduce material in this book. Every effort has been made to trace copyright holders, but where this has proved impossible, the publishers would be grateful for information which would enable them to amend any omissions in future editions.

Foreword

I recently attended a lecture by Professor Khaya Mfenyana, Dean of the Faculty of Health Sciences at Walter Sisulu University in Eastern Cape province. Khaya emphasised the importance of "going deeper in defining family medicine within the context of Africa." This wonderful textbook does just that.

I have been very impressed reading through the chapters of this book. This third edition of the *Handbook of Family Medicine* provides an ideal resource for meeting the needs of family doctors in South Africa, and I expect also in many other nations in Africa. This is an invaluable 'one-stop shop' text covering the breadth of important family medicine issues. It is written by a talented team of authors who combine their extensive practical clinical knowledge with their experience as dedicated and respected educators.

I am convinced that strong primary care and family medicine is the answer to the health care challenges facing every nation. If family medicine is going to meet the health and wellbeing needs of the many diverse communities across the continent of Africa, then it needs to adapt to changing health needs and expectations. Health solutions for Africa need to be developed in Africa, for Africa, by the people of Africa. This textbook is a vital contribution to this process.

Family medicine also needs to focus on equity: equity of access to health care and equity of outcomes of health care. Strong family medicine will enable us to ensure that high quality health care is available to all people in our nations, including those who are disadvantaged and marginalised. I especially welcome the case studies in this book, based on real people, which provide lessons and instruction on how to manage some very challenging clinical situations.

As family doctors we need to have detailed knowledge of the breadth of clinical conditions if we are to provide effective health care and advice to all our patients. The diversity of new findings in all areas of medicine can be overwhelming for the medical student or busy family doctor as we each try to develop a balanced, informed and practical approach to providing up-to-date quality care in our own individual clinical settings. Most importantly, this text addresses the context of providing high quality family medicine care in developing countries, especially in areas of disadvantage and low resources.

The *Handbook of Family Medicine* is an immensely useful contribution to the body of knowledge for general practice. Not only does it deserve to become an essential resource for medical students, but I suspect there will be many copies sitting permanently on desks in front of family doctors across Africa and being referred to on a regular basis as we each strive to provide the best quality service to the people who trust us for their medical care and advice.

In his foreword to the original edition of this textbook, distinguished South African family doctor and past Wonca President, Professor Bruce Sparks wrote, "There is no other book which encapsulates the various aspects of the discipline of family medicine in a South African context in such a concise and understandable way." This new edition lives up to this well-deserved reputation.

Professor Michael Kidd AM
President-elect
World Organization of Family Doctors (Wonca)

Introduction: Family medicine in an African context

Introduction

Previous editions of the Handbook of Family Medicine have drawn heavily on definitions and principles derived from European and North American publications. Since the last edition was published in 2006 there has been an extensive dialogue and a number of publications in sub-Saharan Africa that articulate a clearer picture of what family medicine means in an African context (Mash, 2010).

The African context is broadly characterised by a number of features. African communities are frequently poor, sometimes very rural and remote, and almost always connected to traditional health systems and beliefs (Reid, 2011). District health services are often underdeveloped and struggle for adequate resources to meet the needs of the population. Equipment and medication supplies are often scarce or erratic. Referral of patients with more complicated or serious problems to specialists in the cities is often difficult. The family physician in an African context, therefore, has significant challenges to overcome in his or her daily work. Sub-Saharan Africa is also predicted to have a shortage of 240 000 doctors and 551 000 nurses by 2015 (Scheffler, 2009).

In South Africa there have also been important developments since the last edition of the Handbook. In 2007 the Health Professions Council recognised family medicine as a specialty on an equal footing with other specialist disciplines. This decision has had major implications for the training of family physicians. Doctors who want to specialise in family medicine must now work in a registrar post for a supervised training period of at least three years and in an accredited training complex. Most registrars obtain a Master in Medicine degree from a South African university and in the near future will be required to sit a single national exit examination. This will most likely be offered by the Colleges of Medicine. Once qualified, family physicians will be employed in specialist posts within the district health services at district hospitals and community health centres. Already a number of specialist family physicians have been employed throughout the country.

During this period several departments of family medicine have been involved with the training of a new cadre of mid-level health worker

– namely the clinical associate. Within the next few years we should see clinical associates being employed to assist the health care team at district hospitals.

Currently in South Africa there is political commitment to the introduction of National Health Insurance and if this becomes a reality over the next few years, it will have major implications for the integration of public and private practices within the district health system. The family physician in both public and private settings may see their familiar landscape change dramatically.

The role of the family physician

According to Mash, the family physician has six important roles to play in the district health care system (2008):

Care-provider

The family physician is a competent clinician who is able to deal with the majority of health problems in the community that he or she serves. Family physicians work at the district hospital as well as the clinic or health centre. At the district hospital they need to look after patients with a broad range of diseases and perform appropriate procedures in areas such as anaesthetics, general surgery, obstetrics and orthopaedics. The family physician also needs relational skills and an ability to form effective doctor-patient relationships. These skills include a patient-centred approach, good communication skills and a bio-psychosocial assessment with attention to the patient's family and broader context.

Consultant

In South Africa first contact care in the public sector is usually with clinical nurse practitioners, who remain the lynchpin at clinics and health centres, but will often call upon the family physician as a consultant to see more complicated or difficult patients. Patients may be referred to the family physician within the health centre or from outlying clinics. Patients may also be referred by more junior doctors or other members of the primary care team. Some large health centres may have their own family physician or the family physician may visit weekly. The family physician must be part of a well-functioning clinical team.

Mentor and clinical teacher

Primary care is offered by a team of nurses, doctors and allied health professionals and the family physician is usually the most senior clinician, often mentoring and teaching other health workers who are part of the primary health care team. This role may require particular skills in adult learning and clinical teaching. In many hospitals the role of clinical teacher is driven by the need of the family physician to share clinical responsibilities with junior and often transient staff, such as doctors doing community service.

Supervisor

A more formal aspect of the teaching role is that of an accredited supervisor for medical students, interns and registrars. which often requires more formal educational activities and assessment and responsibilities to the university and Health Professions Council. Again, this role may require additional skills in education and teaching.

Manager

The family physician is primarily a clinician, but in most facilities will have responsibility for co-ordination of clinical services and for improving the quality of those services. Clinical governance may involve organising morbidity and mortality meetings, quality improvement cycles or continuing professional development activities. Often the family physician's clinical managerial role will extend beyond the facility to other clinics or health centres in the sub-district. The family physician is usually a member of the facility's management team and may also be part of the district management.

Community-orientated practitioner

Family physicians are expected to not only think about the individual patients that come to them for health care, but also about the population as a whole within their sub-district. Often the problems presented by individual patients point to underlying issues in the community. An awareness of the patient's context is enhanced by "thinking family" and a holistic bio-psychosocial approach. More than this, however, a community-orientated approach is based on a deeper understanding of the health problems in the community and the underlying social determinants of health. For example, teenage pregnancy may be driven by inadequate recreational activities and underage drinking in local shebeens. Chronic non-communicable diseases may be driven by unhealthy food options at local supermarkets or a lack of access to green spaces for physical activity. While the family physician cannot solve these problems single-handedly he or she can contribute to change through collaboration with community leaders, other health care workers and government and non-government organisations.

Ten principles of family medicine

Principles may be thought of as beliefs that guide thinking and behaviour. While the roles of the family physician are described above, this section looks at the top ten underlying principles (McWhinney, 1997; Mash, 2010).

1   *The family physician is committed to the person rather than to a particular body of knowledge, group of diseases, or a special technique.* The family physician responds to any problem that a patient may present with and draws from the whole body of medical knowledge concerning the patient's needs and remains committed to the patient. That commitment has no defined end point – it continues for as long as they both wish to maintain the relationship. The family physician works in a patient-centred way that allows them to hear and clarify the patient's concerns and to identify why the patient has consulted them. The patient-centred clinical method is described in Chapter 2.

2   *The family physician attaches importance to the subjective aspects of medicine.* The family physician considers both their and the patient's subjective experience. For example the patient's concerns, expectations, beliefs, feelings and experiences may be explicitly acknowledged and elicited. These subjective aspects are not considered as a peripheral interference in the process of assessing and treating patients but are acknowledged as central and important aspects of the process of care. This is discussed further in Chapter 3.

3   *The family physician seeks to understand the context of the illness.* The family physician wishes to understand the context within which the patient's illness has occurred. The biomedical context may include their past medical history, medications, allergies, smoking, alcohol and genetic predisposition to disease. In family medicine, however, the context is expanded to include the family, occupation, and community environment. Chapter 4 looks at the thinking family approach in family medicine.

4   *The family physician sees every contact with patients as an opportunity*

for prevention or health promotion. The family physician recognises that each consultation presents an invaluable opportunity for modifying the course of an illness or preventing future illness. Preventive medicine and health promotion are dealt with in Chapter 5.

5   *The family physician is able to perform most of the common clinical procedures and operations appropriate to the district health system.* The clinical skills required of the family physician at the district hospital, health centre and clinic have been defined (Couper, 2008; Mash, 2006). The family physician should also refer patients appropriately for procedures that are outside their scope of practice

6   *The family physician views their practice as a population at risk.* The family physician is interested in the health needs and priorities of their practice population as a whole. For many this will mean an interest in the population living within their health district. The family physician is alert to these needs and will work in a collaborative way with the community, colleagues, and other key people and organisations to make effective interventions that improve the health of the population. Chapter 9 deals with community-orientated primary care.

7   *Family physicians see themselves as part of a community-wide network of supportive health care agencies.* The family physician understands and uses all available resources in the community and makes themselves available to the greater community as one such resource. In Chapter 10, we look at using available resources to put the principles into practice.

8   *The family physician is an effective clinical manager.* The family physician manages and deploys resources by decision making that is evidence-based, ethical and sensitive to the personal needs of the patient, as well as equitable and fair to the community and health system. The family physician is also committed to improving the quality of clinical services offered by the health care team. This is discussed further in Chapter 10.

9   *Family physicians see themselves as mentors or teachers for other practitioners in the district health system.* The family physician should be trained in educational and teaching skills that support their role. The family physician should also be able to function in and offer leadership to the multi-disciplinary primary health care team.

10 *The family physician is a life-long learner.* Many consultations in primary care challenge the family physician and raise questions about the best practice, the latest treatment, the best advice, or diagnostic tests. Knowledge in primary care is one of breadth more than depth in any particular discipline. It is therefore a particular challenge

for the family physician to have skills in answering the questions that come up and to become a lifelong learner. These skills are described in Chapter 13.

Family medicine, primary health care and primary care

The World Health Organisation (WHO) defined primary health care as "essential health care made universally accessible to individuals and families in the community by means acceptable to them, through their full participation and at a cost that the community and the country can afford. It forms an integral part of the country's health care system, of which it is the nucleus, and of the overall socio-economic development of the community" (1978). Primary health care in its broadest sense is a philosophy or set of values and principles for organising the health system as a whole.

Since primary health care was conceptualised at Alma Ata in 1978, many countries, including South Africa, have attempted to implement health systems based on a primary health care model. The 2008 World Health Report *Primary Health Care: Now More Than Ever* was devoted to re-focusing our attention and commitment to primary health care (WHO, 2008).

The term primary care was first used in 1920 in Britain to distinguish health care given in clinics and general practices from secondary care delivered in hospitals. The term was later expanded to include primary medical or clinical care. In this book, the term primary care will be used to refer to all care delivered at the first or primary level of contact in contrast with care delivered in the hospital. Over the years research has also helped to identify the core components of effective primary care as shown in Table I (Kringos, 2010). The family physician makes an important contribution to the realisation of core dimensions of primary care systems and the principles of family medicine are congruent with the philosophy of primary health care.

In South Africa the family physician is a general practitioner who has completed four years of vocational training, has an additional qualification in family medicine, and is registered as a specialist in family medicine with the Health Professions Council of South Africa.

Table 1 Core dimensions of primary care systems

STRUCTURE

Governance of the primary care system

The governance dimension can be summarised as the vision and direction of health policy exerting influence through regulation, advocacy, collecting and using information. Eight features of primary care governance have been identified:

1. Health (care) goals: The vision and direction of a primary care system depends on explicit health or health care goals at national level.

2. Policy on equity in access to primary care services: Equity in access can be influenced by policy development and regulation of the distribution of human resources and quality of care across geographical areas, by setting policy objectives regarding the duration of waiting time for (specific) primary care services; and by assuring universal financial coverage for primary care services by a publicly accountable body.

3. (De)centralisation of primary care management and service development: This is shaped by the level (national, regional, local) at which primary care policies are determined, the degree in which standards allow for variation in primary care practices geographically, and the development of policies on community participation in primary care management and priority setting.

4. Quality management infrastructure in primary care: This can consist of a number of mechanisms that need to be in place to assure adequate quality of care. These include co-ordination of quality management, quality assessment mechanisms, certification of providers, licensing of facilities, quality incentives, availability of quality information, availability of relevant clinical guidelines, professional competence and standardisation of facility equipment.

5. Appropriate technology in primary care: Medical technology in terms of techniques, drugs, equipment and procedures are crucial in the delivery of primary care. Appropriate development and use can be stimulated at government level by developing a national policy or strategy concerning the application of ICT in primary care, and by organising guidance to government and providers on technology appraisal on the use of new and existing medicines and treatments.

6. Patient advocacy: This can be embedded by primary care-oriented patient organisations, and patient compliance procedures in care facilities.

7. Ownership status of primary care practices: This provides an indication of the level of government involvement in primary care provision.

8. Integration of primary care in the health care system: Integration of primary care through interdisciplinary collaboration between primary care and secondary care, and task substitution and delegation can be promoted by governmental integration programmes, or legislation.

Economic conditions of the primary care system

The economic condition of a primary care system is made up of six features:

1. Health care funding system: The method of financing health care for the majority of the population, such as taxes, health insurance, or private means.

2. Health care expenditures: Total expenditures on health care.

3. Primary care expenditures: Total expenditures on primary care.

4. Employment status of primary care workforce: For example, salaried employed providers, or self-employed providers with/without contract(s) with health service or insurance.

5. Remuneration system of primary care workforce: For example fee-for-service payment, capitation payment, salary payment or mixed payment.

6. Income of primary care workforce: Annual income of primary care workforce, also compared to specialists.

Primary care workforce development

The workforce development dimension can be summarised as the profile of primary care professionals that make up the primary care workforce, and the position that they take in the health care system. The following six features of this dimension were identified:

1. Profile of primary care workforce: The type of health care professionals that are considered to be part of the primary care workforce, and their gender balance.

2. Recognition and responsibilities: Whether the primary care discipline is officially recognised as a separate discipline among the medical disciplines, with recognised responsibilities.

3. Education and retention: Vocational training requirements for primary care professionals, primary care workforce supply and retention problems, and capacity planning.

4. Professional associations: The organisation of professional associations for the primary care workforce.

5. Academic status of the primary care discipline: Reflected by academic departments of family medicine/primary care within universities.

6. Future development of the primary care workforce: Hampering threats to the current development and expected trends in the future development of the primary care workforce, from the point of view of stakeholders.

PROCESS

Access to primary care services

Access to primary care services can be defined in terms of seven features:

1. Availability of primary care services: The volume and type of primary care services relative to population needs.

2. Geographic accessibility of primary care services: Remoteness of services in terms of travel distance for patients.

3. Accommodation of accessibility: The manner in which resources are organised to accommodate access (for example appointment systems, after-hours care arrangements, home visits)

4. Affordability of primary care services: Financial barriers patients experience to receive primary care services, such as co-payments and cost-sharing arrangements.

5. Acceptability of primary care services: Patient satisfaction with the organisation of primary care.

6. Utilisation of primary care services: Actual consumption of primary care services.

7. Equality in access: The extent to which access to primary care services is provided on the basis of health needs, without systematic differences on the basis of individual or social characteristics.

Continuity of primary care

The continuity of care dimension can be summarised as a hierarchy of three features:

1. Longitudinal continuity of care: Having a long-term relationship between primary care providers and their patients in their practice beyond specific episodes of illness or disease between a single provider and a family is stressed.

2. Informational continuity of care: An organised collection of each patient's medical information readily available to any health care provider caring for the patient. This can be reached through medical record keeping, clinical support and referral systems.

3. Relational continuity of care: The quality of the longitudinal relationship between primary care providers and patients, in terms of accommodation of patient's needs and preferences, such as communication and respect for patients.

Co-ordination of primary care

The co-ordination of care dimensions reflects the ability of primary care providers to co-ordinate the use of other levels of health care. The following features were identified from co-ordination of care studies:

1. Gatekeeping system: The level of direct access for patients to health care providers without a referral from a primary care provider.

2. Primary care practice and team structure: For example shared practices, team premises and team size and tenure.

3. Skill-mix of primary care providers: Diversification and substitution of primary care providers.

4. Integration of primary care-secondary care: Care integration can be achieved through specialist outreach models and clinical protocols facilitating shared care.

5. Integration of primary care and public health: The extent to which primary care providers collaborate with practitioners from the public health sector to provide services that influence health.

Comprehensiveness of primary care services

Comprehensiveness of primary care services represents the range of services available in primary care to meet patients' health care needs. A distinction can be made between:

1. Range of medical equipment available.
2. Range of health problems for which first contact care is provided.
3. Range of diagnoses for which treatment and follow-up care are provided.
4. Range of medical technical procedures and preventive care provided.
5. Range of mother and child and reproductive health care services provided.
6. Range of health promotion activities provided.

OUTCOME

Quality of primary care

The quality of primary care resembles the degree to which health services meet the needs of patients, and standards of care. This dimension mirrors the quality of the services provided in primary care:

1. Prescribing behaviour of primary care providers: For example the frequency at which providers prescribe medicine.
2. Quality of diagnosis and treatment in primary care: For example reflected by the occurrence of avoidable hospitalisation for acute conditions.
3. Quality of management of chronic diseases: For example the prevalence of chronic diseases, receipt of treatment characteristics, and the occurrence of avoidable hospitalisation for chronic conditions.
4. Quality of mental health care: For example prevalence of mental disorders, and anti-depressant medication, and continuity of mental care.
5. Quality of maternal and child health care: Reflected for example by maternal mortality rates, occurrence of preventive screening for pregnant women, and infant vaccination.
6. Quality of health promotion: For example obesity, smoking or alcohol use in the population.
7. Quality of preventive care: For example the occurrence of preventable conditions, or cancer screening.

Efficiency of primary care

Efficiency of primary care is the balance between the level of resources in the system used to treat patients to come to certain outcomes. Primary care studies approach efficiency in different ways:

1. Allocative and productive efficiency: Respectively, minimising patient's opportunity cost of time spent in treatment; maximising the patient's outcome, minimising the cost per patient.
2. Technical efficiency: A system is technically efficient if it cannot reduce its resource use without reducing its ability to treat patients or to reach certain outcomes.

3. Efficiency in performance of primary care workforce: Reflected by basic figures relating to the provision of care, such as number of consultations and their duration, frequency of prescription medicines (unnecessary use), and the number of new referrals to medical specialists.

EQUITY IN HEALTH

Equity in health seems to be a relatively small, though important, area of research in primary care. It is the absence of systematic and potentially remediable differences in health status across population groups.

It is approached by the level of disparity for primary care-sensitive health outcomes across population groups.

SOURCE: Kringos, 2010

The new edition

The third edition of the *Handbook of Family Medicine* is written for medical students during their undergraduate training and for those beginning their postgraduate training in family medicine. The Handbook represents the latest thinking in sub-Saharan Africa on family medicine and also includes more clinical material on the most common reasons for encounter and diagnoses made. In addition, we have recognised the established and growing interest in traditional, complementary and alternative medicines amongst our patients and the medical profession. There is a need to look at ways of understanding and integrating different knowledge on health, wellness and disease from these other perspectives with more orthodox bio-medical approaches. We have therefore added a new chapter on integrative medicine which opens a dialogue about this interface.

We hope that this new Handbook will enable you to engage with the concepts and practice of family medicine in your work and to grow as a practitioner who offers a high quality of care to his patients and broader community.

1   A different context of care

Bob Mash
Division of Family Medicine and Primary Care
Department of Interdisciplinary Health Sciences
University of Stellenbosch
Khaya Mfenyana
Executive Dean, Faculty of Health Sciences
Walter Sisulu University

Introduction

The establishment of family medicine as an academic discipline provides a context of learning that is different from that of the traditional teaching hospital. In South Africa, as in many other countries, it is now considered essential to train doctors not only in the traditional academic teaching hospital but also in the district health system, within clinics, health centres and district hospitals (Health Professions Council, 1999). This is to allow medical students to deal with the common problems encountered in all types of settings. If medical students were only exposed to academic teaching hospitals their experience of and preparation for handling typical health problems would be significantly limited. Figure 1.1 shows, during a typical month in the USA, that less than one person in 1 000 is admitted to a teaching hospital, while 217 people consult a doctor elsewhere. This chapter is intended to describe this different context of care and help the student to understand how this context differs from the traditional teaching hospital.

In this chapter, we refer to personal experience of the contexts in which we work. Professor Khaya Mfenyana has worked in rural clinics in the Eastern Cape and Professor Bob Mash in Khayelitsha, a large peri-urban township outside Cape Town. The majority of their patients are poor, use the public health sector, and speak Xhosa as their first language.

Figure 1.1 The ecology of medical care

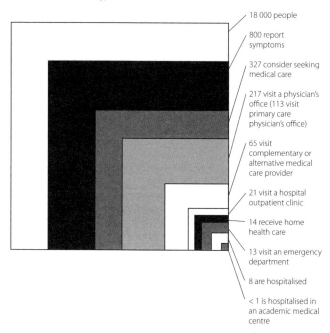

18 000 people

800 report symptoms

327 consider seeking medical care

217 visit a physician's office (113 visit primary care physician's office)

65 visit complementary or alternative medical care provider

21 visit a hospital outpatient clinic

14 receive home health care

13 visit an emergency department

8 are hospitalised

< 1 is hospitalised in an academic medical centre

Common conditions in family medicine

The burden of disease

Recent work in South Africa has defined the burden of disease in our communities (Bradshaw, 2007). The burden of disease is defined in terms of years of life lost due to premature death or disability (sometimes referred to as disability adjusted life years or DALYs). Figure 1.2 and Table 1.1 show the top 20 conditions that cause the greatest burden of disease in South Africa. These conditions can be categorised into four broad groups:

- Conditions related to HIV and Aids (such as TB)
- Conditions related to violence and trauma (such as interpersonal violence and road traffic accidents)
- Conditions related to chronic non-communicable diseases (such as asthma, diabetes, hypertension, heart disease)
- Conditions related to maternal and child health (such as pneumonia, diarrhoea and low birth weight).

South Africa is often said to have a quadruple burden of disease; conditions related to poverty and under-development are often combined with conditions related to the transition to a more urbanised and developed society.

People who consult doctors or nurses in primary care are likely to suffer from common conditions that reflect this burden of disease. Underlying this burden of disease are a variety of risk factors, which have been identified (see Table 1.1) and knowing these risk factors gives us the opportunity to prevent these common conditions. Unsafe sex, interpersonal violence, alcohol abuse and smoking tobacco make up the top four risk factors. Interestingly, being overweight and underweight are both listed sequentially as important risk factors. Disease prevention and health promotion are discussed further in Chapter 5.

Figure 1.2 The burden of disease in South Africa (Bradshaw, D. 2007)

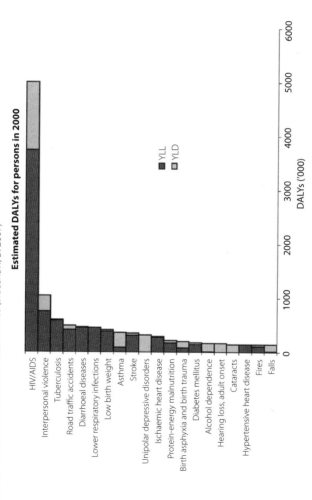

Table 1.1 Risk factors and the burden of disease in South Africa (Bradshaw, D. 2007)

Rank	Risk factor	% total DALYs	Rank	Disease, injury or condition	% total DALYs
1	Unsafe sex / sexually transmitted infections	31.5	1	HIV/AIDS	30.9
2	Interpersonal violence	8.4	2	Interpersonal violence injury	6.5
3	Alcohol harm	7.0	3	Tuberculosis	3.7
4	Tobacco smoking	4.0	4	Road traffic injury	3.0
5	Excess body weight	2.9	5	Diarrhoeal disease	2.9
6	Child and maternal underweight	2.7	6	Lower respiratory infections	2.8
7	Unsafe water, sanitation, hygiene	2.6	7	Low birth weight	2.6
8	High blood pressure	2.4	8	Asthma	2.2
9	Diabetes	1.6	9	Stroke	2.2
10	High cholesterol	1.4	10	Unipolar depressive disorders	2.0
11	Low fruit and vegetable intake	1.1	11	Ischaemic heart disease	1.8
12	Physical inactivity	1.1	12	Protein-energy malnutrition	1.3
13	Iron deficiency anaemia	1.1	13	Birth asphyxia and birth trauma	1.2
14	Vitamin A deficiency	0.7	14	Diabetes mellitus	1.1
15	Indoor air pollution	0.4	15	Alcohol dependence	1.0
16	Lead exposure	0.4	16	Hearing loss, adult onset	1.0
17	Outdoor air pollution	0.3	17	Cataracts	0.9

Presenting problems

The burden of disease discussed above may present in a wide variety of ways at the primary care level. Table 1.2 shows the most common symptoms with which people present to ambulatory primary care in South Africa. These are derived from a study of 19 000 consultations spread across the Western Cape, Northern Cape, North West and Limpopo provinces. Primary care providers must have an approach to the assessment of all these symptoms. South African primary care differs from other countries in America, Asia and Europe in the frequency of generalised aches and pains as a complaint and in the frequency of symptoms that are probably due to HIV/AIDS and TB (weight loss, sweating, loss of appetite, abnormal sputum, respiratory pain and dysphagia) or STIs (genital/pelvic pain, vaginal and urethral discharge and vaginal symptoms).

Cough is usually a symptom of upper respiratory tract infection and this disease is usually self limiting. However, it is a challenge for the family physician not to take things lightly, as cough may be a symptom of a serious disease. The history and physical examination therefore become very important. Could this be pneumonia, tuberculosis, asthma, or cardiac failure, for example?

Headache is a common symptom that can easily be ignored and yet can be a pointer to a serious underlying problem, either psychological or organic. In our context, many patients who say "Doctor, I have a headache" are indirectly saying "Doctor, can you check my blood pressure?" Unfortunately, many headaches tend to be associated with hypertension, not because headaches *per se* are a common symptom of hypertension, but because many hypertensive patients have tension headaches. So. while tension headaches should be diagnosed and treated appropriately, it is the real reason for the headache that is important.

Fever is another common presenting problem. In our context, patients may complain of fever, but when asked what exactly they mean or what they feel, several answers may come up. These may include *ubushushu* (hotness), or *umkhuhlane* (a common cold), or *ingqele* (cold), or *ubugxathu* (pain between the shoulders). When we examine these patients, we may find that they have an upper respiratory tract infection and/or an elevated temperature, or no signs at all. *Ingqele* does not always imply an upper respiratory tract infection. The patient may have a serious illness characterised by fever and rigors, but, on the other hand, the patient may have no signs of any disease or may just have pain between the shoulders. *Ingqele* may be attributed to a certain day when the patient was exposed to rainy or cold weather and this day may not be yesterday or last week. Pain between the shoulders may also be attributed to stress or heavy manual work. Therefore it is always important to find out what the patient thinks about the illness. The other interesting symptom we are picking up in our environment is painful throbbing neck veins. This is usually related to stress.

Abdominal pain is another common symptom, which may be a symptom of conditions such as gastritis, pelvic inflammatory disease, cystitis and so on. Some patients will describe feeling as if something is going up from the abdomen to the chest. Some will talk of *umoya oshushu onyukayo* (hot wind that is going up). These are examples of ill-defined symptoms that can only be left at a symptom level at this stage of our understanding, as putting a diagnostic label on them would be premature, irrelevant, and dangerous. What would be more helpful would be to try to understand what that particular patient means by their description of the symptom. We need to explore patients' thoughts, feelings, beliefs, and expectations carefully in order to unearth the real reason for encounter. If, on the other hand, the feeling that something is going up from the abdomen to the chest is summarised as abdominal pain, there is a danger of reducing the whole interview to only the routine questions of "Is it colicky in nature?", "Does it radiate?", "What relieves it?", and so on. Understanding the culture and language of the people you are serving is helpful in these situations.

Chest pain is a common symptom in our context. It can be a non-specific symptom or a symptom of a serious respiratory or cardiac problem. What is not usually taught at medical school is the common left-sided chest pain or submammary chest pain that has no organic origin, but which is commonly mistaken for angina pectoris. The pain is sharp in nature, unexpected, and usually comes at rest. This pain is real and resembles the pain of pleurisy. Some of these patients are investigated unnecessarily for chest and cardiac problems. A careful history leads to the assessment of submammary chest pain. *Intliziyo yam ibetha kancinci* (my heart is beating softly) is usually a symptom of a person who has an anxiety disorder, but if you are not careful you can end up investigating for or labelling the patient with angina pectoris.

Backache is yet another common presenting problem in our context. Some of the people who present with backache may complain of *izintso* (kidneys). If you are working through an interpreter, you may subject the patient to all sorts of unnecessary investigations and end up assigning the false label of kidney problems. The patients who usually complain of backache in our context are those who do hard manual labour for a living.

Chapter 7 provides a more detailed approach to the assessment of some of the common presenting problem in primary care.

Table 1.2 The most common complaints in primary care (N=31451)

Reason for encounter	N	%
1. Cough	2 821	9.0
2. Headache	1 500	4.8
3. Fever	869	2.8
4. Sore throat	623	2.0
5. Generalised aches or pains	585	1.9
6. Diarrhoea	575	1.8
7. Abdominal pain or cramp, generalised	528	1.7
8. Dysuria	431	1.4
9. Back pain	426	1.4
10. Loss of appetite	419	1.3
11. Vomiting	413	1.3
12. Leg or thigh pain or cramps	366	1.2
13. Sneezing/blocked nose	356	1.1
14. Generalised rash	318	1.0
15. Vaginal discharge	306	1.0
16. Vertigo/dizziness	299	0.9
17. Localised rash	290	0.9
18. Ear pain	281	0.9
19. Weakness/general tiredness	277	0.9
20. Nasal symptoms	268	0.8
21. Pruritus	247	0.8
22. Abdominal pain, localised	232	0.7
23. Respiratory/pleuritic pain	223	0.7
24. Joint pain or symptoms	212	0.7
25. Knee pain or symptom	190	0.6
26. Shoulder pain or symptom	187	0.6
27. Shortness of breath	180	0.6
28. Chest pain	178	0.6
29. Foot and toe pain or symptoms	165	0.5
30. Weight loss	165	0.5

Common diagnoses

Many patients in primary care present with ongoing problems or for preventative interventions when there is no illness. In fact, follow up of hypertension is currently the most common overall reason to attend primary care. This is in part because follow up of patients with HIV/AIDS and TB is done in dedicated and separate antiretroviral or TB clinics. Preventative interventions include visits for growth monitoring, immunisations, family planning and antenatal care. Sometimes patients attend for administrative reasons, for example when they request a disability grant. Table 1.3 lists the top 25 diagnoses encountered in South African primary care and is derived from the same study as Table 1.2. You will note that in some cases a specific diagnosis could not be made and the assessment was listed as cough or muscle pain. A specific diagnosis is not always possible in a single consultation and may require ongoing care and follow up. Even then patient problems are not always easily understood with conventional diagnostic labels, for example *inyongo* implies a problem with bile, but has no equivalent medical concept.

Although injury and trauma represent a large component of the burden of disease this is not seen in the list. This may be because patients generally present to emergency units or hospitals and because interpersonal violence, such as intimate partner violence, often goes undetected in primary care. Likewise birth- and neonatal-related issues that are seen in the burden of disease will more probably present in maternity units. It should also be noted that mental health issues are thought to be under-represented in the burden of disease estimates and also largely undetected in primary care. Their absence from the list therefore demonstrates poor recognition and not an absence of mental health problems in our primary care.

Table 1.3 Top 25 diagnoses in South African primary care (N=24561)

Diagnosis	n	%
Hypertension, uncomplicated	2 957	12.0
Upper respiratory tract infection	1 306	5.3
HIV/AIDS	961	3.9
Type 2 diabetes	946	3.9
TB	862	3.6
Cough	681	2.8
Osteoarthritis	530	2.2
Asthma	485	2.0
Acute tonsillitis	454	1.9
Epilepsy	375	1.5
Sexually transmitted infections	366	1.5
Urinary tract infection	317	1.3
Pneumonia	306	1.2
Acute bronchitis/bronchiolitis	263	1.1
Hypertension, complicated	262	1.1
Gastroenteritis	255	1.0
Diarrhoea	236	1.0
Acute otitis media	233	0.9
Generalised body pain	213	0.9
Headache	209	0.9
Influenza	189	0.8
Muscle pain	183	0.7
Allergic reaction	176	0.7
Dermatophytosis	160	0.7
Chronic obstructive pulmonary disease	140	0.6

Where do family physicians work?

Different levels of care

Family physicians work within the district health system where they are the most senior medical practitioners. The district health system includes the primary level of care, where the patient encounters the health system for the first time (Smith, 1987). Some of these patients may be further managed by family physicians within the local district hospital. Patients who cannot be managed within the district health system can be referred to a higher level of care at the secondary level or to a tertiary level hospital.

Consider the following example:

Mr VM, aged 25 years, sat next to my desk and spoke quickly with rapid hand movements. He complained about burning in his left leg and arm, especially in the joints, and experienced stiffness in the morning. He had recently collapsed while at the funeral of his cousin and had been told by another family physician, who examined his red eye, that he had rheumatism. He appeared quite an anxious personality and was not sleeping well.

The *primary level of care* is where a patient such as Mr VM encounters a clinical nurse practitioner for the first time with a problem that is medically undefined. If the clinical nurse practitioner is unable to fully deal with the problem, he/she may refer the patient to a family physician. The family physician therefore must be able to cope with a broad range of undifferentiated problems, many of which are not strictly biomedical. For example, the family physician might consider the possibility of Mr VM having a mental disorder, as well as inflammatory or reactive arthritis. In this situation the family physician also acts as a consultant to the clinical nurse practitioner and should give supportive feedback.

In the public sector first-contact care is usually offered by a clinical nurse practitioner working on a mobile van, in a small clinic or larger community health centre. Larger community health centres may also have full-time doctors, while smaller clinics may only be visited by a doctor once a week. Doctors may be interns, medical officers, registrars or family physicians. The family physician at the primary level may work in different types of organisations in different situations. For example, she/he may work alone as a private general practitioner, with partners in a managed care organisation, for the local government, or for the provincial administration as a member of a large multidisciplinary team in a community health centre. An overview of these different primary care organisations is given in Chapter 10.

Ideally, the primary level of care should be close to the community that it serves and should offer a comprehensive range of services that are easily accessible under one roof. These services should include curative, preventive, promotive, and rehabilitative activities for both adults and children. Historically, in South Africa these services have been delivered by different organisations, in different places, in a haphazard and fragmented way. For example, children from the same community must attend one clinic to receive immunisations and a different clinic for help when they are sick. However, over the last decade, district health services have been developing and in many places primary care has improved dramatically.

Q While you are studying family medicine, ask yourself if your clinic is offering a comprehensive range of services. If not, are these offered by someone else or simply not available? How easy is it for people to access all the services they require during one visit?

The district health system also includes the district hospital with general wards for men, women, and children, and a maternity ward. If the primary level cannot provide all the help that is required within the community, then the patient may be treated at the district hospital.

Here is an example:

Ms NM arrived at the rural hospital casualty unit with a letter written by a clinical nurse practitioner explaining that she was worried about an ectopic pregnancy. The letter asked the hospital to investigate her for this possibility and, of course, to operate if the diagnosis was confirmed.

Ideally, patients at the district hospital should be seen only if they are referred by another health worker. The referral letter should clearly define the problem and the reason for referral (see Chapter 6). In many rural areas, much of the family physician's time is spent at the district hospital and clinical nurse practitioners are more involved at the primary care level. The special challenges for the rural family physician are discussed in Chapter 11. In urban areas, the family physician is often more involved at the primary level, although in recent times even urban areas have been introducing district hospitals. Over the next few years a new body of health workers, the clinical associate, will be introduced. The clinical associate is trained to work alongside the family physician at district hospitals and to assist with ward work, emergencies and procedures.

The *secondary level of care* is offered by specialists at a hospital with a range of core specialities such as paediatrics, surgery, internal medicine, obstetrics, and gynaecology. The secondary level of care is hospital based and deals with patients who are referred to it from the district health system with a problem that is usually biomedical and already partially defined. Family physicians may spend time during their training at the secondary hospital, but once qualified will work within the district health system. Some secondary level hospitals also provide district hospital-type services to their immediate community and in this situation may also have a Department of Family Medicine and family physicians.

The final layer of the health system, or the *tertiary level of care*, includes all the specialities and subspecialities, such as plastic surgery, urology, haematology, renal dialysis, and cardiac surgery. Family physicians do not work at this level of care, which is often delivered by a large academic teaching hospital. This is where medical students spend most of their time. These hospitals are quite distant from rural communities and situated in large urban areas.

Availability of care

Although access to primary care has improved dramatically over the last 15 years, it remains a challenge in many parts of South Africa. In rural areas, the physical distance of the clinic from home and difficulties with lack of transport and poor roads may limit accessibility to primary care. In peri-urban areas, it may be limited by the number of patients who can be seen with the available staff or by restricted opening times. In some areas, there may be no primary care clinic. After the South African elections in 1994, fees for indigent patients were removed, which made health care more accessible.

The community's perceptions of the quality and acceptability of the service will also have an influence. For example, if the staff is seen as disinterested, aggressive, or rude, this will act as a barrier to care. In some areas, because of poor access to or low acceptability of primary care services, patients have flocked to district or even secondary and tertiary hospitals looking for assistance. For this reason, many hospitals have been overwhelmed with primary level problems and have been unable to focus on the needs of referred patients.

South Africa has a large number of generalists, although relatively few have qualified as family physicians. In 2010 the Health Systems Trust (http://www.hst.org.za/healthstats/15/data) reported that South Africa had 27.3 generalist doctors per 100 000 people or one doctor for every 3 663 people. This ratio is much better than many other African countries, but much lower than developed countries such as New Zealand (82.4 per 100 000) or the United Kingdom (65.7 per 100 000). However, the problem in South Africa has been the severe maldistribution of generalist doctors. In rural provinces such as North West there was only 16.0 generalists per 100 000 population compared to 34.2 in the Western Cape. This uneven distribution of doctors in rural areas is discussed in Chapter 11. The government has attempted to address this problem by shifting certain tasks to nurses, importing foreign doctors, creating compulsory community service for newly qualified doctors and introducing rural allowances.

Health districts

Post-1994 in South Africa, a political decision was taken to move to a district health system for primary level services. The entire country has been divided up into health districts, within which all government health workers will be employed by one health authority. Twelve principles have been agreed upon to guide the development of districts (Naidoo, 1997):

- To overcome fragmentation
- To ensure equity
- To offer comprehensive services
- Effectiveness
- Efficiency
- Easy access to services
- Local accountability
- Community participation
- Decentralisation of management
- A developmental approach
- An intersectoral approach
- Sustainability.

Family physicians play a key role in the health districts, not only in providing individual clinical services but also in supporting district development that meets the needs of the whole community. Family physicians must focus not only on the needs of the individual patient within the consultation but also on the needs of the district or practice population. The challenges of community-orientated primary care are dealt with in Chapter 9. In addition, family physicians are often responsible for clinical governance and the quality of clinical care within a team of health workers, a whole facility or a sub-district.

While you are studying family medicine, ask about the health district you are in and consider to what extent it is meeting the principles outlined above.

Examples of family practice

All this discussion of different levels and organisational structures may sound very theoretical and far removed from the experience of seeing patients and being a family physician. It should, however, be clear that family practice in South Africa varies enormously depending on the geographical setting and type of organisation. To illustrate the enormous variety of practice, we asked three family physicians to describe their work. Each of them works in different settings and approaches family practice in their own way.

One week in the life of.........Zandy Rosochaki

We are a private practice with seven doctors in an urban centre close to Cape Town: four men and three women. All are generalists with special interests. The partner with whom I have worked longest stands out as the family doctor who exemplifies family medicine. He is my strongest inspiration to our core work: that is, good evidence-based general practice, while remaining a patient-centred doctor.

The clinical part of my week involves about 100 consultations that would in all likelihood match the profile of my counterparts in Toronto or Strasbourg. Most of my patients are a bit like vintage cars, generally well made and preserved, but needing meticulous attention and care to keep them on the road.

Many consultations involve acute care, which is superimposed on chronic maintenance; for example coughs, colds and minor injuries present in tandem with fine-tuning glycaemic control in diabetics or pain control for palliative care patients. The specialist care available to my patients is of a high standard. With this goes high patient expectations and associated medico-legal risk. This quality of care is a privilege in South Africa, but can remain up to date with the latest international developments. The part of work that seems arduous is managing staff, patient records, computer systems, accounting systems and keeping the building intact.

Younger patients tend to be more health aware and health promotion and disease prevention activities fall on fertile ground. On the whole this happens opportunistically during any consultation when the presenting complaint is dealt with rapidly (for example, a common cold) or when a clinical presentation begs a response. This is where the unfailing spirit of my partner comes in, for example, at the end of the day when the last patient wants a quick consultation about whether his cold needs an antibiotic or not. My partner would focus on a discussion about smoking cessation.

Stellenbosch university provides me with the opportunity to teach individuals or groups of family medicine registrars online. Teaching is a great gift. It supports my intuition of how the job of growing family medicine must be done: an army, preferably an obedient Chinese army, of well-trained family practitioners must be out there doing what accumulated evidence dictates. Online teaching in chronic disease management or teaching and learning principles is a special ritual that happens uninterrupted at the end of my day. A map of South Africa with geographically placed photographs of fresh faces (my students) with brief biographies hangs on the wall above me. It is my visual classroom guide to the kindred spirits I am communing with in cyberspace.

We have a registrar in the practice, which helps integrate the direction of the practice with ideas generated from family medicine. Supervising her thesis introduces a chronic disease audit to the rest of the practice team. I also have mentoring discussions with her, to reflect on the last five patients seen. Often this re-ignites the pleasures of family practice; how interesting this work is if one allows time for reflection.

Every two weeks a colleague and I meet with a group of twenty registrars to engage in small-group learning. This is mostly an inspiration as it reinforces the belief that the ambitious, expanded role of the family physician is developing in real people. They are raised with potent communication and organisational tools (computers). Their professional world seems increasingly free of racial baggage that may unconsciously have hindered previous generations from achieving a meritocracy to be proud of. They are part of a family medicine network that is young, but vigorous and with vision.

There are other areas of reprieve from consulting: one is selecting the right patient at the right time for a joint replacement and then assisting with the surgery.

As modern doctors we are forced to be technocrats. New drugs and tests come and go, but fragile people in the context of seeking health, remain the most complex enigma we have to deal with. My attempt has been to remain real as a *Mensch* and to stay technologically competent. I do not think I achieve either completely, but both keep me busy.

One week in the life of........Werner Viljoen

I never wanted to be a family physician. In fact, like most students, I also wondered why anybody in their right mind would specialise in something so ill defined and, to be blunt about it, unimpressive and vague. Why waste the time when you could be a paediatrician or a gynaecologist? Better status, better earning potential, much more exciting and intellectually stimulating; this seemed a way better career path to me than just becoming an over-qualified general practitioner.

The question I ask students is why anybody in their right mind would choose to limit their scope of practice when the majority of patients require a broader approach. We are conditioned to think that the natural progression of our career is to specialise. I wanted to specialise in obstetrics until, in 1997, I started as a junior medical officer at Helderberg Hospital. It took only two weeks for me to become addicted to district hospital practice.

Helderberg Hospital is a 162-bed hospital rendering comprehensive acute hospital services to a population of 530 000 people, of whom 76% are under the age of 40 and 10% under the age of 5. Bed occupancy is almost always above 100% with an average of 12 000 patients per month accessing services.

To describe a typical week in this bustling hive of health care is impossible. At Helderberg every day is different and every week a smorgasbord of change. It brings with it new challenges, new goals, learning opportunities galore, and also the laughter, tears, and battle scars associated with growing into the best possible doctor you can be for your patients.

Patients are a fascinating collective. They can be complex, difficult, unco-operative, stubborn, frustrating, but also interesting, inspiring, and humbling all in one. With experience, I have learned that survival depends on mastering five basic principles.

Communication is everything. The power of words to build, direct, and comfort is often underestimated. It is the most valuable tool you have; a well-placed sentence or skillfully applied phrase can make a world of difference.

You need to be fit for mental gymnastics. You need to be able to approach any problem with an open mind and a willingness to change direction in mid-leap. What the patient presents with may not be the real or the only problem present. Consider all the angles.

Never promise patients a cure. Our job is to care, to help, to relieve, and to soothe the sick and suffering, not aid and abet the legal profession. It is impossible to cure every patient, but you can definitely make every patient feel better. .

Paranoia is your friend. Never assume anything. I know they say that if it barks and wags a tail it must be a dog … but sea lions, monkeys, deer and even some birds bark as well.

Be real. It is acceptable to admit that you are human, that you don't know, and that you do not always have all the answers. If you bluff, misdirect, lie, pretend, or evade in any way, patients will sense it and lose faith in you.

Hospital-based family practice is a different kettle of fish compared to primary care. You need to be innovative, adaptable, practically orientated with a wide skill set, and able to think on your feet. You will be expected to constantly manage patients across all disciplines of medicine at a moment's notice, while keeping the family, the broader community, and available resources in mind.

I start every day with a blank page. Anything can happen and probably will. The truth is I cannot wait to be there to learn, to teach, to experience medicine in its entirety. It is why I became a family physician after all …

A day in the life of …George Rupesinghe

Family medicine at Mthatha General Hospital has changed character three times since its inception. At first the doctors only cared for out-patients during the day and ran a casualty section. In 1996 there was a big paradigm shift and family medicine moved out to five community health centres, abandoning the hospital completely. However, in 2004 there was another paradigm shift and it was declared that the seat of family medicine is the level one district hospital. The role of the family physician in the Department of Family Medicine has thus changed over the years. Being a university department makes this a busy hospital, with both service and teaching components. The latest change is an outreach service to the community health centres that were vacated six years ago, once again reiterating that primary health care is the so called bread-and-butter of family physicians.

For the doctors in the Department of Family Medicine the day begins at 7.30 am with a common gathering. Monday is a business meeting where we discuss all the issues of the previous week and plan for the rest of the new one. The management of the hospital complex has decided that these morning meetings should not exceed half an hour and that the doctors should be at their work stations by 8.00 am. Every attempt is made to satisfy the management, but in reality the meetings seldom end by 8.00 am.

The day I wish to share with you began with a morning gathering where a final year medical student presented a patient. The young lady was fluent in her presentation. The patient had multiple clinical, personal and contextual issues, which evoked a healthy discussion from the audience, so much so that the 8.00 am cut off time was far exceeded. This was followed by an hour long meeting of the nine specialists in the department who discussed the MMed, MBChB and Clinical Associate teaching programmes.

After the morning meeting I proceeded to the Gateway Clinic in Mthatha where I have been relocated to render services while also supervising a registrar and an intern. The Health Professions Council has made it mandatory that registrars spend time in the health district as part of their primary care training. The Department of Family Medicine offers an outreach service to three community health centres in the King Sabatha Dalindyebo subdistrict.

Many of the patients attending the Gateway Clinic suffer from chronic illnesses such as diabetes, hypertension, epilepsy and asthma. Most of the patients who consulted me on that day were those for whom I had given review dates. Most of the other patients had minor complaints and so consultations were not long. However many patients were obese and blood pressures and blood sugars were not well controlled. I have the luxury of a health promoter to help me and she educates the patients about diet and adherence to treatment. On average I manage seven to ten patients per hour. The registrar and the intern also consulted me several times about some issues with their patients. While I was busy with my routine work a woman was brought to me as an emergency. She had not been able to close her mouth that morning and was drooling saliva. The nurse who brought the patient was rather distraught and suggested that I transfer the patient to Mthatha Hospital immediately. She said she had already summoned the ambulance. I calmed down both the patient and the nurse, as it was just a dislocated mandible and I had reduced many of them in the past at the hospital with no problems. I made the patient sit and reduced the dislocation. Although it was a simple procedure, I was able to educate three people: the patient, the nurse and the intern. I taught the patient how to avoid a recurrence, I taught the nurse not to panic in such situations and I taught the intern how to perform simple procedures in primary care.

Who do family physicians work with?

The answer to this question is not as simple as it seems and goes beyond a simple list of people likely to be found in any given district hospital or health centre. In looking after an individual patient, the family physician may be working with a diverse group of people, many of whom are unseen and not acknowledged as part of the health care system.

In a study of women with depression and anxiety in Harare (Abas and Broadhead, 1997), it was found that:

- About 65% of patients sought help from family, friends, or church members (29% used only these resources)
- About 55% consulted a traditional healer
- About 29% went to a primary care clinic.

These women saw the cause of their depression as:
- Psychosocial, for example, marital dispute or bereavement (73%)
- Physical disease, for example, high blood pressure (16%)
- Spiritual or supernatural influences (24%).

Family and friends

The process of recognising and defining illness often involves a lay consultation with family members and friends.

In a two-week period up to 90% of adults will experience a physical symptom (McWhinney, 1989) and the family is where these symptoms are first experienced. As doctors we need to understand that experiencing symptoms is an inevitable and normal part of daily life. How many symptoms have you experienced in the last few weeks? Did you take any medicines? Did you ask advice from a friend or colleague? The question is not whether someone has symptoms, but how they react to them and explain them.

The importance and meaning attached to particular symptoms may depend on their interpretation by the grandmother, spouse, or even a family conference. As a result, symptoms may be seen as self-limiting and ordinary or as serious enough to adopt the sick role.

Families may believe in particular remedies, such as gargling with antiseptic, taking "rescue remedy", or the use of laxatives and enemas. Self-treatment may involve traditional remedies, over-the-counter medicines bought at the local shop or chemist, as well as leftover medicines from previous prescriptions and not necessarily their own! In one study, 80% of adults and 55% of children had taken at least one medicine in a two-week period (McWhinney, 1989).

Before deciding to seek help people often ask themselves the following questions (Helman, 1981):
- What has happened?
- Why has it happened?
- Why to me?
- Why now?
- What would happen if nothing were done about it?
- What should I do about it or who should I consult for further help?

Therefore, in deciding to seek help the patient's own explanation of what is causing the illness, what may help the healing process, and how serious the illness is will influence who the patient consults. If the patient decides to consult a family physician, it will be important to understand the patient's own explanatory model and the reasons for the encounter during the consultation. In choosing to see a family physician, what kind of help does the person expect? What were the fears and anxieties that led to the decision to consult? A useful tool to use in assessing the reason for the consultation is outlined at the end of this chapter. Subsequently, the treatment offered by the family physician will be evaluated by the patient together with their family and friends, and in effect the family physician is working alongside these key people.

Traditional health practitioners

For many years traditional medicine was illegal in South Africa. The Witchcraft Suppression Act 3 of 1957, and subsequent amendments to this act, prohibited traditional healers from practising their trade. The Traditional Health Practitioners Act 22 of 2007 finally provided for legal recognition and regulation of traditional medicine in South Africa as per constitutional requirements. Under this Act, which expressly states that it is not applicable to persons who are registered as medical practitioners or dentists, five categories of traditional healers are recognised, including:

- Traditional surgeons, who will perform male circumcision at initiation schools
- Traditional birth attendants
- Herbalists
- Diviners
- Apprentices of traditional healing.

The Traditional Health Practitioners Council, which was established under the same Act, aims to promote public health awareness; ensure quality of services; promote and maintain appropriate ethical and professional standards; encourage research, education and training; promote contact between the various fields of training within traditional health practice and set standards for such training; compile and maintain a professional code of conduct; and, ensure that traditional health practices comply with universally-accepted health care norms and values. Similarly, the Department of Health's draft policy on African traditional medicine (July 2008) recommends that a legal framework be established to regulate and register African traditional medicine and medicinal products; protect African traditional medicine knowledge and intellectual property rights; and protect the rights of persons involved in the practice of African traditional medicine. It has also been recommended that a National Institute of African Traditional Medicines of South Africa and a national pharmacopoeia be established (Mokoena, 2009).

In South Africa, there are thought to be about 200 000 traditional healers and 80% of the black population, in both urban and rural areas, make use of their services (Kale, 1995). Traditional healers are usually highly respected opinion leaders within their communities and are usually seen as allies in the healing process and in combating evil.

Different types of traditional healers would include the traditional doctor or *inyanga/ixhwele*, who is often male and who prescribes a variety of curative and protective herbal and other medicines.

An *igqira/sangoma* or diviner is usually female, works within a traditional religious supernatural context, and acts as a medium for the ancestral shades. In the divining process, the *igqira* often uses dice, which may be collections of bones and other objects. Illness may be explained in terms of witchcraft, pollution, or the relationship with the ancestors. Witches or sorcerers have a mystical ability to cause harm through magic powers, poison, or by sending agents such as the *thokoloshe*. The diviner may identify the witch, who is often a person within the extended family or neighbourhood. It is important to make a distinction between the diviner who attempts to identify the witch and the *igqira* or witch herself. In referring to all traditional healers as witchdoctors, this distinction is blurred and the healing role of the diviner is seen as malicious. Witchcraft may be suspected, particularly when there is a climate of envy, jealousy, or conflict within a family or community. A state of pollution is not caused intentionally but may relate, for example, to contamination during menstruation, after a death, or by handling a corpse. Certain rituals or use of medicines such as enemas or emetics may cure this polluted state. The ancestral shades are responsible for maintaining health and good fortune, and neglect of this relationship may cause withdrawal of their protection. Illness may be seen as a prompting from the ancestors to perform certain rituals or to show respect for your elders. These rituals often involve animal sacrifice and traditional beer.

Umthandazeli/umthandazi are faith healers who operate within independent African churches and who mix Christianity with traditional practices. Spirit possession or sinful behaviour may be seen as the cause of illness. Modes of healing would include the laying on of hands, holy water, prayer, immersion in water, and various non-herbal medicines such as seawater (Hammond-Tooke, 1989).

In one rural study (Hammond-Tooke, 1989), it was found that:

- Witchcraft was interpreted as the cause of about 72% of illness.
- About 8% of illness was seen as a message from the ancestors.
- Non-mystical causes such as accidents were given by about 17% of patients.

Traditional healers may address the whole person by looking not only at the cause of the illness but also at the meaning, whereas family physicians are often primarily concerned with diagnosing the cause. In addition, the traditional healer often deals with the meaning of illness in terms that are closer to the person's own ideas and explanations. People may consult the traditional and other practitioners simultaneously for different reasons, or may see one as more appropriate for certain kinds of illness. The main conditions seen by traditional healers in a study from the North West Province are shown in Table 1.4 (Shai-Mahoko, 1996).

Table 1.4 Conditions seen by traditional healers in North West Province

Rank	Diagnosis	Rank	Diagnosis
1	Infertility	8	Mental illness
2	Septic sore	9	High blood pressure
3	Impotence	10	Palpitations
4	Sexually transmitted infection	11	Tuberculosis
5	Deliveries	12	Alcoholism
6	*Makgome**	13	Diabetes
7	Asthma	14	Cancer

NOTE: *This is a culturebound syndrome described as a funeral sickness where a person might experience symptoms such as nausea, vomiting and diarrhoea.

However, failure to receive help from one practitioner may prompt the patient to try one of the others. Therefore, when a patient consults a family physician, it is highly likely that this person has consulted, is consulting, or will consult a traditional healer. The family physician will in many cases be an unconscious partner with the traditional healer.

Health professions

Health professions are derived from Western, scientific medicine and includes the people usually found in medical schools, hospitals, and clinics. The family physician working at the district level will be only one member of a team of other professionals.

In this professional sector, illness is traditionally seen as the result of a disease or pathology affecting the normal functioning of organs within the body. Treatment is aimed at restoring the function of these organs or preventing progression of the disease. In its simplest form, the body is seen as a machine and disease as the result of a breakdown in some internal component that must be fixed or replaced. This pathological model of illness in the professional sector is the foundation of most medical training but may not always be useful in family practice. In teaching hospitals, the pathological model of illness is usually applicable to the problems encountered, and where no disease is found the patient is discharged. In family medicine, however, disease is not the only cause of symptoms and the interaction with a patient's problems may be more uncertain and more complex. What is required is an alternative approach to the patient and an alternative model of illness that makes more sense of the family physician's experience. In addition, this pathological model may be very different from the magical or moral models that are utilized by families or traditional healers, and the resultant contradictions can lead to problems in the consultation. A more appropriate clinical method for family practice is discussed in Chapter 2.

The *primary health care* team may include certain core people, such as the receptionist, nurse, doctor, and pharmacist, who are involved in most encounters with patients. Even people not professionally trained may be key members of the team, such as the cleaners, porters, and security staff. Patients may turn to them for help and direction; for example, in our context, many of the cleaners are also members of the local community health committee. The team members may vary depending on the type of organisation, for example, in many private practices the family physician also dispenses the medicines and does not use a pharmacist (see Chapter 6). In many areas, the core person at the primary care level is the nurse, who may have received further training to allow consultation with patients. In future the clinical associate will join the team at the district hospital.

In addition, the team can include a broader group of professionals who are required to help with the patient's problems. This broader group, if available, may include the physiotherapist, social worker, counsellor, occupational therapist, dentist, health promoter, psychiatric nurse, and dietician. In primary care settings, patients can also refer themselves directly to many of these professionals. In a large community health centre, the team members may share the same building, but in many areas, they are spread out within the district at a variety of places.

Although the concept of the primary health care team is useful it may also be necessary to reflect on what kind of teamwork is modelled and how effectively the team is working together in your setting. Both interdisciplinary and multidisciplinary teams have been described. Multidisciplinary teams refer to a situation where team members may occupy the same building, but manage patients independently and may only share information afterwards. Interdisciplinary teams refer to a more active process of collaboration where the management plan is jointly developed and negotiated (Coombs, 2004). In terms of management of district hospitals effective teamwork has been described as having the following attributes (Couper and Hugo, 2005):

- Spirit of working together
- Purposeful, participative, and appreciative meetings
- Respectful supportive relationships that value each person's contribution
- Ownership of problems collectively – unity
- Holding a common vision
- Commitment to serving the community
- Effective communication and exchange of information.

What we should keep in mind is that although teamwork is very important, it should not be imposed on patients. Imagine a patient who comes to see a family physician with a problem that is not easy to share, who then goes through the pain of confiding in you. What enables the patient to be candid in a consultation is an effective doctor–patient relationship. When the patient has gone that far, she/he then expects help from you and may feel abandoned or betrayed if you immediately refer her/him to someone else who is a specialist in this area. Care given by a group of health workers may be greater than that given by individual health worker, but check this with the most important member of the team first, that is, the patient.

The family physician often has a leadership function within the team and a number of key qualities have been identified that promote effective leadership (Pritchard and Pritchard, 1994):

- To have the ability to inspire trust
- To be a good listener
- To have the ability to select good staff
- To have the ability to run effective meetings
- To strive to be a good speaker and presenter of information
- To accept responsibility
- To be able to be calm under stress
- To be able to tolerate uncertainty
- To respond positively to failure
- To be able to deal with conflict positively
- To be ready to smile.

In addition to knowing about and working with these other health professionals within the primary care team, it is necessary for the family physician to have a working knowledge of the network of *community based* and *nongovernmental organisations* (CBOs and NGOs) within the health district. These organisations are essential for helping patients with the wide variety of personal, psychosocial, and medical problems seen in family practice. For example, these organisations may work in the areas of job creation, disability, sheltered employment, support groups for HIV/AIDS, counselling, or legal advice. It is worth asking the tutor or staff at your teaching site if they have a list of local community-based resources. If not, then compiling one may be a useful task!

Community health workers

Another group of people who sit on the boundary between the community and professionals are *community health workers* (CHW). They are found in both rural and urban areas where primary level health services have been scarce or inaccessible or where community development is an important concern. They are local people chosen or elected by their communities to receive basic training in health issues. They live in the community that they serve and share the same culture and environment. They may be trained to use a limited range of medications and dressings, and to manage first aid and minor illness episodes themselves. In some areas, community health workers may offer family planning services, assist with the daily observation of anti-tuberculosis therapy or support adherence to anti-retroviral medication. They may also be involved in home-based care for people with advanced HIV or AIDS. In addition, they are often responsible for visiting a group of households or members of a village and screening for health problems. Due to their proximity to the beliefs and problems of the community, they are often seen as ideally situated to communicate health education and promotion messages, especially in the areas of child care, pregnancy, and nutrition. Lastly, they may be seen as having a role in community development and advocating health issues within local community structures, as well as representing the community at broader forums (Frankel, 1992).

At the time of writing the department of health is considering a major "re-engineering of primary health care" and much of their thinking is based on the Brazilian model of family health care teams. Health indicators in Brazil have improved significantly as a result of this model of community-orientated primary care. These teams consist of five to six CHWs, nurses and a doctor who take responsibility for a specific group of households. CHWs spend most of their time in the community, visiting families and identifying health risks or problems. The CHWs work closely with the nurses, who provide primary care at a local clinic and are supported by a visiting doctor. The health care team take responsibility for the health of a specific community rather than the needs of ad hoc patients that present to the clinic.

Allied health professions

The Allied Health Professions Council of South Africa (AHPCSA) is a statutory health body established in terms of the Allied Health Professions Act 63 of 1982 in order to regulate the allied health professions. At this stage, recognised allied health professions include:

- Ayurveda
- Chinese medicine and acupuncture
- Chiropractice
- Homoeopathy
- Naturopathy
- Osteopathy
- Phytotherapy and herbalism
- Therapeutic aromatherapy
- Therapeutic massage therapy
- Therapeutic reflexology
- Unani-tibb.

Many of these allied health professions have very different conceptual frameworks for disease, illness and wellness. Many of these therapies are considered in more detail in Chapter 14.

As with patients who consult traditional healers, patients may prefer to consult an alternative practitioner before or at the same time as a family physician. Some of these therapies, such as acupuncture, manipulation, and homeopathy, have also been incorporated into family practice by interested practitioners.

From this outline it can be seen that, whether they like it or not, family physicians work in parallel with a wide variety of healers and practitioners. The family physician may need to adopt an open and non-judgemental approach to understanding the illness and the involvement of other healers or practitioners in the healing process.

A practical approach for understanding the reason for encounter

From the above discussion you can understand that when you are seeing a patient for the first time it is helpful to explore not only "What is the diagnosis?" but also "Why have you come now and why to me?" The following is a practical approach that can help with this and you can try to place your patients within this classification. This will help you to understand not only why they have come but also their expectations, and it should enable you to use your time more efficiently in the consultation (McWhinney, 1972).

Limit of tolerance

This means that the person just cannot take it any more. An example is backache that has intruded so much into the patient's lifestyle that he/she can no longer perform in his/her daily life. This will vary from person to person; for example, the patient cannot make the bed, or complete a round of golf, or wield a pick. One of the concerns of these patients will be relief of their symptoms.

Limit of anxiety

The person has become too worried about the symptom or problem. Again this limit will vary from person to person and even in the same person depending on what else is going on in her/his life. The symptoms may be relatively minor, but the meaning and significance have created enough anxiety for the person to seek help. A woman with mastalgia may consult because of a fear of breast cancer or a man with chest pain may be worried that it is angina. A mother may bring her infant with a minor cold because of her fear that he/she may have tuberculosis. In this consultation, it will be important to hear the specific anxiety and to address it in your management plan.

Life problems presenting as symptoms

People are led to believe that when you visit a family physician you must have a symptom, which is usually associated with a disease. As a result, they often see symptoms that will justify a visit to the family physician. Life problems and emotional distress frequently present with physical symptoms. Often the patient is aware of the underlying cause but presents the physical symptoms. The underlying problem may be a lack of food, unemployment, intimate partner violence, or financial stress. In these patients, it will be important not to dwell too long on the physical symptoms but to explore the underlying psychosocial issues. Often family physicians feel out of their depth with these problems and do not have an effective approach to dealing with them. The issue is discussed in more detail in Chapter 7.

Administrative needs

People may visit the family physician because they need help with various administrative tasks, such as filling in sick leave forms, applications for disability grants, insurance reports, and so on.

No illness (preventive)

People also present to their family physician in order to prevent illness. This may be a mother bringing her baby for immunisations, or an executive coming for an annual physical examination. However, do not forget that there is always a reason that precipitated the person's decision to come at that time. Are they actually concerned about something else?

2 The consultation – a comprehensive approach to the person

Marietjie de Villiers: Deputy Dean: Education, Faculty of Health Sciences, University of Stellenbosch.

Soornarain S (Cyril) Naidoo: Dept of Family Medicine, Nelson R Mandela School of Medicine, University of KwaZulu-Natal.

Introduction

The consultation is the essence of medical practice, and comprises an encounter between the person who seeks the assistance of the doctor and the doctor themselves. Implicit in this encounter are the core elements of trust, respect, patient autonomy, confidentiality and empathy. It is important to understand and apply an appropriate framework to the consultation in order to function effectively and deliver quality health care.

The objectives of the consultation are three-fold, namely to understand the real reasons for the encounter, to achieve an optimum outcome for the person through a negotiated approach, and to strengthen the doctor-patient relationship. In order to achieve these, a patient-centred doctor needs an array of consultation skills including communication skills, clinical skills, procedural skills, clinical reasoning, integrative skills, counselling skills, health promotion skills and educational skills.

This chapter introduces the family medicine student to the clinical method which family physicians use in their approach to patients. The patient-centred method (also referred to as the bio-psycho-social approach) supplements the standard biomedical approach to the consultation. This includes taking a history, performing an examination and formulating a management plan. The family physician is not only interested in the disease but also explores the patient's experience of the illness. This chapter provides a framework for incorporating the components into a comprehensive clinical approach to the patient. Chapter 3 elaborates on the skills needed to apply the method in the consultation.

The patient-centred clinical method

Patient-centred care can be defined as the philosophy of care that encourages (a) a focus in the consultation on the patient as a whole person with particular values and needs that are contextualised within their own family and community environment (in contrast to a focus in the consultation only on a body part or disease); and/or (b) sharing control of the consultation and decisions about the management plan with the patient (Lewin *et al.*, 2001, Epstein *et al.*, 2008).

Patient-centredness encompasses the important principle of family medicine that the patient and their illness are more important than the biological disease (McWhinney, 1989). It is not merely a tool of the consultation process, but the very essence of the consultation in family medicine (Levenstein, 1994).

Patient-centred care is quality health care achieved through a partnership between informed and respected patients and their families, and a coordinated health care team (Picker Institute, 2004). This links into an increasing acknowledgement of the positive contribution of patient-centred health systems. In South Africa, the patient-centred approach underpins the principles of the Patient's Rights Charter and the *Batho Pele* principles of a caring health system (refer also to Chapter 11).

Evidence for patient-centred care

A number of research studies have found that there is a positive link between the practise of patient-centred health care in clinical settings and health outcomes (Henbest *et al.*, 1992, Stewart *et al.*, 1995, Little *et al.*, 2001). There is clear evidence that the patient-centred approach leads to an increase in patient trust and patient satisfaction, resolution of the person's concerns and a resultant decrease in anxiety, improved quality of life, more appropriate prescribing, increased doctor satisfaction and more efficient practise, resulting in fewer diagnostic tests and unnecessary referrals (Baumann *et al.*, 2003; Epstein *et al.*, 2008) .

There is also fairly strong evidence to suggest that some interventions to promote patient-centred care may lead to significant increases in the patient-centredness of the consultation processes. Training health care providers in patient-centred approaches may impact positively on patient satisfaction with care (Lewin *et al.*, 2001). Further research is needed on the effects of such interventions on patient health care behaviour or health status.

The World Health Organisation's report "Primary health care – Now more than ever" published in 2008 emphasised the role of patient-centredness in health care and provided numerous examples of such strategies being implemented throughout the world with significant positive outcomes as evidence. "Primary care health workers have to care for people throughout the course of their lives, as individuals and as members of a family and a community whose health must be protected and enhanced, and not merely as body parts with symptoms or disorders that need treatment. Each individual has his or her own way of experiencing and coping with health problems within their specific life circumstances; health workers must be able to handle this diversity."

Elements of the patient-centred model

The patient-centred model, illustrated in Figure 2.1, consists of six interconnecting components, namely (Stewart *et al.*, 1995):
- Exploring both the disease and illness experience
- Understanding the whole person
- Finding common ground
- Enhancing the doctor–patient relationship
- Incorporating prevention and health promotion
- Being realistic.

The next section will outline each of these components.

Figure 2.1 The patient-centred clinical method

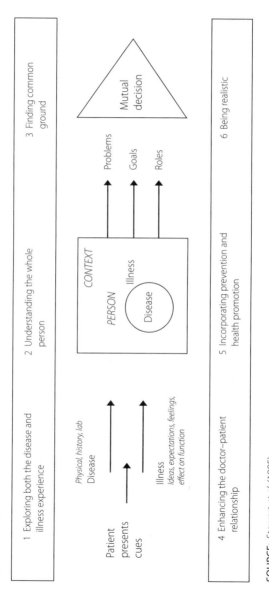

| 1 Exploring both the disease and illness experience | 2 Understanding the whole person | 3 Finding common ground |

Patient presents cues

Physical, history, lab
Disease

Illness
Ideas, expectations, feelings, effect on function

CONTEXT

PERSON

Illness

Disease

Problems

Goals

Roles

Mutual decision

| 4 Enhancing the doctor–patient relationship | 5 Incorporating prevention and health promotion | 6 Being realistic |

SOURCE: Stewart *et al.* (1995)

Exploring both the disease and the illness experience

Disease is the medical explanation of a health problem, whereas illness is more a personal experience of symptoms, feelings, and discomforts. This experience varies in different people, communities, cultures and contexts. To come to a complete understanding of the problem the family physician should understand both the illness and disease.

In the patient-centred approach, we use the terms *patient's agenda* and *doctor's agenda*. The doctor's agenda for the encounter involves identifying the problem and/or making a diagnosis, whereas the patient's agenda involves having their concerns and expectations regarding the illness addressed. For example, the expectations of a person complaining of a recurrent headache may include the performance of a skull X-ray, whilst the doctor's response may simply be to prescribe some medication for an apparently minor complaint. One way that medical staff change from doctor-centred to patient-centred is when they get sick and the roles are reversed. A good example is a professor of surgery who, shortly after his own operation and, having felt so much pain himself and not receiving adequate treatment, changed the whole post-operative pain management protocol. Both agendas are important and the concept is useful in reminding us that we cannot assume that the two agendas will be the same. In a patient-centred consultation, part of the doctor's agenda should be to understand and address the patient's agenda!

Exploring the disease

In exploring the disease we deal with the patient's complaints. The family physician uses critical reasoning skills to make a diagnosis from the presenting symptoms and signs. This is an essential part of any consultation and good clinical practice. The family physician takes a comprehensive but appropriate medical history, always performs a thorough and focused physical examination, supplemented by the necessary side-room investigations, and requests relevant special investigations. To truly practise patient-centered care we should record our findings using a model which includes both the patient's complaints and concerns. Donnelly (2005) proposes the HOAP model incorporating History, Observations, Assessment and Plan.

Exploring the illness

In exploring the illness we deal with the patient's perspective. Failure by the family physician to attend to the illness experience is in part responsible for non-adherence to treatment, patient dissatisfaction with health care, and missing the actual reason for consultation. In exploring the patient's illness experience, we specifically ask about the following:

- The patient's thoughts and ideas on the illness
- The patient's fears and concerns about the illness
- The effect of the illness on the patient's functioning
- The patient's expectations of the consultation.

The key to the patient-centred method is to allow as much as possible to flow from the patient, in order to understand the patient's expectations, feelings, and fears (Ellis, 1994).

Ideas

We all have our own thoughts and ideas on what could be wrong with us when we experience symptoms. For example, a medical student may think that her palpitations are due to a heart condition, but in actual fact after a thorough consultation it transpires that she is healthy but is consuming excessive amounts of coffee. Patients' upbringing, experiences, background, and fears shape their ideas about their illness. Failure to ascertain the patient's ideas about her illness results in poor communication between the family physician and the patient with resultant limited adherence and frustration for both the patient and the physician.

The patient's ideas about illness can be explored in the consultation by using simple questions such as:

- What do you think is the problem with your health?
- Have you any idea about what the cause of this may be?

Fears

When we become ill it is natural to be concerned and sometimes to fear the worst. Could this lump be cancer? Could this cough be tuberculosis? Is this spot a melanoma? If the doctor is not aware of the patient's worries important concerns will remain unresolved.

A consultation is not complete without the family physician exploring the patient's fears. If we do not address this we may find the patient consulting again, as these fears may continue to cause anxiety, and the patient may not improve subjectively despite objective recovery.

Explore your patient's fears with questions such as:

- What is it about your illness that worries you?
- What is the worst thing you think this might be?

Expectations

Patients always have expectations about what is going to happen when they consult their family physician. They may want medication, a sick certificate, reassurance, and so on. It is important to establish what the patient expects from you and the consultation process. Patient satisfaction is linked to the family physician openly considering the patient's expectations, but not necessarily acting upon all of them.

Explore the patient's expectations by asking the following questions:

- What is it that you want me to do for you today?
- What were you hoping we might do today?

The following example illustrates the value of being patient-centred rather than doctor- or disease-centred during the consultation:

A 42-year-old man attends a community-based health screening programme and enters the consulting room walking with an exaggerated limp and significant functional disability. His first utterance is that of disappointment and disillusionment with all doctors, nurses and social workers who have consulted with him previously during the past ten years after he was injured in a motor vehicle accident. The attending doctor's attention is diverted towards the large surgical scars on the patient's lower limbs and she continues to perform a clinical examination. The patient appears irritated and disinterested. The alert doctor then decides to listen more attentively to the patient and his concerns. The patient relates his frustration at not having received a disability grant from the state despite numerous attempts to gain the attention and empathy of a number of health workers previously consulted. He leaves the consulting room smiling broadly, and armed with a well-written referral note to the social welfare department. He is clearly impressed with having been consulted by a doctor who is patient-centred.

Loss of function

Together with any illness, there is usually some loss of function for the patient. For instance, the student missed an important test, the mother was too sick to care for her baby, and the labourer's backache was too severe for him to use his shovel. Exploring the extent of loss of function assists us in understanding the person and the effect the illness has on their life.

Loss of function indicates not only to what extent the patient is incapacitated by the illness, but also whether the functional loss is out of proportion to the disease. Disproportionate loss of function may be the result of individual, family or cultural beliefs, personal coping strategies or even the possibility of secondary gain from illness.

Explore loss of function with questions such as:

- How does this illness affect your daily tasks and life?
- Does the illness make it difficult or impossible for you to do any of your day-to-day tasks?

What patient-centred care is not:

- It is not being a nice guy.
- It is not only having a good bedside manner.
- It is not meeting all of the patient's demands (as opposed to addressing concerns).
- It is not only an academic exercise.
- It does not necessarily take more time.

The patient-centred method may take longer when you are learning it and integrating it into your approach. Once integrated, however, it does not take more time and does in fact make consultations more efficient and improves both the patient's and doctor's satisfaction with the consultation. (See also later in the chapter under Time constraints.)

The patient's context – understanding the whole person

Each person functions within a unique context. We have different backgrounds, upbringings, families, traditions, cultures, and education. The family physician should explore and attempt to understand the full context of the person. This includes understanding the family, the life stage of the patient, employment or lack thereof, cultural background, and the possible influence of the patient's community on their health (Stewart *et al.*, 1995). The case study below shows the importance of knowledge of the family in understanding the whole person:

A 32-year-old female patient presents with a two-year history of fronto-temporal headaches which have become progressively worse. Enquiry reveals that she lives with her husband and two children aged seven and two. Clinical examination is non-contributory. The attending doctor makes a diagnosis of chronic depression and refers this patient to a senior colleague.

The senior doctor who is very experienced in understanding family and contextual issues explores the illness further and, with the assistance of an ecomap (Refer to Chapter 4 for more information on an ecomap) is able to conclude that unresolved conflict between the patient and her husband and underlying extended family issues form the basis for this presentation. The patient and husband are counselled extensively, and the patient later experiences relief of her symptoms.

The same way that the patient has their own context, we should remember that the family physician also brings their own context to the consultation. We also have our own culture, family background, and prejudices. This is more at the level of our personal perspective – the subjective aspect of the doctor's perspective and how our behaviour stems from our own beliefs and fears. Where and how we grew up, how and what education we received, and how we live and are seen in our communities all influence the values that we bring to each encounter with a patient.

Family

Families have a profound influence on beliefs, behaviour, and attitudes. The family physician who understands the whole person recognises the impact of the family in ameliorating, aggravating, or even causing illness in family members. This is explored in more detail in Chapter 4.

The life stage of the patient

We start life as an infant, progressing through the toddler phase, primary school, adolescence, young adulthood, family formation, being parents, children moving out of the parental home, midlife, retirement, and old age. These stages influence and challenge the individual in different ways. Also, within these stages each person develops differently. It is important to identify the current life stage the person is experiencing and to assess to what extent the patient has adapted or is experiencing difficulties with it, as the following case study shows.

A family is in crisis after the sudden death of their father and husband. Mr X has just had a fatal heart attack and Mrs Y and her two children, a boy aged 17 and a girl aged 19 have to adapt very rapidly to this sudden change of circumstances.

Mrs Y is not able to work due to chronic knee pains. She asks her two children to decide amongst themselves as to which of them would be happy to abandon their studies and work in order to support the family. The boy feels compelled to follow his father's example as the family provider, and makes the decision to seek employment as a labourer. He presents at your clinic with complaints of chronic tiredness and lack of drive. It transpires that he performs well at school and has ambitions to become a doctor some day. After a family conference and with the assistance of a social worker a successful application for a disability grant for the mother is lodged, and a scholarship for the boy is obtained which also provides some support for the family.

Work

Employment (or lack thereof), including where someone works, what they do and who they work for, has a potential influence on health. This is not only in terms of finances, but also in terms of physical and mental well-being. Losing or not having a job means that you cannot feed yourself and your family. Consider all the possible occupational health hazards due to a person's particular occupation such as mining, construction, security work, nursing, airline pilots, and so on. Blue-collar workers may suffer anxiety and stress due to administrative work pressures. Being gainfully employed or providing volunteer services can also have a positive effect on health as it provides a sense of purpose, making a contribution, and belonging to a supportive community in the workplace. Well-being in the workplace is a very important concept. Consider the following case study.

A 35-year-old man consulted a family physician at a health centre because of pain in the knees and lower legs. He had visited the health centre a number of times with the same complaint. The family physicians that he saw during these visits had not found much on examination, but told him he had arthritis and treated him with non-steroidal anti-inflammatory medication and analgesics. During this time, he had also been X-rayed and had blood tests, all of which were normal. On this occasion, the family physician eventually asked him "What do you think might be causing the problem?" He responded that he thought it was due to his work, where he operated a forklift truck and spent most of the day using his legs to regulate the controls. It caused a lot of vibration and stress on his legs. The family physician wrote a letter to the man's employer and asked for him to be given other duties for a month. When the man returned a month later, he was pain-free and did not want any more tablets!

Community

The community in which people live and work plays a significant part in their well-being. Each community has its own environment, structures, habits and values. For example, a child from a poor township area is more likely to suffer from infectious diseases, possibly due to inadequate sanitation and the effects of overcrowding. People from rural areas with limited access to clean water, for instance, are more susceptible to gastroenteritis.

The community factor is relevant not only for the poor but also for the middle classes and the rich. The diseases of urbanisation are well known – hypertension, obesity, diabetes mellitus and atherosclerosis, to name a few. Consider the prevalence of crime and violence in some communities and the devastating effect this has on the lives of our patients. The manner in which communities function and are structured, especially in terms of community resources, also influences the health of its people.

The following information might be useful to obtain from your patient in order to explore the community context:

- Housing and household size
- Water supply
- Sanitation and hygiene
- Pests, such as mosquitoes, animals, and rodents
- Indoor air pollution, for example from cooking methods
- Food storage methods and possible contamination
- Community resources such as health and welfare service.

Culture

Our culture has an important influence on our health beliefs and views of our symptoms and illness. In some ways each person is a unique blend of cultural influences and yet may broadly share certain cultural beliefs or practices. Every encounter, in some way, is cross-cultural. A person's culture provides them with ideas about health and illness, the possible cause of the disease, and ideas about and how health care should be provided. These potential differences between the family physician and the patient pose a barrier to patient satisfaction and good health outcomes. Knowledge and understanding of and respect for the different cultures in which the family physician practises is vital (Silverman *et al.*, 1998).

Cultures are never static but keep changing. For family physicians to become culturally competent they move through various stages, from culturally destructive to culturally blind and, finally, culturally skilled. Culturally incompetent family physicians are of the opinion that patients from their own culture are of better health and follow instructions better that others. Culturally destructive doctors talk in a paternalistic way about patients from other cultures, don't feel at ease with people from different backgrounds, and often have exotic ideas or engage in stereotyping people from different cultures.

Mrs FM, a 45-year-old type-two diabetic, visits the family physician with symptoms of headaches and tiredness. The family physician is very upset to find out that Mrs FM has not taken her medication regularly, and warns her about the serious consequences of her actions. Mrs FM says nothing and leaves the rooms. When discussing the case with a colleague, the family physician is reminded that she saw the patient during the Muslim holy month of Ramadan, a factor that she had not even considered and discussed with the patient.

The family medicine student needs to keep in mind that doctor–patient interactions may differ in different cultures. What is considered good manners in one culture may not be understood as such by a person of another culture (Skelton *et al.*, 2001). For instance, in some cultures it is not acceptable to look somebody in the eye when you greet them, whilst in other cultures this would be seen as suspicious. Practitioners should also not be surprised that some patients may not understand or co-operate with your patient-centred approach as they are used to health services where the power vests solely in the health worker.

Finding common ground

Family physicians should reach common ground between the patient's ideas and expectations, and their own ideas, plans, and management goals. Finding common ground mostly involves the family physician and the patient, but wider networks of family members and significant others should also sometimes be included. All parties should be encouraged to participate in the process of finding common ground. Sharing information is a prerequisite for this as people are not able to fully participate in shared decision-making if they are not empowered with the relevant knowledge. In finding common ground the family physician integrates a number of skills, namely effective communication, ethical reasoning and applying evidence-based knowledge into practice (see also Chapters 12 and 13). The process for finding common ground involves the following (Stewart *et al.*, 1995):

- Develop a shared understanding of the presenting problems.
- Understand and agree on the goal of the management plan.
- Explore the expectations of the family physician and patient regarding each other's roles.
- Undertake mutual decision-making in the management of the problem.

There are four key communication skills that can assist you in the process of finding common ground, namely (Stewart *et al.*, 1995):
- The provision of clear information
- Questions from the patient
- A willingness to share (discuss) decisions
- Agreement between the patient and the family physician about the problem and the plan.

It is essential that safe and ample space is provided within the consultation for patients to ask their questions. Often the doctor will ask the patient for any questions and then not provide time and empathy for the patient to respond.

Defining the problem(s)

Stott and Davis (1979) have described a useful four-point framework to achieve maximum benefit from the clinical assessment and subsequent management plan in any consultation and that can assist in finding common ground. See Figure 2.2 for the concept of the exceptional potential in each primary care consultation.

Figure 2.2 The exceptional potential in each primary care consultation

A. Management of presenting problem(s)	C. Modification of help-seeking behaviour
B. Management of continuing problem(s)	D. Opportunistic health promotion

A: Management of presenting problem(s)

There should be agreement on the nature of the presenting problem(s) between the family physician and the patient. The family physician's understanding of the problem(s) should make sense from the patient's perspective. Family physicians often do not relate their explanations to the patient's context and level of understanding, and ignore cues from patients about their ideas. Also, we can get into difficulty in defining the patient's problem by inappropriate use of the conventional medical model and/or using medical jargon (Stewart *et al.*, 1995). A practical way to make sure that patients understand the problem is to ask them to explain their understanding of the problem in their own words.

B: Management of continuing problem(s)

It is important to note that, with the dramatic increase in chronic diseases over the last century, both presenting and continuing problems may co-exist. These problems may or may not be related. For example, a patient presenting with a urinary tract infection may also have type-two diabetes; an HIV-positive patient may present with acute diarrhoea; or a patient with a sore throat is also known to have rheumatoid arthritis. A systematic approach to the management of both the presenting problem and any underlying or concurrent disease is part of a comprehensive approach to patient care. In providing comprehensive primary care the family physician must pay attention to all the patient's health problems as the commitment is to the whole person and not a particular group of diseases, as may be the case in specialist hospital practice.

Barriers to continuity of care (such as patient numbers, excessive demands on the doctor, lack of funding, drugs and equipment, etc) may be overwhelming to many doctors, especially at primary care level. The appropriate strategy to deal with these challenges may vary from place to place, and may include using a different patient record system, increased time allocation to certain patients, as well as the proper and judicious usage of other members of the primary care team, individually and as teams.

C: Modification of help-seeking behaviour

Doctors should identify and analyse the motives behind the help-seeking behaviour of the patient. By addressing this, patients may be better equipped to perform more appropriate self-care. This might avoid unnecessary future consultations or ensure that patients seek help more timeously in future for serious health problems. It is particularly important that every family physician analyses help-seeking behaviour and encourages those that are perceived to be positive and discourages those that are not. For example, patients and their families may be encouraged to initially treat a common cold with over-the-counter remedies in future rather than immediately consulting a doctor; a mother may be taught how to make and administer oral rehydration solution at home if her child again develops diarrhoea and be educated on issues such as monitoring of hydration and when to seek help. A patient just needing a repeat prescription may be informed about how to obtain this without wasting time on a full consultation or a patient with ischaemic heart disease, who experiences angina, is educated on the proper use of sublingual glyceryl trinitrate and when to attend the health centre as an emergency.

D: Opportunistic health promotion

Stott and Davis (1979) also emphasise the goal of attending to health promotion and disease prevention in the consultation. The current burden of disease, with its accompanying morbidity and mortality, has much of its origins in risky behaviour and the lifestyles of individuals (see Table 1.1 in Chapter 1).

The promotion of healthy lifestyles and the early screening for many diseases by both doctor and patient remain an exciting and attractive option within the consultation. The patient is assisted to identify components of their lifestyle that could be changed and therefore positively influence future health outcomes. This could include social and recreational habits such as increased physical activity, healthier eating, smoking cessation and moderate alcohol use. Screening for early disease may, for example, include testing blood pressure and blood glucose, as well as breast examinations and cervical smears,

Together, the promotion of health and the prevention of disease form two of the essential components of the patient-centred clinical approach, and are described in detail in Chapter 5.

Defining the management goals

The management goals in relation to the presenting as well as continuing problems should be discussed with the patient. Firstly, listen carefully to the patient's expectations. The subtext could include a referral for a specialist opinion, and if this is not addressed, the patient will remain dissatisfied with the outcome of the consultation. Some patients respond by declaring; "But you're the doctor and know what the best decision is". These patients may need encouragement to reveal their expectations. In addition, the family physician should be aware of her sweeping decision-making powers that this declaration, by implication, gives to her. If previous treatment plans did not work, explore what happened without becoming defensive.

Defining the roles of the patient and the family physician

Family physicians and patients will have perceptions of each other's roles. Three kinds of relationships can be identified:

1 *Paternalistic.* Some patients will expect the family physician to make all the decisions. The family physician does what they think is best for the patient without necessarily eliciting the patient's preferences.

2 *Consumerist.* At the other extreme, the patient controls the relationship. To keep the patient happy, the family physician may accede to the patient's requests and waste resources with little real benefit to the patient.

3 *Collaborative.* In the third instance, both the family physician and the patient have a high degree of control. There is open negotiation and discussion of goals and plans. The patient's preferences are actively sought and compared with the family physician's thoughts and suggestions. The relationship aims to find common ground and a mutually acceptable plan is the ideal.

Each consultation is different and dissatisfaction or frustration can arise from a mismatch in assumptions about the roles of doctor and patient, for example if the patient would like more participation, but the doctor is grounded in a paternalistic approach or if the doctor would like participation but the patient can only conceive that the doctor knows best. The trend in family medicine is to strive for a more collaborative approach where open dialogue can resolve differences in perspective.

Shared decision-making

Failure to involve the patient in the decision-making process often leads to non-adherence to therapy or management. Shared decision-making means the family physician shares the treatment options with the patient, provides sufficient information on the risks and benefits of each treatment, and acknowledges the patient's preference. This not only increases patient satisfaction, but also increases the effectiveness of treatment modalities, and leads to a reduction in the waste of resources (Elwyn *et al.*, 1999). It is important that the family physician uses her evidence-based practice skills in the process of shared decision-making (see also Chapter 13).

Practical steps that family physicians can follow to attain shared decision-making include the following (adapted from Elwyn *et al.*, 1999):

• Establish an atmosphere in which the patient's views about treatment options are acknowledged and understood.

- Elicit the patient's preferences so that appropriate treatment options can be discussed.
- Transfer technical information to the patient on treatment options, risks, and benefits in an unbiased, clear, and simple way.
- Help the patient conceptualise the process of weighing risk versus benefit, and ensure that their preferences are based on fact and not misconception.
- Provide the patient ample opportunity to ask questions and raise concerns or issues relevant to them.
- Discuss the patient's concerns and establish their understanding following that.
- Establish explicit expression of agreement by both the patient and yourself on the above.

The following is an example of dynamics in a shared decision-making process:

A final year medical student examines a woman who was dizzy and tired. On examination the patient had a cardiac murmur and symptomatic heart failure with a haemoglobin count of four (later proven to be 2.7). The student consulted the physician on call for possible referral, as the woman needed to be admitted, transfused and investigated. Imagine the student's surprise when the patient refused admission! He had omitted to discuss with the patient the management possibilities. She wanted to attend a family funeral on Saturday (now Wednesday). The team then negotiated admission for transfusion, discharge by Friday and follow-up on the Monday to continue the investigations.

Patients often do not ask questions despite being prompted because the family physician uses only closed questions, does not give enough time for the patient to consider the questions, and confuses the patient with an overload of information without checking for the patient's understanding. Other reasons for patients not asking questions include (adapted from Tuckett *et al.*, 1985):
- They believe it is not their place to ask questions or to behave as if their view is important.
- They are afraid that the family physician will form a negative opinion of them.
- They are too anxious to express themselves clearly.
- They are frightened of a negative response by the family physician.
- They doubt that the family physician will provide any more information.

- They forget or wait until the end of the consultation.

The three-stage assessment and management plan– a practical tool

The three stage assessment is an instrument that we use to assess our patients holistically (Fehrsen and Henbest, 1993). It is referred to as an assessment, rather than a diagnosis, as often in family medicine the patient presents too early during the disease process for a definite diagnosis to be made. Sometimes there is no physical disease present or the patient presents with psychosocial problems impacting on their well-being.

The three stage-assessment consists of three components: clinical, individual, and contextual assessment.

The clinical assessment

This is the biomedical part of the assessment, based on the symptoms, signs and investigations related to the patient's disease. This is recorded at the highest level of certainty. For example, a patient could be assessed initially as "jaundice – cause?" or with more certainty as "hepatocellular jaundice" or with complete diagnostic certainty as "acute hepatitis B". It is important to be clear as to one's level of certainty.

The individual assessment

This is the assessment of how the patient is experiencing the illness; it is their perception of the problem. It includes the patient's ideas, emotions, thoughts and fears about the illness. It also includes the person's expectations around the consultation and its outcomes, as well as the possible impact of the illness on their daily functioning.

The contextual assessment

This is the assessment of the person's environment and how it affects them, as well as how the patient's illness impacts on their family, life and work environment. It includes the person's family, support structures, life stage, work, community, environment, and so on. It is a description of where the person finds themselves in the social system. Practical tools to assess the patient's family context are the ecomap and the genogram, which are described in Chapter 4.

The three stage assessment can be used in any consultation. The emphasis may shift with varying presenting problems, but in most patients, such a holistic assessment is useful. Below are examples of how you would use it.

Example 1

A mother presents with her 24-year-old son at the clinic. He has suffered from epilepsy for many years and has had extensive investigations and treatment at the neurology clinic of two different tertiary hospitals. He has not been able to find work although he is otherwise fit and healthy. The mother bursts into tears when the family physician explains that the epilepsy is never going to be cured and that the son will always have to take tablets. See Table 2.1 for a three-stage assessment for this patient.

Table 2.1 Example of a three-stage assessment and management plan

	Assessment	Management
Clinical	Epilepsy – generalised tonic-clonic seizures	• Review anti-epileptic medications following relevant blood tests • Monitor adherence, control and any complications • Promote healthy lifestyle that will minimise risk of seizures, for example alcohol use, adequate sleep, and so on
Individual	• Expectations of cure • Would like to work but anxious about employment • Worries about medications and brain damage • Would not need to continue with medication long term • Worried that he would develop brain damage over time because of condition	• Relevant patient information and counselling (chronic illness and long-term medications, diet and other lifestyle issues, risk exposure, and so on) • Refer to any local support groups
Contextual	• Unemployed • Supportive mother • Financial issues	• Consider referral to SANEL for up-skilling and job creation • Consider eligibility for disability grant • Counsel family regarding the diagnosis and prognosis

Example 2

A 40-year-old man visits the family physician with complaints of central burning chest pain for the past two weeks. He is the manager of a busy supermarket chain and is burdened with a range of responsibilities at work. Furthermore, his wife and two young children have started to feel neglected and they have little time together. He fears that his symptoms could be due to a heart problem and he could face the same fate as his late brother who passed away recently after a heart attack at the age of 44. The patient smokes about ten cigarettes per day. Examination reveals a moderately overweight male with stigmata of hypercholesterolaemia; blood pressure systolic 140 and diastolic 95. See Table 2.2 for a three-stage assessment for this patient.

Table 2.2 Example of a three-stage assessment and management plan

	Assessment	Management
Clinical	• Elevated blood pressure • Overweight • Possible metabolic syndrome • Possible ischaemic heart disease or gastro-oesophageal reflux • Smoker	• Investigate for ischaemic heart disease, ECG and maybe stress ECG • Trial of treatment for gastro-oesophageal reflux and gastroscopy if indicated later • Explore risk factors: fasting glucose, lipogram • Follow-up blood pressure • Behaviour change counselling: diet, exercise, smoking cessation, moderate alcohol use
Individual	• Concerns about family life • Worries about dying and leaving family without income • Concerns about cardiac status	• Acknowledge and address concerns • Explore work/life balance
Contextual	• Family dysfunction • Family history of cardiovascular disease • Business executive	• Include wife in behaviour change counselling and consider seeing them as a couple

Example 3

A 37-year-old male presents to the local clinic with symptoms of urinary frequency and burning on micturition for the past one month. He is employed and married, but admits to having several sexual partners. He smokes fifteen cigarettes a day and drinks a couple of beers every night. Clinically, he has small penile ulcers and a yellowish urethral discharge. Urine dipstick test shows 3+ blood, nitrite positive and protein 1+. See Table 2.3 for a three-stage assessment of this patient.

Table 2.3 Example of a three-stage assessment and management plan

	Assessment	Management
Clinical	• Genital ulcer syndrome • Urethral discharge syndrome • Possibility of HIV • Smoker • High alcohol intake	• Syndromic management of genital ulcer and urethral discharge and counselling • Offer HIV and RPR test with consent • Modify help-seeking behaviour • Consider behaviour change counselling: safe sex, smoking cessation, moderate alcohol use
Individual	• Worried which sexual partner caused his disease • Feels entitled to have multiple sexual partners • Does not want his wife to know about this	• Culturally-sensitive counselling on risky sexual behaviour and his sexual choices
Contextual	• Multiple sexual partners • Cultural and community background	• Discuss contact-tracing as well as future protection, including his wife

The three-stage assessment is a practical tool to use as a framework when we assess our patients and also to integrate a holistic approach into our routine practice. Initially the family physician may record a three-stage assessment in full in the clinical notes, while later on they will use this framework to reach a comprehensive assessment of the patient without necessarily writing it all down.

The doctor–patient relationship

The importance of establishing and maintaining a good doctor–patient relationship cannot be too strongly emphasised. Often both accurate diagnosis and effective treatment are directly dependent on a functioning doctor-patient relationship.

The biggest failure of modern medicine is the breakdown of a caring relationship with our patients. Students sometimes view abuse of patients by health care workers and feel helpless in dealing with it. First and foremost, it is the ethical duty and privilege of all health professionals to care for vulnerable, powerless and compromised patients. Values such as integrity, respect, honesty, humility and unconditional positive regard should reflect in all our actions in providing health care services to our patients and communities. Refer to Chapter 3 for an in-depth discussion of these.

Being realistic

Being realistic is about understanding that we live in an imperfect world, where the theory and the realities of practice sometimes differ vastly. Being realistic is included in the patient-centred approach so that the family physician understands how to work within the specific constraints, challenges and opportunities offered by the setting of their practice. In South Africa, we have to deal with a particular set of realities. In other countries there may be different realities as students returning from international electives often attest to.

> **Q** In the following case study, identify factors that influence reality in health care before you continue with the rest of this section. What are the realities that we are dealing with here?

You work in a rural clinic about 150 kilometres from the nearest hospital. The clinic has a limited supply of medicines and no X-ray facilities. It serves a huge area and there are many patients waiting to see you. You do not feel well today as your 18-month-old baby has a cold and you had to get up in the night to attend to her. The patient sitting before you is Mrs SG (29-years-old), who had to walk for two hours to reach the clinic. It is the third time she has come to the clinic as the previous times she was too late because she walked slowly and there were too many patients before her. She has had a cough for about three months, has lost weight and feels weak and is not able to fetch water for her household every day. Mrs SG has a two-year-old daughter and her husband works on the mines in Johannesburg.

Time constraints

In busy health services, time is at a premium. Mrs SG has already been turned away from the clinic twice before because of the patient load, and you are the only doctor there. If she is not attended to today her health problem may escalate into complications.

The family physician should plan each day to make optimal use of time. Focusing on the patient's agenda, using ongoing consultations, and proper clinical note-keeping are things that you can practise to save time. Concentrate on the most important problem and deal with that first. However, keep in mind that the first complaint is not always the most important problem. Two simple questions to ask in this regard are (Epstein *et al.*, 2008):

- Is there something else you are worried about?
- Is there anything else you would like to tell me about?

The family physician must be able to prioritise problems and, if necessary, negotiate an agenda for the consultation with the patient. You can for instance ask: "Which of these issues would you like us to start with today?"

Not all areas of patient concern need to be explored in every consultation; you can use further consultations to explore issues over a number of visits. In our case, however, Mrs SG had to walk for two hours to reach the clinic. Therefore, you may have to maximise your opportunity with some patients and do as much as possible for them during the one visit.

The family physician must be able to recognise which patients might need more time. Such patients include:

- Those with multiple symptoms or several concerns
- Where there is difficult disclosure of a problem
- Those whose safety is at risk
- Those with a potentially serious problem.

Mrs SG most likely will need to have an HIV test, and therefore more time will be needed to explain this to her and to do pretest counselling.

The patient's context

Mrs SG comes from a traditional, rural Zulu culture. She grew up with her family relying on traditional healers to keep the family healthy, as no other services were available. To her the traditional healer is a respected and well-loved person in the community. If you do not understand this background you may easily react paternalistically to the patient's help-seeking behaviour.

Mrs SG also speaks only Zulu which is not the same as your own home language. You have learnt to use some Zulu phrases, but cannot speak the language fluently. If you need to explore her individual and contextual issues or provide counselling you may need to find a suitable interpreter or refer to a Zulu-speaking counsellor.

Resources

In a rural clinic, you have fewer facilities and resources available than in hospital, and you have to be resourceful so that you can provide the best and most appropriate treatment for the many patients that you see.

To refer a patient to a higher level of care is not always feasible because of the cost factor and the disruption this causes in your patient's life. In Mrs SG's case, you will have to decide whether it is really necessary to refer her for a chest X-ray in addition to the HIV and tuberculosis tests you have requested.

It is important that you know what resources are available to your health service, both in terms of other health services and practitioners to refer to, the NPO sector, as well as resources in the community. Make sure that your health service has a comprehensive list including contact numbers for these resources. If such a list is not available, do a little investigation of what is available and draw up the list yourself.

Costs

Health care costs have spiraled with limited budgets available for health care delivery. In the case of Mrs SG, several cost factors must be considered, for example special investigations, possible treatment including anti-tuberculosis and antiretroviral treatment, as well as management of complications she may encounter with or without treatment. Considering cost implications may interfere with the doctor–patient relationship, as it presents a disparity between what the patient wants or needs, what is affordable, and what the health system can provide. This illustrates the importance of management skills and an understanding of health care financing (see Chapter 10). Part of being realistic is to constantly be aware that you have to make these choices and weigh up the odds correctly. You should use your professional judgement in this process, so that a decision is not made by default but as a result of an active reasoning process, which includes ethical considerations (see Chapter 12).

Being realistic about your own abilities and context

A family physician has their own needs and life at a personal as well as professional level. It is important that you develop self-awareness and are able to identify your own strengths and weaknesses. In the case of Mrs SG, you are tired and worried about your sick baby girl at home. You also feel extra sympathy for Mrs SG as she also has a young daughter to care for whilst she herself is not well. It is good to acknowledge this to yourself and the people you work with rather than to try to be everything to everybody all the time. You serve your patients best when you also take your own welfare and health into consideration. The first step to appropriate help is to admit that there is a possible problem.

Self-awareness – the family physician's context

When we examine our patient, we cannot escape examining ourselves (Balint, 1996). The purpose of self-awareness is to know what is going on inside and to recognise how it has an influence on the consultation. Feelings such as anger, fear, helplessness, and frustration could all impact on your relationship with the patient.

How do we develop this self-awareness? A starting point is to reflect on our experiences within the doctor–patient relationship. Make time to think about what happened in the consultation. How did it make you feel, what thoughts and memories did it evoke in you, and why? Recognise the ambivalence that often forms part of your relationship with patients and deal with it in a responsible manner. Question your ideas and feelings. For example, if you feel anger or fear, explore this:

- What is it that is making me angry right now? Is it something about the patient or is it something about myself?
- Does it tell me something about what is going on?
- Does it interfere with my communication with the patient?
- Does it interfere with my reasoning and decision-making?
- Should I share it with the patient or not?

Do not hesitate to seek help for yourself and/or your family when needed. The patients and community you serve need you to be well, healthy and well-adapted to care for their well-being.

Conclusion

This chapter introduces the student to the patient-centred clinical method. This holistic approach takes into account patients' ideas, concerns, expectations and life situations in addition to their symptoms and signs. The approach encourages the patient to participate in the consultation and decision-making process. The patient-centred approach focuses on the person as opposed to the disease. By using the three-stage assessment tool, you should be able to make a more comprehensive assessment and formulate a management plan that is practical, cost-effective and extends beyond a simple theoretical approach.

Recommended reading

1. Stewart, M, Brown, JB *et al.* (1995). *Patient-centred Medicine. Transforming the Clinical Method.* Thousand Oaks, California: Sage.
2. Fraser RC. (2003). *Clinical Method: A general practice approach.* Oxford: Butterworth-Heinemann.
3. Stott NCH, Davis RH. (1979). The exceptional potential in each primary care consultation. *Journal of the Royal College of General Practitioners.* 201: 201–205.
4. The World Health Report (2008): Primary Health Care – Now More Than Ever. Geneva: WHO.

3 Communication skills

Julia Blitz
Division of Family Medicine
University of Stellenbosch

This chapter describes the communication skills that are effective within the patient-centred clinical method discussed in Chapter 2. It offers a framework in which you can integrate the patient's needs and perspective with the biomedical history by using effective communication skills to get accurate information. In other words, to both discover the patient's unique ideas and concerns and take a focused and accurate biomedical history.

This chapter places communication skills within a comprehensive clinical method by incorporating patient-centred medicine into both process and content aspects of the medical interview.

A strong, therapeutic and effective relationship is the *sine qua non* of physician-patient communication. The Kalamazoo Consensus Statement endorses a patient-centred, or relationship-centred, approach to care, which emphasises both the patient's disease and their illness experience. This requires eliciting the patient's story of illness while guiding the interview through a process of diagnostic reasoning. It also requires an awareness that the ideas, feelings, and values of both the patient and the physician influence the relationship. Further, this approach regards the physician–patient relationship as a partnership, and respects patients' active participation in decision-making. The task of building a relationship is also relevant for work with patients' families and support networks. In essence, building a relationship is an ongoing task within and across encounters: it encompasses the more sequentially-ordered sets of tasks identified below.

Open the discussion
- Allow the patient to complete their opening statement
- Elicit the patient's full set of concerns
- Establish/maintain a personal connection

Gather information
- Use open-ended and closed-ended questions appropriately
- Structure, clarify, and summarise information
- Actively listen using non-verbal (for example eye contact) and verbal (for example words of encouragement) techniques

Understand the patient's perspective and context
- Acknowledge and respond to the patient's ideas, feelings, and values
- Explore beliefs, concerns, and expectations about health and illness
- Explore contextual factors (for example family, culture, gender, age, socio- economic status, spirituality)

Share information
- Use language the patient can understand
- Check for understanding
- Encourage questions

Reach agreement on problems and plans
- Encourage the patient to participate in decisions to the extent they desire
- Check the patient's willingness and ability to follow the plan
- Identify and enlist resources and supports

Provide closure
- Ask whether the patient has other issues or concerns
- Summarise and affirm agreement on the plan of action
- Discuss follow-up (for example the next visit, a plan for unexpected outcomes)

FROM Essential Elements of Communication in Medical Encounters: The Kalamazoo Consensus Statement. *Acad. Med.* 2001; 76: 390–393.

Doctors with good communication skills identify patients' problems more accurately; have greater job satisfaction and less work stress. Their patients adjust better psychologically and are more satisfied with their care (Maguire and Pitceathly, 2002). Therefore, perfecting your communication skills will be beneficial not only to your patients, but also to you and to the success of your practice.

It is difficult to learn communication skills from reading about them. The best way is to be observed and get feedback on your skills in a real consultation. Audio-tape, video-tape, or direct observation are all methods you can use. Role-play of consultations and rehearsal of skills in a safe environment can also be useful. You may like to discuss your answers to the questions posed throughout the chapter with some of your colleagues, or with a tutor.

Before progressing to the full-blown consultation, you may like to practice three core techniques: invite, listen and summarise (Boyle, Dwinnell and Platt, 2005). That is, invite the patient to talk (allow the patient to tell their story), listen actively (concentrate on the task of listening, observe their verbal and non-verbal cues) and summarise (respond to what you have heard and seen and express empathy).

Remember that the first impression that you and the patient have of each other is where the communication starts. You cannot know what impression you may give the patient, but it is worthwhile to start the consultation attempting to convey a professional, friendly and concerned approach. This can be conveyed by your body language, the nature of your greeting and your overall appearance. The first impression that the patient gives you can be valuable if you are able to tune into the patient's emotional state. However, be careful of making assumptions about the patient based on their initial appearance.

From the start, you need to bear in mind your goal of collaboration with the patient and to do all you can throughout the consultation to facilitate this outcome.

Kurtz et al. (2003) have given us a framework of tasks for the consultation that covers both the process of relationship building and the structure of information gathering. This is summarised in Figure 3.1.

Figure 3.1 Objectives and tasks to be achieved within the medical interview

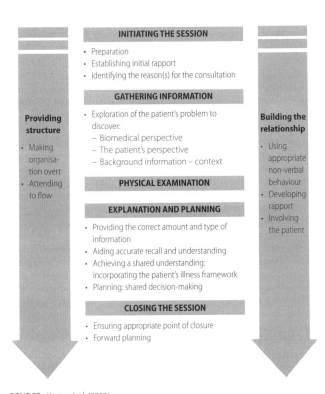

SOURCE: Kurtz *et al.* (2003)

Prior to the consultation

Prepare yourself to be of help to this particular patient, by being open to their agenda and their health belief model. Ensure that you will have no avoidable interruptions (telephone, receptionist, cleaner, and so on) to your consultation. It is equally important to establish whether you have an agenda for this particular consultation. Scan the patient's record and problem list briefly, to reconnect with their last visit. There may be an opportunity for health promotion, or education, or to address an issue that needs following up.

The first half of the consultation

The first half of the consultation extends from the initial greeting to the end of the physical examination, when the family physician reaches their initial assessment and considers an appropriate management plan.

The specific tasks and communication skills needed in the first half of the consultation are listed in Table 3.1 below.

Table 3.1 Communication tasks and skills for the first half of consultation

Building the relationship

- DEMONSTRATES GENUINE INTEREST AND RESPECT: appropriate non-verbal be-haviour (eye contact, posture, position, movement, facial expression, use of voice), reads or writes in a way that does not break flow or damage rapport, avoids or deals with inappropriate interruptions

- ACCEPTS LEGITIMACY OF PATIENT'S VIEW: shows difference between acceptance and agreement, avoids arguing with or judging patient, unconditional positive regard

- DEMONSTRATES EMPATHY AND SUPPORT: reflective listening, expresses concern, willingness to help, acknowledges coping efforts and appropriate self-care

- IS SENSITIVE TO EMBARRASSING AND DISTURBING TOPICS: includes examination

- APPEARS CONFIDENT: reasonably relaxed

Initiating the session

- GREETS patient: checks patient's name

- INTRODUCES SELF: clarifies role as medical student

- DEMONSTRATES INTEREST AND RESPECT: attends to physical comfort

- IDENTIFIES AND CONFIRMS PATIENT'S PROBLEM LIST: for example "So headache, fever – anything else you'd like to talk about?"

- NEGOTIATES AGENDA: if necessary, introduces other issues on doctor's agenda, negotiates which issues to prioritise

Gathering information

Exploration of problems

- ENCOURAGES PATIENT TO TELL STORY: relate problem(s) from when first started to the present in own words (clarifies reason for presenting now)

- APPROPRIATELY MOVES FROM OPEN TO CLOSED QUESTIONS: uses both open and closed questioning techniques. Obtains sufficient information to enable safe and effective decision-making. Avoids an interrogation style of questioning

- LISTENS ATTENTIVELY: allows patient to complete statements without interruption and leaves space for patient to think before answering or go on after pausing

- CLARIFIES MEANING: by reflective listening statements or questions of clarification, for example "Could you explain what you mean by lightheaded"

- FACILITATES PATIENT'S RESPONSE VERBALLY AND NON-VERBALLY: use of encouragement, silence, repetition, paraphrasing

- USES EASILY UNDERSTOOD LANGUAGE: avoids or adequately explains jargon

- ESTABLISHES DATES

Understanding the patient's perspective

- DETERMINES AND ACKNOWLEDGES PATIENT'S IDEAS: for example beliefs regarding cause

- EXPLORES CONCERNS: for example worries, effects on lifestyle, fears regarding each problem

- DETERMINES PATIENT'S EXPECTATIONS: for example particular types of investigation, treatment, referral, and so on regarding each problem

- ENCOURAGES EXPRESSION OF FEELINGS AND THOUGHTS

- PICKS UP VERBAL AND NON-VERBAL CLUES: body language, speech, facial expression, affect

- CHECKS OUT: appropriate acknowledgement

Understanding the patient's context

- DETERMINES SIGNIFICANT PAST MEDICAL HISTORY

- DETERMINES CURRENT USE OF MEDICATION: both prescription and non-prescription and any allergies

- EXPLORES PATIENT'S LIFESTYLE: smoking, alcohol use, exercise, diet

- EXPLORES THE FAMILY STRUCTURE: household members, draws genogram, key illnesses and psychosocial information (ages, deaths, relationships, abuse, and so on

- EXPLORES occupational history, current employment and work environment

- DETERMINES PHYSICAL ENVIRONMENT: type of housing, services available, location

Structuring the consultation

- SUMMARISES AT END OF A SPECIFIC LINE OF INQUIRY: verify own interpretation of what patient has said to ensure no important data was omitted

- PROGRESSES USING TRANSITIONAL STATEMENTS: explain rationale for change in topic

- STRUCTURES INTERVIEW IN LOGICAL SEQUENCE

- ATTENDS TO TIMING: keeps interview on task, avoids repetition

Physical examination of the patient

Complete internal hypothesis-testing

SOURCE: Adapted from the Calgary-Cambridge Observation Guide (1998)

Building the relationship

Use appropriate non-verbal behaviour

Touch is a very powerful non-verbal means of conveying the family physician's feelings of care, concern, and support. In the role of doctor, we are given permission to touch patients when we examine them. However, touch outside of the examination, if used sensitively and genuinely, can help the patient when they find it difficult to express feelings. Be aware of the fact that you are invading the patient's personal space when you do this and be prepared to retreat if they do not respond positively. Be aware of how you use other forms of non-verbal behaviour, such as eye contact, posture, facial expression, position in the room, clothing and hand movements. When writing notes or using the computer, be careful not to break the flow or lose contact with your patient.

Developing rapport

Continue to develop rapport with your patient by displaying genuine acceptance and respect for them as a unique individual. Development of this rapport allows the growth of a doctor–patient relationship within which communication is effective, but which is in and of itself a therapeutic relationship. A number of attributes have been identified that are associated with a therapeutic doctor–patient relationship (Silverman *et al.*, 1998).

Respect

An American psychologist, Carl Rogers (1967:63), referred to respect as "unconditional positive regard". For the family physician, this means having the skill to accept the patient as a person who may be very different from you and to acknowledge the patient's feelings, experiences, and meanings. We cannot develop the relationship if we ignore or judge the person's thoughts, fears, feelings, and expectations. If a family physician can display this kind of non-judgemental acceptance, it fosters a very valuable sense of safety and trust for the patient.

Any behaviour by family physicians that betrays the trust that patients place in them leads to a feeling of betrayal in the patients (and often their families), which is usually irreversible. Once patients lose the confidence that they may securely share information, thoughts, fears, and feelings with their family physician, the relationship will be broken.

Empathy

This has been referred to as "walking with" the person, or listening with understanding. In other words, it means seeing things from the patient's point of view and having an idea of what it means to them and what it feels like for them. This should not be confused with sympathy, which is to be simultaneously affected by the same feelings as your patient. Rather than being angry when your patient is angry, understand why it is that they have reacted in this way and acknowledge how that reaction makes them feel.

Honesty

This does not necessarily mean brutal honesty, where the patient needs to always and immediately be told the truth, the whole truth, and nothing but the truth. Rather, it refers to an attitude of integrity and fairness. We also can express what we feel in the consultation. In other words, the patient needs to know exactly where they stand. Again, this attitude fosters a secure relationship. Never tell your patient something that is not true. However, in the words of Richard Clarke Cabot (quoted in Wilkins, 1991:34), "Before you tell the truth to the patient, be sure you know the truth, and that the patient wants to hear it". Avoid offering premature reassurance because if your assumptions are not confirmed by your further history-taking and examination, you may turn out not to be in a position to offer any reassurance at all. Wait until you know sufficient facts before starting to make a plan.

Tolerance

This means tolerance of emotionally disturbing things. This is the skill to be able to deal with things that we hear from patients that may arouse a range of emotions in us, from anger to disgust and from fear to revulsion. Despite evoking these emotions in us, they remain our patient and we need to find ways of dealing with our feelings. How do we feel about the man who brings the woman he has just finished beating to casualty for us to look after her wounds? How do we feel when we need to treat someone who is brought to us on suspicion of drunk driving after having run over a pedestrian? How do we feel when the HIV-positive person continues to have unprotected sexual intercourse? Our emotional responses depend to some extent on our personal prejudices, values, and assumptions, as well as the prevailing societal response to such issues, but also may be modified by our knowledge (or lack thereof) of the patient.

Support

Express your willingness to help the patient in an ongoing partnership. This is not taking on patients' problems as your own, but confirming your commitment to help with them. Acknowledge the efforts that the patient has already made to cope with their problem and affirm appropriate attempts at self-care, as this will build the patient's self-efficacy, sense of partnership, and communicate your genuine respect for what they have done.

Sensitivity

Be aware of questions, topics or activities during the consultation that may be embarrassing or distressing to the patient. Handle these topics or events with sensitivity.

Initiating the session

Establish initial rapport

It is important to establish rapport with the patient from the beginning of the consultation. Rapport is defined as a relation of mutual understanding or trust and agreement between people. This will be facilitated if you aim to begin the consultation by communicating your respect, interest, and care for the patient. Give the patient your full attention – do not be tempted to write notes at this stage. The patient could interpret this as a lack of interest. Greet the patient appropriately (preferably by name) and introduce yourself if you do not already know the patient. This also gives you a chance to check that the patient's identity corresponds with the medical record and if necessary to explain your role as a student.

Identify the reason(s) for the consultation

Establish from patients what they would like to achieve by the end of the consultation – their agenda. Allow patients to complete their opening statement without interruption. If necessary, negotiate with the patient to pursue your own agenda for the consultation and then establish a mutually agreed-on plan that will cover both your needs and those of the patient. When the patient presents many apparent problems, it can also be helpful to ask which one should be tackled first or even which ones should be tackled today or deferred to a later visit. This allows patients to prioritise their problems with you. This prioritisation is based on the patient's level of concern and therefore helps you to ensure that if you tackle the patient's top priorities, you are more likely to achieve some level of patient satisfaction, than if you determine the level of priority for the patient yourself.

The opening question should encourage patients to state the reason(s) for their visit. Different opening questions can elicit different responses. For example, to the question "What brought you here today?" patients have often answered "The bus"! It seems to be easier for patients to tell their story if you start the consultation with a more open question, such as "What can I do for you today?", rather than a specific question, such as "What is the problem?".

Not interrupting the patient's opening statement is perhaps the most important skill. One study of consultations showed that on average patients were allowed to talk for a grand total of 18 seconds before the doctor interrupted them (Beckman and Frankel, 1984)! Sometimes the interruption may be to clarify what the patient has said, but delaying that interruption often allows the patient to complete their opening statement and identify all their problems. In the same study it was found that most patients who were allowed to complete their opening statement without interruption took less than 60 seconds to tell their story. Also, it was found that most patients had more than one problem and that the serial order in which these problems were presented was not related to their clinical importance. Patients therefore should be encouraged to express all their reasons for coming, before the doctor starts to explore any particular one in detail.

Gathering information

Information should be gathered from three different areas as shown in Table 3.2, namely the patient's biomedical problem, the patient's perspective and the patient's context or background.

Exploration of the patient's biomedical problems (disease)

In order for us to hear the patient's story, we need to be able to facilitate the telling of it. Facilitation skills that the family physician can use include the following:
- Make eye contact.
- Nod appropriately.
- Make encouraging noises such as "uh-huh", "um", and "go on".
- Allow waiting time or silence.
- Give specific encouragement, such as asking "Anything else?".

Silence in a consultation is quite difficult for most of us to tolerate, because we seem to think that we need to be busy. However, it often helps the patient enormously if you indicate by your silence that you are interested enough to wait for what they have to say. Pay attention and respond to the patient's silence. For example, do not busy yourself by writing while they are silent or quickly fill this sort of gap in the conversation with another question. Patients generally do not rehearse what they are going to say before they see a doctor and sometimes need the time to respond with care and accuracy to the questions that you ask. Sometimes they need the time to pluck up the courage to tell you something.

The doctor should also use appropriate questions to explore the problem. This is best done initially by asking open-ended questions that the patient can elaborate on and not by asking closed questions that require only yes or no answers. For example, here are three responses to a patient who says "I am so dizzy":

- Closed question – "Do you ever get dizzy when you stand up?"
- More specific question – "What makes your dizziness better or worse?"
- Open question – "What is your dizziness like?"

Having established an understanding of the problem, the family physician may need to gather further specific information from a medical perspective in order to test a specific hypothesis or suspected diagnosis (see also page 159). This usually means moving from open to more closed questions.

It is helpful to the patient if the doctor avoids using jargon or more than one question at once. Patients may find it difficult to indicate that they have not understood the question or the words that you have used. This may result in an inaccurate answer.

It may be helpful to remember why patients might not disclose their problems. See Table 3.2.

Table 3.2 Reasons why patients might not disclose their problems

· They may believe that nothing can be done.
· They may be reluctant to burden you.
· They may not want to seem pathetic or ungrateful.
· They may have a concern that the particular problem is not a legitimate "medical" problem.
· They may worry that their fear of what is wrong may be confirmed.
	· You may be using blocking behaviours by:
	  – offering premature advice and reassurance
	  – explaining away symptoms as "normal"
	  – attending only to physical aspects
	  – switching the topic
	  – not reacting with appropriate seriousness and respect to a presented symptom or problem.

SOURCE: Maguire and Pitceathly, 2002

Clues that a patient may give are not always verbal. We must develop awareness of the body language that our patients use. We should doubt the value of the answer "No" to the question "Is there anything wrong at home?" if the body language suggests that the patient is feeling sad, depressed, or oppressed. If you perceive an apparent cue, check with the patient whether your perception might be correct.

Clarification is a useful tool that helps us to avoid misunderstanding and ensure that we are not misinterpreting what the patient says according to our own terms of reference. It involves saying something along the lines of "So, if I understand you correctly, you are saying that …" or "When you say … , what do you mean?"

Patients and doctors may use the same terms and concepts but mean different things. To a doctor, flu conjures up an image of a particular collection of signs and symptoms that result from infection with the influenza virus. For the patient, it may mean simply body pains or a cold feeling between the shoulder blades. Clarification also allows patients to make their story clearer when they may have left out or censored key information.

Simple reflective listening statements can serve the same purpose as clarification, avoids the need to ask a question and encourages elaboration by the patient. A reflective listening statement summarises the meaning that you have heard and demonstrates listening, as well as checking that you have understood correctly. For example:

Patient: I worry sometimes that I may be drinking too much for my own good.
Practitioner: You've been drinking quite a bit.
Patient: I don't really feel like it's much. I can drink a lot and not feel it.
Practitioner: More than most people.
Patient: Yes. I can drink most people under the table.
Practitioner: And that's what worries you.

At the end of a particular topic or line of inquiry, summarising your understanding of what the patient has explained (including the sequence of events) is a powerful communication tool (Silverman *et al.*, 1998). The benefits of summarising are as follows:

- It confirms that you have been listening. The patient is not left wondering if you have understood.
- It enables the patient to elaborate further, and thus to add to or correct your understanding.
- It demonstrates your interest and concern for understanding the patient.
- It encourages collaboration and participation in the consultation.
- It allows you space to order your thoughts and review what has been covered.
- It provides structure in the consultation. It indicates that this part of the consultation is at an end.

An example of summarising is shown below:

If I understand you correctly you have been feeling short of breath doing chores about the house, sweating at night and losing weight since last month, not sleeping at night, thinking too much, and you are worried that this could be TB, as the symptoms are similar to when you had TB before.

Table 3.3 Example of interrelationship between content and process (gathering information)

GATHERING INFORMATION	
Process skills for exploration of the patient's problems	
Patient's narrative	
Question style: open to closed cone	
Attentive listening	
Facilitative response	
Picking up cues	
Clarification	
Time-framing	
Summary	
Appropriate use of language	
Additional skills for understanding the patient's perspective	
Content to be discovered	
The biomedical perspective (disease)	*The patient's perspective (illness)*
Sequence of events	Ideas, beliefs and concerns
Symptom analysis	Expectations
Relevant systems review	Effects on life
	Feelings
Background information – context	
Past medical history	
Drug and allergy history	
Family history	
Personal and occupational history	
Physical environment	

SOURCE: Kurtz *et al.* 2003

Exploration of the patient's perspective (illness)

Apart from eliciting information about the medical problem, try to establish the reason why the patient presented now. Many consultations are precipitated by fears that patients have about their illness. In Chapter 2 we discussed the need to explore and understand both the disease and the illness. Here we look at how to explore patients' ideas, concerns, feelings, expectations, and experience of the illness. They may make this clear or give you clues as they tell you their story. You may simply have to listen and clarify the clues that patients give you. Sometimes, however, you may also need to ask specific questions, for example:

- Questions about ideas – "What do you think is causing the problem?"
- Questions about concerns – "What was the worst thing you were thinking it might be?"
- Questions about feelings – "How did that leave you feeling?"
- Questions about expectations – "What were you hoping we might be able to do about this?"
- Questions about experience of illness – "Tell me how you are coping."

If you have not developed a sufficiently trusting and non-judgemental relationship with patients, they are often not confident enough to divulge their own explanation and may reply by saying "You tell me, you're the doctor!".

Exploration of the patient's context

In traditional medical school teaching the background or contextual information that is gathered includes past medical history, medications, allergies, family history of diseases, social habits (such as smoking and alcohol use) and work.

In family medicine a more holistic and functional assessment of the patient's context may be useful. For example, it may be useful to understand who lives together, what sort of relationships they have and what important psychosocial events have taken place. This is described further in Chapter 4. The family physician understands that the illness may impact on the patient's family and occupational functioning. In some instances the illness may be a manifestation of problems in the family or related to their occupation.

Structuring the consultation

Making the structure of the consultation overt throughout may involve explaining to the patient the logic or rationale behind changes in topic or lines of questioning. This can be done, for example, by summarising the preceding content (as above) and then stating that you are moving on to the next area. This allows the patient to understand the purpose of a question or why there has been a change in the topic.

Physical examination

Your communication with the patient does not stop at this point. You need to continue to build the relationship by continuing to display respect and empathy and conducting the examination in a sensitive manner. Remember that your patient needs to give you tacit consent to be examined, so ensure that you continue to inform the patient of what you are doing and why. The information gathering at this stage needs to search for useful positive and negative findings that may help with making your assessment.

The second half of the consultation

The second half of the consultation starts when the physical examination is complete and the family physician shifts from gathering information to making their assessment and ends with the successful closure of the encounter.

Efficient use of time is important for overall management of your day. Avoid unnecessary repetition, ask only what is necessary and focus on the real reasons for the consultation.

The specific tasks and communication skills needed in the second half of the consultation are listed in Table 3.4.

Explanation and planning

By now, you will have assessed the patient's problems, perspective and context. As discussed in Chapter 2, this would be in the format of a three-stage assessment. You must now explain your three-stage assessment to the patient and formulate a three-stage management plan.

Providing the correct amount and type of information

It is worth thinking about *how much* the patient wants to know and *what* the patient wants to know because doctors usually tend to give too little information (although too much is also not helpful). Also, doctors tend to give information about the diagnosis and treatment, whereas patients are also interested in what caused the problem (aetiology) and what will happen in the future (prognosis) (Silverman *et al.*, 1998).

Guidelines for the family physician are as follows:
- Find out what the patient already knows as a starting point.
- Ask the patient what other information would be useful to them.
- Give information in small chunks and check for understanding.

- Use the patient's responses to your information as a guide to how much more is needed and how much is understood.

Table 3.4 Communication tasks and skills for the second half of consultation

---

Explanation and planning

Providing the correct amount and type of information

- INITIATES: summarises to date, determines expectations, sets agenda of what topics are important to patient

- ASSESSES PATIENT'S STARTING POINT: asks for patient's prior knowledge, discovers extent of patient's wish for information

- CHUNKS AND CHECKS: gives information in digestible chunks, checks for understanding, elicits or observes response as a guide of how to proceed, elicit-provide-elicit

- ASKS PATIENT WHAT OTHER INFORMATION WOULD BE HELPFUL: for example aetiology, prognosis

- GIVES EXPLANATION AT APPROPRIATE TIMES: avoids giving advice, information or reassurance prematurely or while patient is distracted

- OFFERS A CLINICALLY APPROPRIATE EXPLANATION / DIAGNOSIS: the apparent diagnosis is clinically appropriate according to the subjective and objective evidence

Aiding accurate recall and understanding

- ORGANISES EXPLANATION: divides into discrete sections, develops a logical sequence

- USES EXPLICIT CATEGORIES OR SIGNPOSTING: for example, "There are three important things that I would like to discuss. First … now shall we move on to …"

- USES REPETITION AND SUMMARISING: reinforces information

- LANGUAGE: uses concise, easily understood statements, avoids or explains jargon

- USES VISUAL OR WRITTEN METHODS OF CONVEYING INFORMATION: diagrams, models, written information and instructions

- CHECKS PATIENT'S UNDERSTANDING OF INFORMATION GIVEN: for example by asking patient to restate in own words and clarify as necessary

Incorporating the patient's perspective – achieving shared understanding

- RELATES EXPLANATION TO PATIENT'S ILLNESS FRAMEWORK: to previously elicited beliefs, concerns and expectations

- PROVIDES OPPORTUNITIES / ENCOURAGES PATIENT TO CONTRIBUTE: to ask questions, seek clarification, personalise information, express beliefs, reactions or feelings, doubts, physician responds appropriately

- PICKS UP VERBAL AND NON-VERBAL CUES: patient's understanding, agreement and feelings may be expressed covertly through non-verbal or minimal verbal clues

Planning – shared decision-making

- NEGOTIATES AN APPROPRIATE MANAGEMENT PLAN: based on scientifically sound evidence and is appropriate for the diagnosis. Plan is mutually acceptable to both doctor and patient

- SHARES OWN THOUGHTS: ideas, thought processes and dilemmas are shared

- INVOLVES PATIENT: making suggestions rather than orders or directives

- OFFERS CHOICES: encourages patients to make informed choices and decisions to the level they wish

- CHECKS WITH PATIENTS: if patient accepts the plan, if concerns have been addressed

Closure

- SUMMARISES session briefly

- CONTRACTS WITH PATIENT regarding next steps for patient and doctor

- DEMONSTRATES APPROPRIATE SAFETY NETTING and explains possible unexpected outcomes, what to do if plan is not working, when and how to seek help

- CHECKS THAT PATIENT AGREES and is comfortable with plan and ASKS IF ANY FINAL QUESTIONS OR CONCERNS

SOURCE: Adapted from the Calgary-Cambridge Observation Guide (1998)

When information is given with the intention of motivating lifestyle or behaviour change it can be useful to avoid advice giving such as "what you must do is ..." which provides the information along with a recommended solution or behaviour change. The natural response to being told what to do is to explain why it is not possible. Instead, information can be shared in a neutral way and the implications of the information elicited from the patient. For example:

Practitioner [Elicit]: Would you be interested in discussing how to take the antiretroviral medication?
Patient: Yes, that would be good.
Practitioner [Provide]: Well, one of the things that we know is that in order to be effective a patient must take more than 95% of the tablets. That means, for

example, that if you are taking tablets twice a day for two weeks, at the very most, you can only miss one of the doses. We also know that people struggle to take tablets on a regular basis and often only manage to take half of what they should be taking. [Elicit] How do you think you would cope with this?

Patient: Well, that sounds difficult, but I can ask my daughter to help me remember.

Aiding accurate recall and understanding

Try to make information easy for the patient to remember and understand in the following ways (Silverman *et al.*, 1998):

- Organise your explanation logically.
- Use clear categorisation. For example: "Now, I would like to talk about treatment."
- Use repetition and summarising to reinforce the message.
- Use concise and easy language, without unexplained jargon.
- Use visual information such as leaflets, drawings, models, and written instructions.
- Pitch the complexity of your explanation with the ability of the patient to comprehend.
- Check for understanding. For example, ask the patient to restate the information in their own words. You may be perceived by the patient as a bit aggressive if you ask "Do you understand me?"

Aim for a shared understanding of the problem

The patient needs to hear that their agenda has been incorporated into your understanding and explanation of the problem. For example, the patient may think that his gastritis is due to the issues that he has at work with his supervisor. You may think that it is due to the alcohol that he is abusing in his attempt to cope with the work situation. If you only tell him about your understanding of the problem, the patient is unable to negotiate a plan with you, as his viewpoint has not been addressed. Similarly a patient with obvious symptoms of TB who expects a chest X-ray, but is offered a sputum investigation, may leave dissatisfied if his expectation is not addressed. Expectations do not necessarily have to be fulfilled, but should be acknowledged and addressed.

As in the earlier phase of exploring the patient's problem (you are now exploring the patient's understanding of that problem), continue to be aware of the patient's reactions – both verbal and non-verbal. Patients with a language barrier between them and the doctor may respond positively to all explanations as they are unwilling to admit they do not understand. However, their body language may indicate their real lack of genuine understanding and agreement. Continue to address the patient's thoughts, fears, feelings and expectations. Check how the patient is responding to suggestions that you make. You may be convinced that you are offering patients some positive information about their problem, but if this is counter to their expectations, they may seem inappropriately negative about it. Remain tuned into your patient so that you will not miss the clues that allow you to check that you have achieved a shared understanding of the problem.

Aim for shared decision-making

This is where the patient's agenda and the doctor's agenda need to be reconciled in order to develop a mutually acceptable management plan. Shared decision-making implies that the patient is informed enough of the different options and associated risks and benefits to participate in a final choice. The doctor as the expert in these matters will need to convey this information in an understandable and practical format. This can be challenging especially when the evidence is vague, the patient speaks another language, or is used to a paternalistic approach. Negotiation is defined as "conferring, with a view to reaching an agreement or compromise." Compromise is defined as "coming to a joint agreement by concessions on both sides" (Fowler and Fowler, 1964). In other words, negotiation is not about trying to get the patient to agree with your instructions! It is not always easy for patients to express their disagreement with a doctor. You need to check your perception of the patient's agreement. When we start the negotiation process around the management plan, we need to remain congruent with our belief in, and practice of patient-centred care. It is not appropriate to revert to telling the patient what to do and how to do it. We need to continue to build the relationship and its implicit partnership.

It is often helpful when dealing with lifestyle changes to ask the patient if they have any preferences or specific ideas. For example, for a patient who is ready to address a weight problem, ask: "What ideas have you had about losing weight?" Motivational interviewing and motivating lifestyle change are discussed in more detail in Chapter 5. The patient's own ideas may be more realistic than your ideas. Ownership of an idea by the patient is more likely to lead to action. However, it is appropriate to make suggestions of your own as you have expertise in what is known to work and how you think this particular patient might deal with their problem. Make an offer or suggestion to give the patient some options. If this negotiation process is followed through, you should be able to agree on a mutually acceptable plan. There is evidence that patients will be more likely to adhere to a negotiated management plan than if they feel that they have not participated in the formulation of the plan and that it has just been foisted upon them.

This is where implementation of the three-stage management plan needs to be discussed. It is important to set realistic goals to avoid disappointment and distrust on both sides if the plan is not implemented. Questions to ask are:

- How much can medication achieve? For example, how rapidly will the anti-inflammatory medication be effective in the relief of the pain?
- How motivated is the patient to make a lifestyle change? For example, how well will the business executive be able to stick to his new cholesterol-lowering diet?
- What are the constraints of the home circumstances? For example, how will the poverty-stricken woman with diabetes be able to adhere to the diet and exercise regime?
- What are the effects that the problem will have on this patient's daily activities? For example "You will have difficulty getting up and down stairs for the next few weeks" or "Avoid any alcohol because this would interfere with the medication." Remember, a teacher with laryngitis may well need time off from work but a clerk with a similar affliction can still manage their duties.

As will be discussed in Chapter 9 a home visit is often a good learning experience in terms of developing realistic advice.

Closing the session

Safety netting

It is worthwhile to have a final check that you and the patient are in agreement regarding the management plan. Check that you both understand the roles, tasks, and the expectations that you have of each other.

Safety netting involves asking yourself a number of questions (Neighbour, 1987):

1 How sure am I of my assessment? Could it be something more serious? What kind of response to treatment is expected? What are possible side-effects of the planned investigation or treatment?
2 How will I know if things do not go according to plan? Under what circumstances should the patient contact me or go to the emergency room? When do I need to see him or her again?

3 What will I do then? If things do not go according to plan what further investigation, treatment or referral might be appropriate?

Having asked yourself these questions you should then decide what to tell the patient about the expected response to the management plan, what to do if things do not go according to plan, and when to see you again.

For example, the mother of a young child with acute otitis media will be better able to cope if you warn her that the pain and fever may not settle within the first 36 hours of starting the medication.

Closure

The easiest way to end a consultation is to give the patient something tangible to do, such as a prescription to fill, a request for an investigation, or a referral to a specialist. Although this is obviously sometimes necessary, it is also often a way of passing the buck when we do not really know what else to do. Doctors often justify this action by saying that patients are more satisfied if they have something to take away from the consultation – after all, what have they paid for otherwise? It seems much less easy or justifiable for us simply to have chatted or listened to the patient!

We certainly need to make sure that the patient takes something away from the consultation, but we need to think a little more broadly as to what this something might encompass. The consultation needs to end with the family physician and the patient having reached a mutually acceptable, clearly understood, and negotiated management plan. This may involve medication, investigation, or referral, but could equally involve a lifestyle modification, a plan to address a difficult family relationship, a follow-up appointment to address the issue more deeply, or an appointment with a community-based resource organisation.

We need to be sure that we end the consultation in a way that enables patients to return whenever they may have the need. Make the closure clear by using a final summary and offering a last opportunity for corrections or additions.

Reflection

Larson *et al.* (1997) end with a final task for the doctor, after the patient leaves, namely time for reflection. An important part of the end of the consultation is for the family physician to take time to reflect on the way the consultation went and to check their stress levels. Every consultation is an opportunity for learning, as discussed further in Chapter 13.

It is important to be aware of and take into account your feelings in the consultation. McWhinney (1997) says that family physicians attach importance to the subjective aspects of the consultation, that is, not only in the patient, but also in themselves. There will be consultations in which you know that you have connected with the patient, heard them, met their expectations, and reached a viable, mutually acceptable management plan. You need to think about why it went well, so that you can use these positive outcomes to improve your level of skill in communicating with other patients. But there will also be consultations in which you do not feel that you have made that connection. Somehow, the story that you have heard and your questions and examination do not result in an assessment with which you are comfortable. Something is missing. Be aware of this feeling because what is missing is often the real reason why the patient came to see you. The sooner you tune into this feeling, the sooner you can turn the situation around and establish the real reason for consulting by trying again to conduct a patient-centred consultation.

Family medicine can be stressful with a stream of highly varied problems and competing demands for attention. It is important to develop awareness of your own stress levels and ways of coping. Here are some ways that you can reduce or relieve stress during and between consultations (Neighbour, 1987):

- Use relaxing rituals, such as drinking a cup of tea, taking a short walk, making a telephone call, reading for a brief while, and so on.
- Talk to a colleague or co-worker.
- Do not exceed your concentration span without a break.
- Incorporate a variety of activities in your day.
- Place icons in the room that are associated with peace and well-being.
- Be aware of how you project your feelings onto the patient. Ask: "Who does this person remind me of? When else have I felt like this?"
- Be aware of your stereotypes and attitudes towards patients from particular cultural, political, or religious backgrounds.
- Be aware of your own posture, muscle tone, and breathing. Adjusting this can help alter your mood.
- Be aware of your own negative thoughts and how they affect your mood.
- Practise here and now awareness. Become fully aware of the present moment and cut out past and future worries.
- Tell the patient how you are feeling!

Remember also to look after yourself outside of work time and develop the ability to reflect on, acknowledge, and work on your own rewards and challenges.

If you attempt always to be true to all these different aspects of communication, you stand a better chance of effectively communicating with your patients in a way that will allow a therapeutic doctor–patient relationship to develop during the consultation process. There is a better chance of a more satisfying outcome for both the family physician and the patient if there is a relationship in which both parties are able to share an understanding of the other's point of view.

Q Read the following case studies and identify the skills and attitudes that the family physician should display:

Mr Sipho Z is complaining of a chronic cough. After examination and investigation, you establish that he has a treatable malignancy. You tell him that you will refer him to a tertiary centre for treatment. He, however, opts to go to the traditional healer first and chooses to go back to KwaZulu-Natal to consult with his family.

Mrs Barbara W (the mother of two young children) comes back to see you after missing her follow-up appointment. She was diagnosed as having idiopathic epilepsy a few months ago and you put her on an anti-epileptic agent. She says that she did not want to come back for her pills because they make her drowsy.

Mr Rakesh N comes to see you complaining of severe, acute gastritis. He is not your patient, but his wife is. You have been helping her to deal with the physical abuse that Mr N submits her to whenever he has too much to drink.

Miss Zanele M has just been told that her HIV test is positive. She cries quietly into her hands.

Communication with children

In a consultation in which a child is the patient, the dynamic of the doctor–patient relationship becomes a dynamic between the family physician and two others – the child and their caregiver. Do not forget the third relationship that encroaches into this sort of consultation – that between the child and the caregiver. An observation of this relationship can reveal an enormous amount of information about the family dynamics. Have you ever been in a consultation with the mother of a six-year-old boy? He volubly insists on picking up and trying out every piece of equipment in your consultation room. How does his mother react? She either ignores him completely, or says a token admonishment, or reprimands him harshly (which the child ignores), or threatens him with physical violence, or gets up and gives him a hard smack across the back of his head. These reactions may give you some indication of what happens at home in this family, but be aware that your observation is occurring in the unusual setting of the consultation.

All children seem to respond well when treated with respect. They enjoy developing a relationship with the family physician, as long as they have the escape of easy return to the safety of their caregiver's arms. Also, do not forget that even young children will notice the relationship between you and their caregiver, so it is worth ensuring that you have the trust of the caregiver before you start talking to, or examining, the child.

Most people find it very threatening to have a stranger looming over them. As family physicians we are given the privilege of invading our patient's personal space. With children, we need to be aware of the fact that we are not only invading their space, but we are much bigger than they are and use strange-looking equipment. We may well be seen as one of the strangers that they are not supposed to talk to or as the person who will give them an injection if they are naughty. It helps if we physically come down to the child's level whenever possible, so as not to appear to be some kind of looming giant.

However, children respond very well to genuine interest and concern with their problems. They are very quick to perceive a tense atmosphere in a conversation and a lack of genuineness from adults, so guard against these things. For example, you will jeopardise the development of a long-term trusting relationship if you tell a child that an injection is not going to hurt when you know that it probably will.

Non-verbal communication can enhance, lessen, or even destroy any trust the child might have in us before we start talking or listening.

2 How would you deal with a four-year-old who refuses to open his mouth to let you check for what you suspect is follicular tonsillitis?

Communication with adolescents

The relationship between the family physician and adolescent is unusual in that it is one of the few times the family physician does not interact with an adult. In younger children the adult parent is usually the one to give consent or negotiate with the doctor. The family physician should be aware of the particular social and cognitive developmental issues in adolescence. Adolescents are in the phase of their life cycle where they are trying to achieve autonomy from their parents, initially in their peer group and later on in small groups or couples. In addition, they are transforming from concrete to more abstract and complex thought processes, with associated changes in identity and body image. We need to respect and support their development and to work at building a relationship of trust. It is often difficult to walk the fine line between treating the parent and treating the adolescent patient, as there are often serious issues of confidentiality, privacy and autonomy (McPherson, 2005).

Commonly, an adolescent is brought in by a concerned parent. They are thus often resentful of the perceived interference in their life. They are often not interested in being there and may be embarrassed by the fact that they are unable to stop their parent from controlling their life in such a way. You need to try to decide on a general principle of when you would include the parent in the consultation and when you would not. It is certainly easier to see the adolescent alone initially and call the parent in later, rather than trying to get the parent to leave once you come across a problem in the consultation. However, you need to be sensitive to cultural and gender issues that may play a role in how your actions may be perceived or what the response may be. You need to ascertain the accepted norms in the community in which you work.

On the other hand, the adolescent may initiate the appointment. This may then turn out to be a consultation for an issue with which they need help, such as contraception, sexuality, eating behaviour, domestic violence, or concern about drugs or sexually transmitted infections. In these cases, the family physician needs to be upfront and clear about issues such as consent to treatment and confidentiality. There is often a very clear power differential in these consultations, in which the family physician can easily take on the parental role. Again, we need to think of the long-term benefits for the patient, and their health, and of developing a trusting relationship with the patient.

Q How would you deal with a 14-year-old who comes to see you about having missed her period? She is sexually active with her 19-year-old boyfriend and neither of them uses contraception. She tells you that she has not and will not discuss any of this with either of her parents and she wants to know if you will maintain confidentiality and help her.

Communication with an interpreter

In South Africa, with 11 official languages, the family physician and patient often have different first languages and are forced to communicate in a second language or with an interpreter. The effects of a poorly managed language barrier can be profound for a number of reasons (Schlemmer, 2005):

- It interferes with working efficiently when nurses, cleaners or porters are co-opted as interpreters or when the doctor must go hunting for an interpreter.
- It causes uncertainty in the family physician about the accuracy of interpreting.
- It is enhanced by a lack of education, for example, when a cleaner is used as an interpreter and they do not understand the medical terms that the doctor is using.
- It causes ethical dilemmas as confidentiality may be broken through the use of neighbours or relatives as interpreters or consent is not truly informed due to poor communication.
- It negatively influences attitudes with, for example, patients feeling discriminated against when they are not understood or forced to communicate piece-meal in a second language.
- It decreases the quality of patient care as, for example, the diagnosis, use of medications and follow-up arrangements are not clearly understood.
- It decreases patient satisfaction with care.
- It causes cross-cultural misunderstandings, for example, one of the doctors reported the severe reaction of his patient when he jokingly asked if the "gremlins" took his plaster cast off and it was translated as "Did the *Tokoloshe* take your plaster off?"

The need to bridge this language barrier by working "with" trained interpreters is clear. The term "with" is used in order to convey that in a consultation where an interpreter is needed, the dynamic of the consultation changes because there is another person and relationship to take into account. Although often the term "through" is used, this implies that the interpreter is simply an empty vessel used to transmit information. In South Africa, where we do not have trained translators but commonly use nursing personnel, this concept of an inert body in the consultation process is not helpful.

Remember that you should ask the patient's permission to introduce this new person into the consultation. It is helpful to introduce the interpreter and patient to each other, to describe the role of the interpreter to the patient and to assure the patient that the interpreter is required to respect the confidentiality of all that is discussed. To forget to do this may prevent the patient from developing sufficient trust with the participants in the consultation to divulge everything that they would like to.

Most interpreters have been accustomed to the role of the traditional mode of systematic interrogation and disease-centred care. They are often quite perplexed by a family physician who wants to ask all sorts of questions about how the patient feels and what they understand by their illness experience, sometimes to the point of not being able to adequately translate your questions in an open manner. Your translated question may also provoke a very long, voluble, and dramatic answer, not one word of which you understand but which conveys a sense of great importance and significance. The interpreter then turns round to you and says: "The patient says yes, Doctor!" In other words, observation of non-verbal communication becomes even more valuable when we do not understand the verbal communication. This may help us to understand the depth of feeling expressed, as well as the congruence between verbal and non- verbal communication.

The family physician should acknowledge and use the expertise of the interpreter not only in language, but also in providing information about local culture, health belief systems, and community-based support systems (Wood, 1993). This sort of partnership works well if the family physician and the interpreter are also able to develop a working relationship in which they support each other in coming to a clearer understanding of how best to help the patient. It would be helpful for you to gain some understanding of the language used by most of your patients, so that you can assess for yourself the nature of the communication between the patient and the interpreter. Both the interpreter and the patient can help you to learn a new language and culture (Ellis, 2004).

An important consideration when consulting with an interpreter is the seating arrangement. Be wary of having a seating arrangement that would facilitate the development of the family physician's relationship with the interpreter instead of with the patient. It is so easy to look at the interpreter and say: "Ask him if he uses condoms" while you scribble down the answer to the last question. Imagine the non-verbal responses that you would miss! The family physician and the patient still need to talk to each other. In other words, it remains important for the family physician and the patient to watch each other and to be able to pick up each other's non-verbal cues. A way of facilitating this is for the family physician and the interpreter to sit alongside each other, with the patient sitting opposite them both (see Figure 3.2).

Figure 3.2 Seating arrangements for a consultation with an interpreter

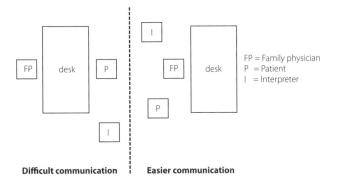

Difficult communication | Easier communication

Communication with the disabled

It seems surprisingly difficult to remember that people who have problems speaking or hearing may still be able to understand normally. How often have you seen someone talking more loudly to a person who appears not to understand? How often have you seen someone talking in a more simplistic if not baby-like manner to someone in a wheelchair? Remember that Stephen Hawking, one of the greatest living theoretical physicists, has amyotrophic lateral sclerosis (Lou Gehrig's disease) and is in a wheelchair and cannot speak without his voice synthesiser.

Deaf people need to be able to watch you speak, so remember to position yourself accordingly and make sure that you have attracted their attention by something other than sound when you want to start speaking to them.

Blind or poor-sighted people may need some assistance in getting around the unfamiliar territory of your consulting room. It is also less scary for such patients if you warn them about exactly what you are doing in your examination. Remember they cannot see the cold stethoscope coming and thus cannot brace themselves.

Conclusion

This chapter has outlined the communication skills necessary at each phase of the consultation to understand and manage our patients' problems. Our aim should be to aid patients in solving their problems by conducting a functional consultation in which the patient is treated with dignity, respect, and honesty.

Recommended reading

Boyle, D, Dwinnell, B and Platt, F. (2005). Invite, Listen and Summarise: A Patient-Centered Communication Technique. *Academic Medicine* 80:29–32.

Ellis, C. (2004). *Communicating with the African Patient.* Pietermaritzburg: University of KwaZulu-Natal Press.

Fraser, RC. (ed). (1999). Leicester Assessment Package: *Clinical Method: A General Practice Approach* (3rd ed). Oxford: Butterworth-Heinemann.

Kurtz, S, Silverman, J, Benson, J and Draper, J. (2003). Marrying Content and Process in Clinical Method Teaching: Enhancing the Calgary Cambridge Guides. *Academic Medicine*, 78:802–809.

Larsen, J, Risor, O and Putnam, S. (1997). P-R-A-C-T-I-C-A-L: A Step-by-Step Model for Conducting the Consultation in General Practice. *Family Practice* 14:295–301.

Makoul, G. (2001). The SEGUE Framework for Teaching and Assessing Communication Skills. *Patient Education and Counselling* 45:23-24.

Silverman, J, Kurtz, S and Draper, J. (1998). *Skills for Communicating with Patients.* Abingdon: Radcliffe Medical Press.

Stewart, M, Belle Brown, J, Weston, WW, McWhinney, IR, McWilliam, CL and Freeman, TR. (1995). *Patient-Centred Clinical Method: Patient-Centred Medicine: Transforming the Clinical Method.* Thousand Oaks, California: Sage.

4   Family-orientated primary care

Graham Bresick
Division of Family Medicine
School of Public Health and Family Medicine
University of Cape Town

A person is a human being by virtue of other human beings
(African proverb)

Treatment that focuses on individual pathologies in isolation
from the context of a person's life is inadequate
(Jongbloed, 1994)

Introduction

The family is the immediate physical, psycho-social and economic
context for the interplay between health and illness. It is here that
complex interactions between the factors determining health and illness
play out, and where recovery takes place. **Family-orientated health
care** recognises that family and other significant relationships affect
health. It also recognises that culture and religion impact on the health
of families by influencing health-related beliefs, behaviours and decision-making. Health care that ignores these and other relational factors
risks making an incorrect diagnosis as well as missing opportunities for
a deeper understanding of health and illness. It also risks not identifying
family-related factors that promote health and provide support or those
factors that may undermine the care plan.

The causes of many lifestyle diseases can be found in the family or
group of origin. Genetic factors are well known; the science and research
of these factors continues to grow and improve and genetic tests and
counselling are well established. Risky beliefs and behaviours however,
get less attention but may have a greater impact in determining lifestyle
diseases; consider smoking, eating and exercise habits.

The shift in the burden of disease from curable acute infectious, often self-limiting disease to chronic, incurable, lifestyle disease increases the need for family-orientated care. Families have to adapt to living with the disease along with the affected family member. Adaptation may include difficult lifestyle changes and the re-allocation of resources within the family. HIV/AIDS has become a major part of the disease burden, impacting the life and wellbeing of families in unprecedented ways. Factors, such as longevity and the trend to reduce the length of hospital stay, also make greater health care demands on families.

Rolland and Walsh (2005) have noted the increased number of courses offering training in family-orientated health care. This increase shows the growing recognition of the importance of working with families to improve health outcomes. There is also a growing interest in identifying and strengthening factors that increase a family's resilience to ill-health instead of focusing only on the problems. As a result, the doctor–patient dyad is shifting to a more triangular relationship that includes other family members. Family-orientated interventions can guard against disease and promote health.

Thinking family

Thinking family is the central, distinguishing feature of family-orientated primary care. Practising family-orientated care does not necessarily mean having family members in the consulting room or doing a home visit – although it includes these on occasion. Thinking family is an approach to the routine primary care of individual patients that considers the **family or household** as an integral part of information gathering, clinical reasoning, and patient care. The preceding chapters have drawn attention to the importance of communication skills, patient-centredness, and the principles of family medicine. They form part of the core knowledge and skills required for family-orientated primary care and will not be repeated here.

This chapter addresses the role of the family in health and illness, highlights the knowledge and skills needed to practice family-orientated primary care, and outlines the theoretical basis for this approach. Six studies illustrate the importance of thinking family in primary care practice and include practical exercises to consolidate your knowledge and essential skills. The answers to some of the exercises are contained in the text; others are meant to encourage reflection and self-directed learning. Many common primary care problems do not have one correct response only. Your interventions will be influenced by your level of interest, knowledge and skill, the preferences and values of your patients and their families, and the availability of resources. Discuss your answers with tutors and other experienced practitioners to maximize your learning.

Note that the use of the term family in this text includes any group of origin, that is, an intimate, nurturing group sharing a past, a present, and a future – bound biologically or legally or socially (McDaniel *et al.*, 2005). In some instances it may be better to consider the household rather than the nuclear family only.

Study 1: Learning to think family

Consider the following complaints made by doctors.

From a family physician:

People come in with persistent physical complaints which I cannot explain. Others come in apparently wanting to be pronounced healthy; but when this is done they become upset and appear to want a diagnosis of some clear-cut physical illness instead, which could explain their distress to them and to their families. Other people come in repeatedly for medical appointments, but it is not clear to me why they come, why they keep coming back, and what they want from me. It is as if I am supposed to discover why they continue seeking my attention (Glen, 1984, in Crouch and Roberts, 1987:1).

Consider also the following public complaints about doctors:

Doctors don't communicate well, they don't really listen, they seem insen-sitive to personal needs and individual differences, [and] they neglect the person in their zeal to pursue diagnostic and treatment procedures (Engel, 1980).

It seems that doctors are often more interested in getting answers to their questions than addressing patients' fears and feelings.

Now read and reflect on the patient study below:

Ms VF (aged 22) presents with a 2-week history of non-specific abdominal pain and "feeling shaky" at work. Your notes reveal that you saw her a year ago when she presented with headaches. The examination findings then were normal; you noted, however, that she smoked ten cigarettes a day and she seemed overly anxious about her health. You prescribed simple analgesia and had not seen her until this visit. Again, the systemic enquiry and examination are normal although she seems to want you to find a physical cause for her symptoms. You reassure her that "there is nothing wrong". She is smoking more heavily now; as before, you advise her to stop the smoking, suggesting that it may be precipitating her abdominal pain. You prescribe antacids and ask her to return in two weeks if the pain fails to resolve itself. At her request you give her a sick leave certificate for two days.

 Critically reflect on your diagnosis and management of this patient:

- Was your diagnosis comprehensive?
- Did you gather all the important information?
- Did you enquire about any underlying concerns she may have had?
- Was your approach doctor-centred or patient-centred?

Five helpful questions when thinking family

The following five questions will help you to think family in all contexts (adapted from Cole-Kelly, 2005)

1. *Has anyone else in the family had a similar problem?* Information on family history is important. Have there been similar illnesses in the family and how did the family cope? Are the patient's responses, for example adherence to treatment, being shaped by the family's past experience?

2. *What do family members believe caused the problem and how do they think it should be treated?* This question might help to reveal the family's explanatory model of the illness and how it may influence the resolution of the illness.

3. *Who in the family is most concerned about the problem?* A visit to the doctor is sometimes driven by the concern of another family member. Knowing something about that family member's concern may be important to understanding your patient and the family.

4. *Have there been any other recent changes or stresses in your life? Are you or any members of your family experiencing any difficulties at present?* This question may uncover information about the reasons for the illness, as well as problems that may hinder recovery. Here is a useful taxonomy of common social stressors and contextual problems to use; inquire specifically about:
   - *recent losses*, for example bereavement, loss of employment; loss of important possessions
   - *family conflict*, domestic violence, emotional, verbal or sexual abuse
   - *substance abuse* in the family
   - *recent major change*, for example a change in employment status,

separation, change in health status
— *isolation*, for example following bereavement, the onset of a disabling illness, or having to care for a family member with chronic illness or disability
— *entrapment* – for example being dependent on someone who is abusive where the consequences of leaving may be perceived as worse than enduring the abuse
— *financial hardship; unemployment; poverty* – can have many consequences including those already mentioned
— *poor housing*; overcrowding
— *stress* from any other cause.

5 *How can your family or friends assist you with this problem?* This question helps to identify those who may work with you and the patient in the caring and healing process.

Symptoms without accompanying physical signs and a definable organic cause are a common presentation in primary care. The common stressors and problems listed above are frequently associated with symptoms that prompt a visit to a family physician. Frequent consultations, patient and doctor dissatisfaction, multiple diagnostic labels, unnecessary investigations and prescribing, and inappropriate referrals are common outcomes of a disease-centred approach in the face of such problems. Knowledge of common presenting patterns and the impact of the family on health and illness is important for accurate diagnosis and proper management, and avoids unnecessary expense. It enables early diagnosis and intervention, preventing serious consequences and the need for more costly interventions later.

Your reflection on Ms VF should have noted that:
• You did not identify a cause of your patient's symptoms
• You did not inquire about any personal and family factors that might explain her symptoms
• Your clinical search was limited to organic causes only (a strictly biomedical approach)
• You did not formulate a comprehensive (three-stage) assessment of the problem.

Here is some essential information you would have obtained had you inquired about your patient's family and context:

Ms VF lives with her father (65) who has well-controlled CCF, and her brother (32) who has moved back home after his recent divorce. Her mother died nearly two years ago at age 55 from complications following a mastectomy for carcinoma of the breast. She still feels angry about this and blames the hospital for her mother's death. Since her mother's death she does all the cooking, runs the home and takes care of her father. She feels guilty that she is not doing enough for him though: "My mother did everything for my father and took very good care of him". She does not seem to see the need for time for herself. She was coping well until recent events at work. She works as a salesperson in a clothing store. Sales have been poor and one salesperson has had to be retrenched. This has left her with extra duties, including working longer hours and more weekends. A friend told her that she may have a thyroid problem and so she thought she should have blood tests. She was concerned that her symptoms were interfering with her work performance and that she may lose her job. She cannot afford to lose her job given the high rate of unemployment.

The limitations of a biomedical model

Similar illnesses affect individuals differently; such differences include the interpretation of illness and the ability to cope with and adapt to illness. These factors result in a wide variation in expression of illness and help-seeking behaviour. In response to the family dynamics in Study 1, the patient may have responded with any of a number of stress-related conditions such as depression, anxiety, epigastric pain, chest pain, palpitations – to list only a few. Some patients will seek help, some will self-medicate and yet others may do both or do nothing at all until an advanced stage has been reached. The decision to seek medical advice is the result of complex attitudes and behaviours which often appear to be irrational and difficult to change (Becker, 1979). Neither the presence of a symptom nor the degree of disability seem to determine which symptoms will prompt the decision to seek help (Robinson, 1971). Factors influencing individual health actions are mainly social and psychological rather than biomedical (Zola, 1973; Wileman, May and Chew-Graham, 2002). Whether an otherwise tolerable symptom is interpreted as a threat that results in a decision to seek help is largely determined by beliefs and norms in the family or group of origin and the culture (Helman, 2001).

Figure 1.1 (see Chapter 1) shows that the overwhelming majority of illness presents and is fully managed in primary care. It has been known for some time that a narrow application of the biomedical approach is inadequate in primary care because it is unable to explain a significant proportion of presenting problems. A significant percentage (the majority in some studies) of patients using primary care services do not have an identifiable organic cause for their symptoms (Wileman, May and Chew-Graham, 2002). Research shows that in some instances fewer than one in five patients had an organic basis for their illness; most of the investigations were unhelpful and the cost was considerable (Kroene and Mandelsdorff, 1989; Reid and Wessely, 2002). The medical response in these situations is often: "There is nothing wrong with you". This invites the usually unexpressed response "So you mean it's all in my head, doctor" or "Do you think I'm imagining things?"

Thinking family is the ability to see the person in the family and the family in the person. Considering the family in the diagnostic and management process is not unique to family medicine. The distinguishing features of family-orientated health care are determined by the extent to which knowledge of the person and the family is necessary for accurate diagnosis and proper management. Failure to grasp this will undermine your ability to deliver cost-effective and quality care to your patients.

Formulate a three-stage assessment from the information provided (see Chapter 2).

How does it alter your earlier assessment and the care of this patient?

Would you summarise this important information diagrammatically to make it more accessible to you and your patient? What are the enabling or supportive, and disabling factors in her family and wider context?

Study 2: The importance of the genogram

The genogram is an essential tool in the practice of family-orientated primary care. Did you use a genogram to summarise the information in the question above?

Figure 4.1 is the genogram of the family in Study 1.
- Study and interpret the genogram with the help of Figure 4.2 before continuing.
- What additional information does it provide that is not given in the case study above?
- How will the information help you in the care of your patient?

Figure 4.1 The genogram of Ms VF's family (September 2005)

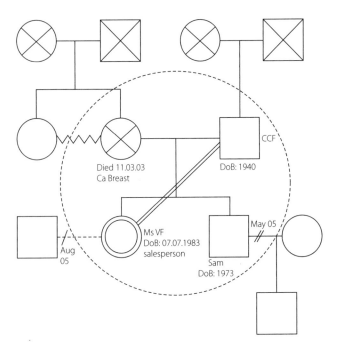

Figure 4.1 indicates that a potentially supportive relationship has ended recently, probably following some conflict – perhaps the result of what is happening in the family – and another possible reason for her symptoms. Her brother has a young son; his recent divorce and having to pay maintenance may well leave him with fewer resources to assist in the home. Her father is an only child and has no surviving family members to provide support. You wonder how father and brother understand the problem and what support may be available from the maternal side of the family, and whether your patient has tried to engage them in assisting.

Drawing a genogram

A key to the symbols used in genograms is given in Figure 4.2.

Figure 4.2 Genogram conventions

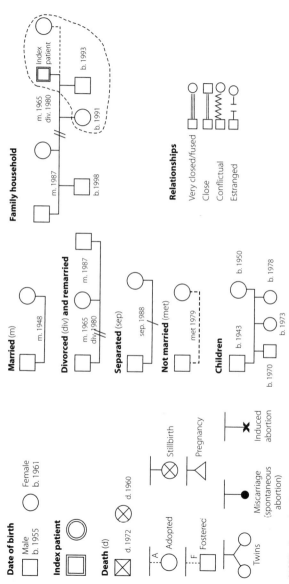

NOTE: Enter the data of the genogram and family name clearly

- Use a clean page and begin near the centre.
- Draw a skeleton genogram at the first visit and record the information needed at that stage.
- At subsequent visits, add information as needed.
- At least three generations should be represented.
- Enter birth dates rather than age, and the date of the genogram.

The value of a genogram

The genogram, if used well, has a number of benefits for the doctor, the patient and the family. Sometimes the information recorded may not be immediately useful, but may be helpful later in continuing care and when seeing other family members. It can serve as:

- A systematic method of recording important information
- An easily understood summary of the patient's context readily accessible to the doctor and patient (use the list of common family problems in the question on page 100)
- A means to identify patterns of organic as well as psychosocial and interpersonal problems
- An aid to explain the origin of symptoms to patients
- A therapeutic tool, assisting patient and family involvement in identifying causal factors and intervention options
- A preventive tool by drawing attention to the consequences of health risks in previous generations
- An aid to identifying complex family problems that need referral to a counsellor or family therapist.

Healthy human development requires the fulfilment of a number of physical, psycho-social, emotional, and spiritual needs in the process of attaining mature adulthood (Figure 4.3). A healthy, well-functioning family is the best-known and most studied social group able to meet these needs. Sadly, it is often responsible for these needs not being met. Drawing a genogram can help to reveal underlying causes such as family conflict, substance abuse, unemployment, poverty, poor parenting, family skeletons, family dislocation, and separation. Outcomes of such social stressors include mental and physical illness, poor school performance, antisocial behaviour, interpersonal violence, and many others. These patterns may be repeated in the next generation if timely identification and intervention are not made. The well-trained family physician is equipped with the knowledge and skills needed to recognise when problems may originate in the family and to intervene appropriately at this level in collaboration with others.

Figure 4.3 The pyramid of human needs

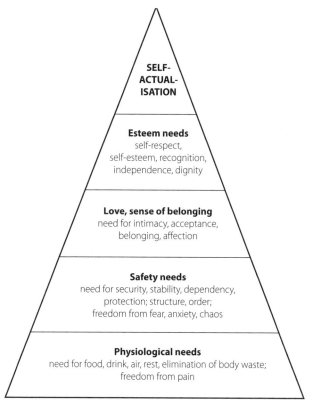

**SELF-
ACTUAL-
ISATION**

Esteem needs
self-respect,
self-esteem, recognition,
independence, dignity

Love, sense of belonging
need for intimacy, acceptance,
belonging, affection

Safety needs
need for security, stability, dependency,
protection; structure, order;
freedom from fear, anxiety, chaos

Physiological needs
need for food, drink, air, rest, elimination of body waste;
freedom from pain

Study 3: The family within a larger system – use of an ecomap

The family can be conceptualised as a biological system that is itself part of a hierarchy of other systems as shown in Figure 4.4. Biomedically-focused practice concentrates on pathological changes in cells, organs and physiological systems while a more holistic practice has a wider lens that includes the whole person and family. Systems theory holds that each level in the hierarchy of systems is semi-autonomous but also interdependent upon the levels above and below and influence each other both positively and negatively. The patient studies in this chapter illustrate how this can happen. Well-functioning systems such as well-functioning families, are flexible and able to adapt to new challenges utilizing their own resources. Dysfunctional systems/families have difficulty adapting and mobilizing resources and break down earlier. This may result in one member of the family presenting with stress-related symptoms.

In Figure 4.4 the broader community outside the family is represented as a higher system in the hierarchy. This system may include extended family groups, networks of friends, as well as occupational, religious and recreational organisations. Health and welfare organisations will also be part of these broader social systems in our patients. In the same way as the genogram is a tool to explore and diagrammatically represent the family system, the ecomap is a tool to understand and document these broader social systems.

Miss T, a 15-year-old girl in Grade 10, presented with vague headaches and dyspepsia after school, usually towards suppertime. This had started about one month previously and there was no nausea, vomiting or disturbance of bowel and bladder function. On further questioning, she denied having any problems at school, had many friends and enjoyed spending time with her two best friends, both of whom were girls. I asked her how things were at home, and her face immediately dropped and she became more serious.

She said that things were pretty awful and that lately she dreaded going home, because her parents were constantly arguing about her elder brother, either at him, or at each other about him. She said that her brother was 21 years old, unemployed, and recently they found out that his girlfriend was pregnant with his child. To make matters worse the girlfriend belonged to a different religious group. They felt that his behaviour was totally irresponsible and that he needed to grow up, find work, and get married to this girl, provided that she convert to their religion. If he was not willing to make these changes, they were not going to support him, and would not want anything to do with his girlfriend or the child.

Figure 4.4 The systems hierachy

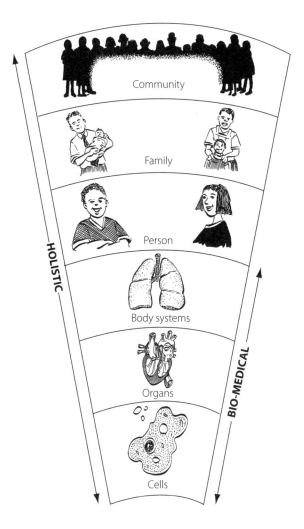

Because of this situation, Miss T admitted, her parents had suddenly become very suspicious of her own whereabouts, and even accused her of having a boyfriend and being involved with bad company. They constantly told her that she was their only hope and warned her about how angry they would be if she got pregnant or if she did badly at school. She said that she felt very tense at home, angry with her brother, and also very angry with her parents. She felt hurt that they would accuse her of keeping bad company, as she felt that they never took the time to find out who her friends were.

She admitted that she had thought about sex and boys, and had heard a lot about teenage pregnancy and AIDS at school. However, she had already made up her mind that she would wait until much later before getting intimately involved with a boy. Even though she would not allow herself to get pregnant, she felt she could not talk to her parents about boyfriends or sex.

Miss T was also quite driven; she wanted to become a nurse, and was planning to work towards that goal.

For these reasons, she felt that her parents were unjustified in their accusations against her. She also said that she did not think they deserved to be reassured by her, as they just assumed that she was getting up to mischief. Although she could see how much her brother's behaviour hurt and upset them, she felt that they did not have faith in her or enough trust in her to know that she would make different choices for herself.

On examination, she was a healthy-looking 15-year-old, with normal secondary sexual characteristics appropriate for her age, with normal vital signs and an Hb of 14. She had tense temporal muscles and mild tenderness in the epigastrium. Nothing further was found on clinical examination.

Use of the ecomap to assess the larger system

The ecomap is one way of diagrammatically assessing the larger system within which a family operates (Figure 4.5) and helps to ensure a community-orientated view of patient care (see Figure 4.4 and Chapter 9 on COPC). The household is placed at the centre and drawn within a circle using genogram symbols as learned in Study 2. Around the household circle are a number of other circles that represent typical parts of the larger system, as well as blank circles that can be filled in with other people or groups that are unique to this family. Next, the connections are drawn between the systems and the household by the use of lines to portray a strong, weak, or stressful connection. Text can be added if necessary to describe the nature of the connection and in addition arrows are added to indicate the flow of resources and energy from or into the household. Connections can be drawn to the family as a whole or particular people within the household. In Miss T's case the ecomap (Figure 4.6) reveals clearly the strong role of religion in this family and the crisis created by the son and his pregnant girlfriend.

Figure 4.5 Ecomap conventions

Name...

Date...

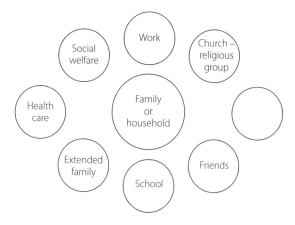

Fill in connections where they exist. Indicate nature of connections with a descriptive word or by drawing different kinds of lines: _____ for strong, --------------- for tenuous, ⫿⫿⫿⫿⫿⫿⫿⫿⫿⫿⫿ for stressful. Draw arrows along lines to indicate flow of resources and energy from or into the household. Identify people and fill in empty circles as needed.

SOURCE: Hartman A (1978)

Draw an ecomap of your own family.

Drawing an ecomap with your patient and understanding the larger system surrounding the family can be helpful in:

- Changing the perception of and level of insight into how a family functions for both patient and doctor and establishing what is influencing the family either positively or negatively
- Building collaboration between patient and doctor
- Building confidence and self-efficacy
- Identifying ways of improving family functioning
- Monitoring change in the way a family functions.

Figure 4.6 Ecomap for Miss T

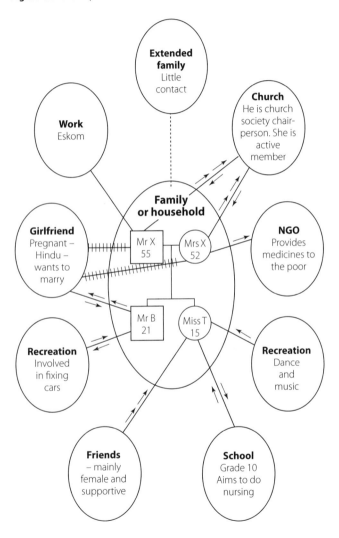

With support, the patient and the family are able to mobilise their own resources and restore equilibrium. The ability of the family physician to move beyond explaining the cause of symptoms and to operate at a higher level of involvement will depend on his/her level of interest, knowledge, and skill in working with families.

Q
- Formulate your assessment of the presenting problems in this family.
- What levels in the systems hierarchy are impacting this family?
- Find out what resources are available to assist such families in your area – such as parenting courses and family counselling services.

Study 4: Chronic illness and disability – supporting family caregivers

Mrs J, a 65-year-old pensioner, sees you regularly for the management of her hypertension, which is well controlled on a beta blocker. Today, she has come for her three-monthly blood pressure check. You find her blood pressure is significantly raised. Knowing that she is very good at adhering to her treatment, you ask her whether she has any idea why her blood pressure is raised. In tears, she explains that her recently retired husband had a stroke four weeks ago. He was discharged from the hospital in the past week and has a left hemiparesis. He was told that although he may have some return of function, he will be left with a significant disability. They live in a temporary structure provided by the local authority while they wait for a new house to be built for them. You acknowledge her plight by saying: "These last few months must have been very difficult for you, Mrs J. How are you managing at home?". "Doctor", she cries, "What must I do?" At this point she breaks down and is unable to continue. You offer her a glass of water and some tissues and sit quietly while she regains her composure. While waiting, you wonder how you should proceed.

Q
- Formulate a three-stage assessment of the problems.
- How would you proceed in this consultation? List your options.

The impact of chronic illness and disability on families

The family of a patient who suffers significant permanent loss of function experiences major disruption and has to adapt to avoid a negative spiral (Figure 4.7). Family members may also experience loss, such as the loss of hopes and dreams for the future or plans to enjoy retirement. The caregivers of stroke patients may experience a range of emotions, such as anxiety over whether they are providing the best care, frustration that they cannot restore function, and anger at the disruption of their lives. There is a strong relationship between adapting to disability and a number of psychosocial variables in the family, such as the quality of relationships and family support. These factors are as important as the level of physical functioning in determining the patient's quality of life after a stroke (Jongbloed, 1994).

Figure 4.7 The negative spiral

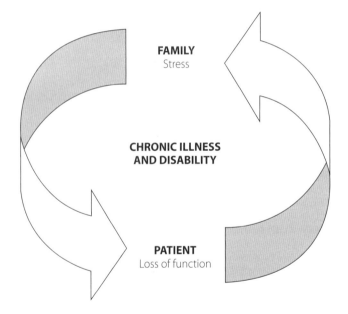

Dependence may result not only from the disability itself, but also from the effect it has on relationships in the family. Family members have defined and familiar roles, which may be disrupted. Normal patterns of interdependence, such as in a marriage, have to be restructured. In their desire to care for their loved one, caregivers may over-compensate and unintentionally encourage further dependence by performing tasks that the patient should be doing (Jongbloed, 1994; McWhinney, 1989:221). Caregiving is associated with deterioration in mental health and caregivers experience above-normal levels of chronic anxiety (Jongbloed, 1994). Low levels of family support are associated with less effective coping responses and poor social support has been found to be a significant predictor of depression among caregivers (Bull et al., 1995). Many families lack the financial resources to meet basic needs such as food and shelter. Meagre resources are strained further by the cost of rehabilitation and care, especially if the breadwinner has been disabled, as in families dealing with HIV. The focus on the patient may leave the caregiver's needs unacknowledged. The more time caregivers have to take care of themselves, the longer they can continue giving care.

The effect of differences in health beliefs

The period immediately following discharge from hospital is known to be particularly stressful for the family. Early discharge increases the strain on caregivers. Previously hidden differences between the health beliefs of the family and those of the health care team may surface at this time (Rolland, 1993). The medical investigations and treatment associated with rehabilitation may unintentionally encourage the family's belief that recovery will be complete. When their hopes are not realised, they may become frustrated and angry. Differences in health beliefs regarding the sick role may also appear within the family. Family members may differ in their views as to how the person should be managed and who should do the caring. Following discharge, the family may be divided on whether the patient should return home or be placed in convalescent care (if they are fortunate enough to have a choice), or they may differ as to what the patient should be allowed to do and conflict may arise. These factors may impact negatively on rehabilitation. You will facilitate successful rehabilitation by being aware of such potential risk factors and intervening early.

In caring for Mrs J, one of your options is to determine what support the couple has. You inquire further and she reveals the following:

Mr and Mrs J are pensioners who live alone. They have a supportive daughter, but she is a single parent (divorced) with two school-going children and she only has casual employment. She lives in a wooden, backyard structure. Mrs J says: "She tries her best to help, but she has her own problems." There are two married sons. "They don't come near to help," she says. "We had good neighbours but that's all gone now." (You recall that most of the neighbourhood was destroyed in a freak storm and her neighbours have been scattered throughout the community.) Mr J has not attended the hospital for physiotherapy because transport is costly. Mrs J has to deal with the consequences of the loss of their home on her own and is finding it very stressful. The local authority has been slow in providing the promised relief; much has not materialized. She finds it difficult to attend meetings on the re-housing plans and has been told that, although they rented the old houses, they will have to buy the new ones. The couple attends a local church. "Our priest is very helpful but he has to help many others too," she says.

Q
- Assess the level of support that Mrs and Mr J have.
- What constraints can you foresee in caring for your patient?
- What interventions would you discuss with Mrs J?

Supporting the caregiver and family in the early phase of disability

Early intervention and treatment strategies that include the family have been shown to improve outcomes (Crouch, 1987). The family physician is well placed to anticipate areas of possible stress in the family and to intervene early by providing information and support, and involving other resources. A home visit will help to gain firsthand knowledge of the family and to develop a comprehensive management plan together with them. Applying principles of family practice such as continuous, comprehensive, and co-ordinated care will facilitate family-centred care and the participation of other members of the primary care team (when present), such as the occupational therapist, physiotherapist, social worker, district sister, and community rehabilitation worker. The challenge is to provide quality care to chronically ill or disabled persons and their families, whose lives are also disrupted (Bresick and Harvey, 1997).

Around the time of hospital discharge

- **Collaborate** with the hospital team.
- **Anticipate differences** between the carer/family's health beliefs and those of the team. A clear explanation for investigations and referrals will help to avoid unrealistic expectations.
- Consider a **phased discharge** that gradually increases the amount of time spent at home, helps to bridge the gap between hospital and home, and enables early identification of problems.
- **Regular contact** with the carer/family after discharge helps to anticipate and prevent problems before they occur, such as the caregiver's health being compromised. Information can be given and

questions answered when the family is ready.
- **Provide information** about available resources such as rehabilitation workers, support groups, respite care and adaptations that reduce the patient's dependence on caregivers. (In many communities access to support services is limited and waiting lists are long. You will have to be innovative and may have to take on an advocacy role – see later.)
- **Home visits** help to balance the medical agenda with the family's agenda. The family is more at ease in the home environment and will take more initiative and responsibility in the rehabilitation process. Joint problem-solving helps the family to maintain some control over their quality of life.
- **Strengthen resolve** by acknowledging progress and affirming the efforts of the patient and the family.

Q Think of a family you have encountered who are dealing with a disability. Which of the above interventions apply? Draft a management plan from the information you have and include a list of additional information needed to provide support for the main caregiver.

Study 5: Working with family members

Experiences common to all families may put members at risk of serious illness. Consider the following study:

Mr L is a 66-year-old patient I know well. He is hypertensive, attends the clinic regularly for blood pressure monitoring, and is well controlled on a diuretic and beta blocker. He recovered well after an uncomplicated myocardial infarction ten years ago and stopped smoking then.

At a recent visit, he presented with emotional distress. His granddaughter, NL, had been killed in a car accident in the early hours of that morning. She lived with Mr L and his wife from birth, together with her single-parent mother. Understandably, his blood pressure was raised. He needed to express his grief and anger at the unnecessary loss of a promising life. NL had worked hard to matriculate and had just started working – no easy achievement given the high rate of unemployment in the community.

I provided supportive counselling, advised as much rest as possible under the circumstances and arranged a follow-up visit in a week to review his blood pressure and how he was coping. A few days later he presented with symptoms of acute myocardial infarction and had to be admitted to a coronary care unit.

Mr L returned for continuing care after being discharged. I reviewed what had happened and learned from a family member that he had not been able to rest during his bereavement. He lives with his wife and daughter (NL's mother) in a two-bedroom council house and sleeps in the lounge so that two grandsons (weekday boarders) can use his room as a study. He has no privacy and could not rest as visitors came to sympathise with the family during their bereavement.

On reflection, I had not considered the risk of a second myocardial infarct due to the stress of bereavement in an already strained family; nor had I considered any interventions to reduce these risks. Given his cardiac risk, it would have been useful to involve the family in reducing the impact of the loss by conducting a family conference as a preventive measure – see below.

As noted earlier, families may influence health negatively and be a causal or precipitating factor in illness. Families can also have a detrimental effect on treatment and rehabilitation and they can hasten relapse. Treatment plans can significantly affect the family; adherence to treatment may be impossible without the co-operation of at least one member of the family. Many common management challenges require involving the family for success. Consider the following examples:

- Adherence to a healthy diet in a diabetic may depend entirely on the co-operation of the family member who does the cooking.
- It is more difficult to stop smoking if other family members continue to smoke.
- The management of a stress-related disorder will be undermined by ongoing conflict in the patient's family.

The family can also have a positive influence on health by choosing a healthy lifestyle, acting as a resource for preventing illness and, in the presence of disease, providing support and enhancing adherence to treatment and rehabilitation. Our responsibility as family physicians includes helping families to mobilise their own resources, providing information, and involving available support services.

Involving the family in patient care

There are a number of levels of involving or working with the family (Figure 4.8). Conducting a family conference requires special skills and is uncommon in most practices. Patients, however, are often accompanied by a family member when visiting the doctor, making it relatively easy to involve the family at this level.

Figure 4.8 The family physician's level of involvement with the family

5 Conduct family therapy where appropriate
(if you have the necessary training)

4 Perform a systematic assessment of family functioning,
identify family dysfunction, and plan a family
conference where appropriate

3 Encourage the family to express feelings, assess the family's
level of functioning with respect to the patient's condition,
and assess the need for family support

2 Exchange relevant medical information on an
ongoing basis (e.g. communicating information
about treatment and obtaining feedback)

1 Minimal involvement. Communicate with the family
for practical and medical/legal reasons only
(e.g. obtaining consent) without engaging with the
family as an integral part of patient care

Each level beyond level 1 requires additional knowledge,
personal development, and skills

SOURCE: Adapted from Doherty and Baird (1986)

Accompanying family members may be directly involved in the patient's care – especially in the case of the elderly or chronically ill – and can provide information that may be useful in developing the care plan. They can be drawn into the consultation (with the patient's consent) to provide a deeper understanding of a problem, to help determine what resources the family has to offer, what aspects of family functioning may impact on patient care, and to enlist their help.

In Study 2, at a follow-up visit, Ms VF happened to mention that her brother Sam had driven her to her appointment and was waiting outside in the car. With her consent, the doctor invited him to join the consultation and inquired about his understanding of the problem. What emerged proved very helpful. Sam felt that his sister was overanxious about their father, that trying to compensate for their mother's death was causing burnout, and that she needed time out. He reported that his father was capable of caring for himself – including preparing meals – but Ms VF insisted on doing everything herself. He appreciated what she was doing to manage the home and did not want to interfere as he may be misunderstood as being unappreciative. Ms VF became tearful and admitted that Sam was correct. Sam agreed to convene a discussion with Ms VF and his father to discuss household duties and offered to be more involved himself. He suggested that Ms VF go away for a weekend. A weight seemed to lift from Ms VF's shoulders; she left with a smile.

On the day Mr L reported the death of his granddaughter he was accompanied by one of his daughters. An opportunity to inform her of the risk to her father's health, obtain her views on how best to reduce the impact of the loss on her father, and to enlist her support, was missed.

Types of family interviews

Engaging a family member is more easily achievable in daily practice. Cole-Kelly and Seaburn (in McDaniel and Campbell et al 2005) note that: "A family orientation has more to do with how one thinks about a patient than it does with how many people are in the exam room. A family-orientated approach does not always require the clinician to meet with the family in their practice." In a review of the literature, Campbell, McDaniel and Cole-Kelly (2002) note three general types of family interviewing in family practice.

The most common is a family-orientated interview with an individual patient and differs from a patient-centered interview only in that the emphasis is on the family rather than the individual; it includes obtaining a family history or genogram and discussing family issues.

The second most common family interview involves interviewing a family member accompanying a patient. Although it occurs in 33% of all visits in the studies reviewed, there are few guidelines on how to conduct such interviews.

The family conference or meeting, while the least common, is the focus of most of the literature on family interviewing. Although uncommon, they are well accepted by patients, may reduce overall health care costs, and have been found cost effective in the management of some chronic diseases.

Home visits which address the health care needs of the whole family may also be cost effective, though this needs further research. See Lang and Marvel *et al.* (2002) for helpful descriptions of the core skills needed when family members are present in the consultation.

Conducting a family conference

A family conference is a specially convened meeting of key family members with specific goals – such as obtaining a deeper understanding of a problem from family members, enlisting their help, determining what resources the family has to offer and assessing aspects of family functioning (McDaniel *et al.*, 2005). It is more complex to set up and therefore not common. However, it is worth knowing something about it as an important tool in family-orientated care. Many of the tasks are applicable to engaging single family members in the consultation; applying them will maximise the benefit of the exercise.

Before the conference

- Identify a person who will contact family members and assist in setting up the conference – normally the patient, if an adult, although it may be another family member who is concerned about the patient's wellbeing.
- Agree on who should attend.
- Set a date and venue.

Ideally the venue should be user-friendly, quiet and where you will not be interrupted. In the public sector this may be a tall order. You may have to use your room although it may be better to use a more neutral, non-clinical venue. Although conducting the conference in the patient's home may have its own limitations, it can reveal useful information about the family in their own environment and the limitations they face. It will help to keep your goals realistic!

Conference tasks

- Connect with each member of the family present by finding out something about them; create a safe environment that encourages participation.
- Clarify the aim of the conference; communicate appropriate information about the medical problem and avoid jargon.
- Ask the family how they understand the problem.
- Establish clear, mutually agreed goals for the conference.
- Gather relevant information from each person (use this later to update the genogram or ecomap).
- Allow the family to generate their own solutions and then add your own; select a suitable option together.
- Identify support services to assist with implementation, for example a social worker.
- Agree on a clear plan for implementation: decide on tasks – who will do what and when; leave a written copy; set a date for follow-up.

After the conference

- Update your genogram/ecomap and revise your hypothesis if necessary.
- Record your findings and the plan.
- Contact the family after an appropriate time period to assess progress; beware of encouraging dependency (keep some distance).
- Affirm the family's efforts even when not successful; acknowledge their difficulties, but encourage action and be willing to reset goals if they prove to be unrealistic.

In our context, it is more reasonable to ask key family members to attend the consultation at the practice with the patient for a longer discussion.

- Make a three-stage assessment of Mr L.
- Use the information provided to draw a genogram.
- What factors may have acted together to precipitate a myocardial infarction? Your genogram should show these clearly.
- Outline your goals for a family conference.
- Who would you choose as the contact person? Where would you prefer to conduct the conference and why?
- At what level of family involvement is conducting a family conference suitable? (see Figure 4.8).

An example of a home visit and family conference

The following case study illustrates the usefulness of a family conference.

A 43-year old domestic worker, Mrs BT, consulted Dr KMH for type 2 diabetes. The doctor noted that her diabetes had never been controlled despite attending regularly for medication over a 5-year period. It was clear that BT had a poor understanding of diabetes and struggled to eat a healthy diet as her children did all the cooking. Dr KMH decided to address the problem by calling a family meeting. Mrs BT agreed that the doctor could visit the family at home, as long as she did not report the illegal shebeen that her husband was running in the house! Mrs BT, her husband and 3 daughters were present at the meeting.

Important issues that emerged in the meeting were:
- None of the family members really understood diabetes. Mrs BT had believed it was due to "evil spirits" and the family wanted to know if it was hereditary. Mr T made a connection between stress and raised sugar levels.
- Mrs BT was functioning well and had no complications so the importance of changing her diet was not a priority.
- The family felt that BT was quite defensive about her eating habits and said "Mom doesn't listen to us when we tell her not to drink Coke."
- They had previously tried to cook separately for her, but this had not worked.
- They felt that they could not afford the special food on the diet sheet.

Dr KMH was able to address the following issues with the family:
- Provide information on diabetes, including risk factors, complications and the basics of blood glucose control.
- Obesity was a significant problem in the family as Mrs BT her husband and at least one of the daughters was obese. The family as a whole therefore were at risk of diabetes and needed to take action collectively rather than just focus on separate meals for BT.
- That portion size was an important issue and that they did not necessarily have to eat different foods. Increasing the amount of vegetables and decreasing the amount of starch and fat would make a difference.
- Physical activity was discussed but safety was a concern in the local area

At the end of the meeting the family were committed to collectively changing their cooking and eating habits.

Although such an investment of time and other resources does not guarantee success, this story shows that using a systems approach to the care of this patient and her diabetes provided helpful insights for the family and the doctor. It also offered a foundation on which to build. The first consultation with a patient is only the start of developing a long-term therapeutic relationship. Similarly, this family meeting can be seen as the first step in building an ongoing partnership with this family. Good relationships are at the centre of cost-effective primary care as trust forms the basis of such relationships and takes time to build. The evidence for the benefits of such partnerships based on the principles of family medicine is well described.

Make a few reflections of your own and formulate appropriate learning needs. The questions below may assist you:

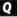

- Why did Dr KMH decide to do a home visit and conduct a family meeting?
- What opportunities did this provide that may not be possible in a clinic consultation?
- Are there any potential risks?
- How does this account differ from the usual understanding of a home visit?
- How would you classify the outcome of this family meeting - successful or unsuccessful? What are the reasons for your answer?
- Review again the steps involved in setting up a family meeting. Were any steps omitted? How may they have made a difference in your view?
- What would you have done at this patient's follow-up visit regarding matters arising from the family meeting?

Study 6: Identifying the family at risk

Family physicians play an important health promotion role. Attending to personal and family health needs shifts the focus from illness and disease to maintaining and promoting health. A helpful, functional under-standing of health is found in the Ottawa Charter for Health Promotion (WHO, 1986) which refers to health as the individual's or family's ability to identify and realise aspirations, to satisfy needs, and to respond to challenges of the environment. Diagnosing health (McWilliam, 1993) in relation to a family's needs, aspirations, and challenges means antici-pating threats to health, intervening to reduce risks, and encouraging healthy choices and a healthy environment.

Ms DB, a 17-year-old girl from Khayelitsha, comes to see you with a sore throat that requires symptomatic treatment only. During the consultation you ask about the family and the following picture emerges.

Her mother passed away six months ago from AIDS and she is looking after her 12-year-old sister. Their baby sister has been taken in by their aunt, but there is no space in the aunt's house for the older siblings. Finances are difficult as they only get the one child support grant and ad hoc gifts from the aunt. They are often dependent on the goodwill of neighbours when they run short of food, which is embarrassing. DB is worried about new clothes for her sister and school fees for next year.

DB's sister is struggling with her schoolwork and is doing really badly, even though she used to love school. Her teachers are often critical of her poor performance and she has been hurt by nasty comments from her classmates about her mother dying of AIDS. Ms DB has a boyfriend, who is 22 and is pressurising her to become sexually active, she doesn't want to lose him, but knows that she will if she doesn't give in to what he wants.

You realise that this is a family at risk and that her presentation with a sore throat is an opportunity to try and support this family before matters deteriorate further. Options that you consider in terms of increasing psychosocial support are to refer her to Fikelela, a church-based organisation, which offers food parcels and financial help for school fees and uniforms. In addition, you ask the social worker to explore ways of accessing the foster care grant, which might have to be applied for by the aunt as Ms DB is too young. You also think about calling a family conference with the extended family members and offering Ms DB counselling to help with decisions regarding her boyfriend.

This encounter illustrates how thinking family can identify families at risk, even during apparently straightforward consultations, and small interventions may prevent future harm and illness in the family.

Questions to assess family health and identify the family at risk

The following questions help to identify the family at risk and to make a family health assessment (McWilliam, 1993):

- What does health mean to this family?
- What does this family need to maintain or restore its health?
- Are there any physical, psycho-emotional, or socioeconomic threats to the health of this family? How can I help this family to overcome them?
- What capacity does this family have to make healthy choices?

- What does this family need from society to optimise its health?
- How can I promote a balance between the family's needs and expectations and the constraints of the health care system?

Q   Apply these questions to the family in Study 6. How many can you answer?

All families are at risk in some way due to internal or external threats; however some families are more vulnerable that others. (Review the list of common problems in Study 1.) HIV/AIDS has increased the burden of illness on many families; isolation due to social stigma, loss of income, loss of both parents, and child-headed households with no adult role-model or supervision are huge challenges. Many of these problems are hidden in a somatic primary care presentation. They will remain hidden and undermine the management of the presenting complaint if a systems approach is not used.

Health promotion includes encouraging families to use the available resources to protect their health. To evaluate the family's effectiveness at using available resources and the outcome of family-orientated interventions (McWilliam, 1993), ask questions such as:

- Does the family use available resources to overcome constraints and improve their health and quality of life?
- How effectively do they do this?
- Do they feel more in control of their lives?
- Do they experience better quality of life?

Some of these questions may be difficult to answer. They depend on subjective assessments and many outcomes are not easily measurable. View the exercise as a challenge to be innovative and an opportunity for research!

Q   Formulate a "health diagnosis" (McWilliam, 1993) for the families in Studies 1 and 3. What are the threats to their health? How can you intervene to reduce risks, encourage healthy choices and a healthy environment?

Further reading and tools to assist you in thinking family

You should also be aware of instruments that assess aspects of family functioning to aid decision-making. These include The Family APGAR

(Smilkstein, 1978) and The Family Circle (Thrower *et al.*, 1982). These will not be discussed here; you are referred to the relevant texts. The acronym PRACTICE is a guide to considering key aspects of family functioning: **P**resenting problems; **R**oles; **A**ffect; **C**ommunication patterns; **T**ime in the life cycle; **I**llness history; **C**oping with stress; **E**cology and culture (Christie-Seely 1984). The five questions listed in Study 1 cover much of the same ground and you may find them easier to use. Knowledge of the family life cycle helps to identify periods when families are at higher risk of stress and illness as they move from one developmental stage to the next, for example as children enter adolescence, parents need to become more flexible and allow more independence. Study 3 shows how parental rigidity can result in the breakdown of relationships and behavioural problems.

Recommended reading

Campbell TL, McDaniel SH, Cole-Kelly K *et al.* (2002) Family Interviewing: A Review of the Literature in Primary Care *Family Medicine,* 34:312–8

Crouch, MA and Roberts, I (eds) (1987) *The Family in Medical Practice: A Family Systems Primer.* New York: Springer-Verlag.

Griffiths F, Byrne D. (1998) General practice and the new science emerging from the theories of 'chaos' and complexity. *British Journal of General Practice,* 48:1697–1699.

Helman, CG (1994) *Culture, Health and Illness.* Oxford: Butterworth and Heinemann.

Helman, CG (2001) *Culture, health and illness.* Oxford University Press, New York.

Lang F, Marvel K, Sanders D, *et al.* Interviewing when family members are present. *American Family Physician* 2002;65:1351–4

McDaniel, SH, CampbellL, TL, Hepworth, J and Lorenze, A (2005) *Family-Oriented Primary Care.* New York: Springer.

McWhinney, IR (1989) *A Textbook of Family Medicine.* New York: Oxford University Press.

Reid S, Wessely S (2002) Frequent attenders with medically unexplained symptoms: service use and costs in secondary care. *The British Journal of Psychiatry,* 180:248–253

Wileman L, May C and Chew-Graham CA. (2002) Medically unexplained symptoms and the problem of power in the primary care consultation: a qualitative study. *Family Practice,* 19:178–182.

5 Disease prevention and health promotion

Gboyega A. Ogunbanjo
Department of Family Medicine and Primary Health Care
Medunsa Campus
University of Limpopo

Introduction

Prevention is concerned with the removal or reduction of risks, early diagnosis, early treatment, the limitation of complications, including those of iatrogenic origin, and maximum adaptation to disability. In preventive practice, the family physician's attitude implies that s/he understands and can use the preventive potential in each consultation. Opportunistic health promotion and case-finding mean that apart from attending to the specific problems of the consultation, the family physician seeks to promote the health of the patient in other areas. Consider the following example where a case-finding activity is unrelated to the reasons for consultation:

A 40-year-old man consults a family physician because he has backache and asks for a sick certificate to stay off work for three days. The family physician issues the certificate, but also measures the patient's blood pressure.

Family physicians are among the first health professionals to recognise that multitudes of factors in illness are preventable. In their contacts with their practice population, family physicians are uniquely placed to promote health and practise preventive medicine. They can intervene with individual patients and thus have an impact on the communities they serve, and they can also influence wider political and social issues.

Prevention – some useful definitions

Primary prevention

This means to remove the causal agents of disease. A few examples of this would be:
- The provision of clean drinking water

- Immunisation programmes (see the appendices at the end of this chapter)
- Anti-pollution measures, including discouraging cigarette smoking.

Secondary prevention

The family physician identifies subjects before they develop symptoms of disease. The most obvious example is hypertension, which we begin to treat long before there are any sequelae.

Screening by definition is a form of secondary prevention since the family physician is involved in systematically investigating a total population at risk with the aim of identifying pre-symptomatic disease. Screening the female population for the early stages of cervical cancer by the use of a cervical smear is an example of this.

Case-finding is also a form of secondary prevention. Here the family physician is involved in opportunistically investigating patients as they consult with the aim of identifying pre-symptomatic disease. Measuring the patient's blood pressure during the consultation is an example of case-finding.

Tertiary prevention

The family physician focuses on limiting the complications of a disease process and thereby limiting disability in patients with established disease. The family physician does this by *regular surveillance* – for example, in the case of a diabetic, this would include blood glucose testing, examination of the fundi, and foot care. The principles of caring for patients with chronic disease are discussed in Chapter 6.

Health promotion

The promotion of optimal health is the ultimate goal of family physicians. To achieve this, they need to actively participate with the communities they serve in to promote good health.

Definitions of health have proved elusive and singularly unsuccessful. The World Health Organisation (WHO) defines health as the "complete physical, mental and social well-being in the absence of disease and infirmity" (WHO/UNICEF, 1948). However, Morrell (1988) adds the following: "From the point of view of therapeutic goals, health is more conveniently thought of as the optimum adaptation of the individual to his environment, physically, psychologically and socially."

Health promotion aims to improve the health of the whole population.

In other words, this approach goes beyond the classical preoccupation with individual health education and lifestyle and includes a consideration of social and economic conditions, which can have an important influence on health. These broader societal issues include legislation, economics, social class, the environment, and development. Family physicians need not become political activists, but they should be aware of all of the important factors that may affect health promotion. Within the health district, the family physician may be able to promote health at a broader community level (see Chapter 9).

Activities that promote health would include the following:

- The creation of healthy environments, for example through tobacco legislation
- The provision of health information, for example through the mass media
- Debate on the socioeconomic causes of ill health, for example through a focus on reconstruction and development programmes.

Promoting health at a community level does not mean that advising the individual about lifestyle, alcohol consumption, and cigarette smoking has no impact. As family physicians, we can have an impact on individual health, but we should acknowledge our limitations.

How do family physicians motivate behaviour change?

A family physician spends a lot of time encouraging and motivating patients to change their behaviour. Cigarette smoking, for instance, is notoriously difficult to stop, but one study (Russell *et al.*, 1974) showed that one in 20 patients gave up after they were given simple advice. Many patients, however, do not change and this can be frustrating for the family physician, who feels that the patient is non-compliant, and for the patient, who becomes fed up with hearing the same lecture repeatedly.

Motivational interviewing (MI) recommends a guiding more than a directing style and is usually more effective than giving advice (Rubak *et al.*, 2005). It has been shown to be effective with topics such as alcohol and substance abuse, diet, exercise, tobacco smoking, and risky sexual behaviour (Lundahl, 2009). MI can be used as part of a patient-centred consultation (see Chapter 2) in sessions as brief as five to ten minutes when behaviour change is addressed. It has been found practically useful by family physicians in the South African context (Mash and Allen, 2004).

The spirit of the approach is as important as specific communication skills or techniques (Rollnick, 2010). The spirit or style of MI is outlined in Table 5.1.

Foundational communication skills include the ability to actively listen and make reflective listening statements or summaries, ask open-ended questions that encourage elaboration and collaboration and the ability to inform by establishing what information is wanted or needed before giving information, and then asking what the implications might be for the patient.

Doctors may use the structure shown in Figure 5.1 as a map to build on their communication skills, structure their attempts at behaviour change counselling and to practice certain techniques that may be helpful.

Table 5.1 The spirit of MI

Collaborative	The relationship between the patient and the doctor is a partnership. The patient's point of view is valued and key decisions are negotiated. The doctor's point of view is not imposed on the patient and coercive and confrontational approaches are avoided. Power is shared in the interaction.
Evocative	The doctor evokes the patient's own goals and solutions as motivators for change rather than seeking to argue with or persuade the patient to accept the doctor's goals and solutions. The doctor believes in the patient's potential to change. The ability to ask open-ended questions is important.
Respectful and supportive	The patient's right and ability to make independent and informed decisions is encouraged. The doctor does not inappropriately shoulder the responsibility for change, but sees it as the patient's legitimate responsibility to make choices and take control of their life.
Empathic	The doctor attempts to understand the patient's perspective and makes this understanding explicit through reflective listening statements and summaries
Direction	The doctor and patient decide together on the topic to be discussed and the doctor keeps the conversation aligned with this purpose. The interaction is focused on a specific behaviour change topic and may have a clear structure that is facilitated by the doctor.

Figure 5.1 Structure of an MI session

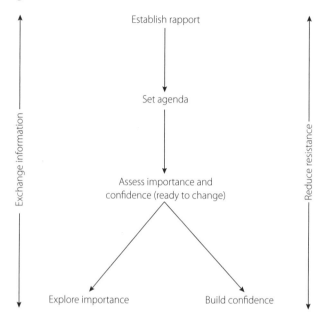

The practical application of MI in a brief behaviour change counselling session can be envisaged in Figure 5.1. Each of these tasks has a number of specific skills which are more fully described by Rollnick, Mason and Butler (1999). A few examples are given here.

Agenda setting may involve simply asking permission to discuss a particular topic or may involve the negotiation of which topic the patient is ready to discuss. Bear in mind that patients may have their own ideas and priorities. For example, in diabetes an agenda-setting tool has been suggested (Figure 5.2) that illustrates the topics that could be discussed and leaves blank circles for other topics raised by the patient. Agenda setting with an HIV-positive mother might look like this:

Dr: There are a number of things we could talk about today, such as your medication, feeding your baby or reducing risky sexual behaviour. I'm wondering if you are ready to discuss any of these, or if there is something else that is more important to you which we should discuss.

Pt: My problem, doctor, is that, if I am going to bottle feed my baby, I have to tell my family why I am different.
Dr: So, how to tell your family that you are HIV-positive is most important to you right now.
Pt: Yes, I'm not sure if I can do it.

Figure 5.2 Agenda setting tool for diabetes

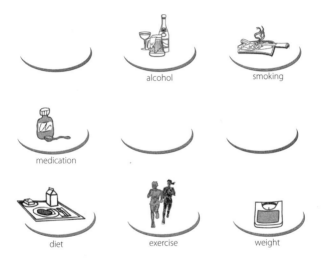

Readiness to change may involve assessing the person's overall readiness or exploring more specifically the dimensions of importance and confidence. The readiness to change ruler (Figure 5.3) may be a useful tool. For example in the same dialogue:

Dr: I am wondering how ready you are right now to tell your family. If you look at this ruler you can see that this end represents not being ready and this end represents being ready – where would you place yourself?
Pt: About here. [points to two thirds along]
Dr: I see. What makes you place yourself here and not at the beginning [not ready]?

Figure 5.3 Readiness to change rule

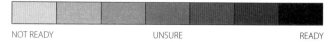

NOT READY   UNSURE   READY

Explore importance. It may help to develop discrepancy by reflecting the difference between the patient's expressed goals and values and current behaviour. Exploring the pros and cons of change or exchanging critical information may be useful.

Build confidence. Support self-efficacy by believing in and helping the patient to believe in the possibility of change. We literally talk ourselves into change and enabling the patient to articulate their desire, ability, reasons, need or commitment to change is helpful. Brainstorming ways of changing, learning from past attempts and imagining what life would be like if you were successful in changing may be useful.

Reducing resistance requires the doctor to see resistance as a product of the interaction that signals the need to modify the strategy being used by the doctor, rather than a fixed trait of the patient. For example, the doctor may be talking about concrete action when the patient is still ambivalent about the need for change and therefore elicits resistance. Another common mistake, called the righting reflex, is when the doctor feels the need to strongly express the argument for why the patient should change so that they can fix the problem. When the doctor argues for change in this way it often has the effect of making the patient explain all the reasons why change would be difficult and may even reinforce the patient's resistance as the doctor elicits from them the argument not to change.

Exchange information carefully by sharing only relevant information that the patient is interested in, in a neutral way. Elicit the implications or interpretation of this from the patient. Asking permission to share information with the patient may be important. This is in contrast to typical advice which provides unsolicited information together with a prescription of what to do about it.

Screening in South Africa

Currently, there are few clear national guidelines for population screening in South Africa. A great deal of research is needed to identify relevant screening programmes. Factors that may hinder screening, particularly in South Africa, are:

- Poverty-related issues such as no fixed addresses and constant mobility in search of work or housing, make a recall system unworkable
- The lack of a structured registration system of patients with a family physician or health care centre
- The lack of financial, human, and organisational resources
- The lack of public awareness (for example, this is one reason why many qualifying women have never had a cervical smear).

The criteria for screening

A number of criteria can determine whether a suggested population screening activity is worthwhile (Wilson, 1976):
- It must be an important health problem.
- It must be a common health problem.
- Resources for further diagnosis and treatment must be readily available.
- There must be an effective intervention for the condition.
- Protocols are needed with a clear statement as to when to treat the condition.
- The condition you screen for must have a latent or early pre-symptomatic phase.
- A suitable and acceptable test must be available with adequate specificity and sensitivity.
- The outcome of the condition must be improved by early detection.
- The natural history of the condition must be clearly understood.
- Screening should be continuous and should incorporate quality improvement cycles.
- Screening should be cost effective.

As yet, we do not have sufficiently researched material in South Africa with regard to what may or may not prevent patients from coming forward for a screening programme. However, a number of studies in other countries have shown that culture, lay beliefs, and ideas affect the numbers of patients who may come forward (Smith, 2004). In addition, participation in screening programmes may have significant psychosocial sequelae; for example, a study of screening for human papilloma virus found that participation "had the potential to communicate messages of distrust, infidelity and promiscuity to women's partners, family and the community" (McCaffery *et al.*, 2003).

Sensitivity and specificity

Sensitivity and specificity are two measures of the validity of a screening test.

Sensitivity by definition means the probability of testing positive if the disease is truly present. A high sensitivity means that almost all people with the disease tested positive. A low sensitivity means that many people with the disease tested negative (false negatives). In a screening test, a low sensitivity will result in people with the disease being falsely reassured that they do not have it.

Specificity is defined as the probability of screening negative if the disease is truly absent. A high specificity means that almost all people without the disease tested negative. A low specificity means that many people without the disease tested positive (false positives). In a screening test, a low specificity will result in many people being unnecessarily subjected to worry and further investigations.

Figure 5.4 shows the formulae for calculating sensitivity and specificity, and Figure 5.5 gives a practical example of the formulae.

In the evidence-based medicine (EBM) approach to diagnostic tests, the concepts of sensitivity and specificity are being replaced by that of the likelihood ratio. The likelihood ratio is calculated from the sensitivity and specificity, as shown in Figure 5.4. This *likelihood ratio*, when multiplied with the estimated pre-test probability of having the disease, can give a more useful measure of the actual likelihood of having the condition. Thus, if the pre-test probability of having breast cancer is estimated as 0.6%, then the pre-test odds are calculated as 0.6/99.4 = 0.006 (see Figure 5.5). If the likelihood ratio of the test is 21.6, then the post-test odds of having the condition are calculated as 0.006 × 21.6 = 0.13. The post-test probability of having the condition is therefore 0.13/1.13 × 100 = 11.5%. In this population, if you screen positive, you have an 11.5% probability of actually having breast cancer. In essence, a more useful screening test will have a higher likelihood ratio (Sackett *et al.*, 2000).

Figure 5.4 Formulae for calculating sensitivity and specificity

a = The number of individuals for whom the screening test is positive and the individual actually has the disease (true positive)

b = The number for whom the screening test is positive but the individual does not have the disease (false positive)

c = The number for whom the screening test is negative but the individual does have the disease (false negative)

d = The number for whom the screening test is negative and the individual does not have the disease (true negative)

Results of screening test (T)	Actual disease		
	Positive	Negative	Total
Positive	a	b	a + b
Negative	c	d	c + d
Total	a + c	b + d	

Sensitivity (sens) %	=	$a/(a + c) \times 100$
Specificity (spec) %	=	$d/(b + d) \times 100$
Positive likelihood ratio	=	$sens/(1 - spec)$
Negative likelihood ratio	=	$(1 - sens)/spec$
Positive predictive value	=	$a/(a + b) \times 100$
Negative predictive value	=	$d/(c + d) \times 100$
Prevalence (prev) %	=	$(a + c)/(a + b + c + d) \times 100$
Pre-test odds	=	$prev/(1 - prev)$
Post-test odds	=	$pre\text{-}test \times likelihood\ ratio$
Post-test probability	=	$post\text{-}test\ odds/(post\text{-}test\ odds + 1)$

Figure 5.5 The sensitivity and specificity for breast cancer screening by mammography

Screening test (mammography)	Breast cancer		
	Cancer confirmed	Cancer not confirmed	Total
Positive	413	3026	3439
Negative	22	65309	65331
Total	435	68335	68770
Sensitivity	$= 413/435 \times 100$		$= 94.9\%$
Specificity	$= 65309/68335 \times 100$		$= 95.6\%$
Positive likelihood ratio	$= 0.95/0.044$		$= 21.6$
Negative likelihood ratio	$= 0.05/0.956$		$= 0.052$
Prevalence	$= 435/68770 \times 100$		$= 0.6\%$
Pre-test odds	$= 0.6/99.4$		$= 0.006$
Post-test odds	$= 0.006 \times 21.6$		$= 0.13$
Post-test probability	$= 0.13/1.13 \times 100$		$= 11.5\%$

SOURCE: Mushlin *et al.*, 1998

Opportunistic health prevention and promotion

In South Africa, most preventive measures in the health sector are opportunistic. Every consultation should be seen as a potential opportunity for health prevention and promotion (Stott and Davis, 1979). Table 5.2 lists possible opportunistic activities that family physicians could undertake in South Africa (Kibel and Wagstaff, 1991; McWhinney, 1989; US Preventive Services Task Force, 2010). The list is not exhaustive and does not include high-risk groups (for example, those susceptible to travel-related illness) or specific diseases (such as diabetes, tuberculosis, asthma, and so on).

Table 5.2 Age-related preventive measures for family physicians

Newborn (≤ eight weeks)

Immunisation

Height and weight (growth) assessment

Breastfeeding assessment

Examine for/check:
Anterior fontanelle and head circumference

Eye movements, cataracts

Cleft palate

Heart

Back (spina bifida occulta)

General tone, movements, and head control

Testes and genitalia

Skin (birthmarks, haemangiomata, and so on)

Hearing (Does the baby startle to sound?)

Eyesight (Do the eyes follow the mother's face?)

Newborn to two years

Immunisation

Height and weight (growth) assessment

Diet, injury prevention (for example paraffin poisoning), dental hygiene, passive
smoking

Examine for/check:
Tooth decay

Signs of neglect or abuse

Eye movements, squint

Hearing defects

Development of speech (baby should babble at nine months, acquire language at 18
months)

Motor development (baby should sit without support at nine months, walk by 18
months)

Tone (do heel to ear test), pincer grip (at nine months), co-ordination and balance
(baby should get from lying to standing without holding on by 18 months)

Heart, skin, hips

Age two–12 years

Immunisation

Height and weight (growth) assessment

Diet, injury prevention (for example safety belts, firearms), dental hygiene, passive smoking

Problems with vision, hearing, language

Skin protection from ultraviolet light (if relevant)

Examine for/check:
Tooth decay

Signs of neglect or abuse

Heart and femoral pulses

Testes

General skeletal development and co-ordination of movement

Age 13–18 years

Immunisation (consider tetanus–diphtheria booster, rubella)

Height and weight (growth) assessment

Diet, injury prevention (for example, safety belts, firearms)

Smoking, alcohol, drug use

Safe sex and need for family planning

Sexually transmitted infections (chlamydia, gonorrhoea, syphilis, HIV) in those at risk

Dental health

Skin protection from ultraviolet light (if relevant consider skin examination)

Age 19–39 years

Immunisation (consider tetanus-diphtheria booster, rubella)

Blood pressure

Obesity

Smoking, alcohol, drug use

Safe sex and need for family planning

Sexually transmitted infections (chlamydia, gonorrhoea, syphilis, HIV) in those at risk

Domestic violence

Depression

Dental health

Non-fasting total blood cholesterol

Cervical smear (especially for women over 30 years)

Skin protection from ultraviolet light (if relevant consider skin examination)

Age 40–64 years

Immunisation (consider tetanus-diphtheria booster)

Blood pressure

Obesity

Smoking, alcohol, drug use

Safe sex and need for family planning

Sexually transmitted infections (chlamydia, gonorrhoea, syphilis, HIV) in those at risk

Domestic violence

Depression

Dental health

Non-fasting total blood cholesterol

Discuss aspirin chemoprophylaxis in those at increased risk of coronary heart disease

Cervical smear (for women)

Faecal occult blood for colo-rectal cancer (>50 years)

Mammography for women

Skin protection from ultraviolet light (if relevant consider skin examination)

Ages 65 and over

Immunisation (consider tetanus–diphtheria booster, influenza, and pneumococcal vaccines)

Blood pressure

Obesity

Osteoporosis in women

Smoking, alcohol, drug use

Depression

Dental health

Non-fasting total blood cholesterol

Discuss aspirin chemoprophylaxis in those at increased risk of coronary heart disease

Abdominal aortic aneurysm in men who have never smoked

Mammography for women

Vision and hearing

Functional status at home

Skin protection from ultraviolet light (if relevant consider skin examination)

Pregnant women

Genetic and obstetric history

Diet and breastfeeding

Smoking, alcohol, drug use

Sexually transmitted infections (chlamydia, gonorrhoea, syphilis, HIV)

Blood pressure

Haemoglobin

ABO/Rhesus typing

Rh(D) antibody screen

Hepatitis B surface antigen

Rubella

Urinalysis

Need for maternal serum alpha-fetoprotein test, ultrasound scan, amniocentesis

Need for blood sugar or glucose tolerance test

Q Consider what opportunistic health prevention and promotion would be appropriate in the following consultations:

A woman visits her family physician for her regular contraceptive injection. She tells the family physician that this is likely to be her last injection as she has decided to become pregnant.

A mother brings her one-year-old baby to see the family physician because the child has had a cough for two weeks. The child is not feverish and the family physician detects no abnormality apart from a runny nose.

A 14-year-old girl consults a family physician about a vaginal discharge.

A 70-year-old man presents with a seborrhoeic keratosis.

A 40-year-old man presents with epigastric pain. From the man's description of the pain, the family physician considers an early peptic ulcer as the cause. A physical examination reveals no abnormality and the family physician decides to prescribe an antacid and to review the patient in a week.

A 52-year-old woman, who rarely attends the practice, consults the family physician because she needs immunisations for a foreign holiday.

Specific diseases and high-risk groups

The previous section outlines possible opportunistic interventions in patients of different ages that may be considered in the consultation. Many specific diseases have well-documented strategies for prevention; some diseases are only worth preventing or case-finding for in particular high-risk groups. We will not give a comprehensive outline of all these diseases and high-risk groups here, but have selected a few specific diseases because of their importance in South Africa. This section will focus on intimate partner violence, alcohol abuse disorders, HIV/AIDS, tuberculosis and malaria.

Intimate partner violence

Despite new rights under the Constitution and new legislation (such as the Domestic Violence Act, No 116 of 1998), domestic violence still poses a very serious challenge in South Africa (See Chapter 8, page 263). Family physicians should actively enquire about and participate in the education of their practice populations against violence just as they do against alcohol, drug abuse, and cigarette smoking. The use of a question such as "How are things going on in your relationship?" is recommended, particularly in women who present with the following cues (Joyner and Mash, 2010):

- Vague non-specific symptoms
- History of mental illness or medication
- Fatigue, sleep problems, unexplained somatic complaints
- Symptoms of depression
- Feeling anxious/dizzy/thinking too much
- Chronic pain syndromes
- Repeated sexually transmitted infections or HIV
- Assault or trauma
- Suspected alcohol or substance abuse.

Alcohol use disorders

In South Africa, alcohol is relatively affordable. In many episodes of violence, the use of alcohol and other addictive drugs appears to be a contributory and aggravating factor. One study in a rural South African town found that "[t]he high prevalence of alcohol dependence (56%) in this community, and the possibility of comparable results in many similar rural South African communities, reflect a startling reality that should be addressed" (Claassen, 1998). South Africa has one of the world's highest prevalence of foetal alcohol syndrome (May, 2005). The CAGE and AUDIT are useful screening or case-finding tools for alcohol use disorders (see the appendices at the end of this chapter). CAGE is shorter, but the AUDIT is more sensitive to harmful alcohol use without physical dependency.

HIV/AIDS

A key message from the International AIDS Conference in Barcelona in 2002 was that the successful management of HIV and AIDS hinges on an ongoing interplay of therapeutic and preventive interventions. Health promotion at the community and societal level and health education at the clinic level are vital in preventing HIV/AIDS. Key people and organisations, such as the mass media, business, trade unions, opinion leaders and political leaders, must contribute towards greater openness, awareness, and behaviour change. Issues of poverty, migrant labour, unemployment, and so on that may contribute towards the transmission and progression of HIV/AIDS are also important. The need to particularly empower women and focus on the relationship between HIV, poverty and gender inequality has been emphasised (Kim and Watts, 2005).

At the clinic level, no opportunity should be missed to educate and influence people when they consult. Physicians should treat sexually transmitted diseases, provide condoms, and offer HIV Counselling and Testing (HCT) services. These activities, at the clinic level, are further described in Chapter 8.

The typical components of a district health plan to prevent the spread of HIV/AIDS would be as follows (Health Systems Trust, 1997):

- Raise awareness through local media and community events.
- Offer education programmes through schools, the workplace, and non-governmental organisations, and for special high-risk groups such as sex workers. Avoiding multiple concurrent partners is thought to be particularly important in reducing rapid spread of infection through sexual networks.
- Encourage the control and syndromic management of sexually transmitted diseases (Grosskurth *et al.*, 1995).
- Supply condoms.
- Reduce blood transmission through a safe blood supply, universal precautions, and needle-stick injury policy.
- Reduce mother-to-child (materno-foetal) transmission.
- Address socioeconomic factors that contribute to the spread of HIV/AIDS.

The district must also address the needs of those already infected by HIV/AIDS and attempt to reduce the impact of the infection. Typical aspects that must be addressed include the following:

- Develop primary health care, district hospital care, and tuberculosis services.
- Develop counselling services and support groups.
- Provide antiretroviral therapy and monitor compliance
- Provide and encourage home-based and hospice care.
- Provide welfare support and address the needs of disrupted families where children or the elderly may be left unsupported.

Understanding sexuality

Although not all HIV is transmitted by means of sexual intercourse, understanding sexual behaviour is important in understanding the HIV epidemic in South Africa. Sexual behaviour can be understood in terms of the personal, interpersonal, and contextual factors which are all closely interconnected (Matthes, 2005). For example, low self-esteem is associated with becoming sexually active at a younger age, more sexual partners, and negative attitudes towards condom use.

Inability to negotiate about sex and condom use with one's partner increases the risk of HIV. Negotiating power is further reduced by intimate partner violence or a male partner more than five years older (Matthes, 2005).

Contextual aspects include traditional views that support gender inequality and perceptions that sexual conquests are a mark of masculinity. Migrant labour and poverty (sex may be exchanged for material goods) are also risk factors (Matthes, 2005).

Multiple concurrent sexual partners

Having multiple sexual partners at the same time results in the exponential spread of HIV. This can be explained by the fact that HIV is most infectious during sero-conversion when viral loads are very high and the person is unaware of their status (an HIV test may still be negative at this stage). Assuming a woman is infected by her partner, she will now be sero-converting and any other partner/s will have a far higher risk of infection due to the high viral load associated with the sero-conversion process. They in turn will then be sero-converting and are very likely to infect their partners.

In contrast, if a person practices serial monogamy and is infected with HIV, he can only infect his new single partner. When she is sero-converting, she is only highly infectious for her current partner and less infectious for future partners.

Therefore messages promoting one partner at a time are even more important than messages promoting fewer lifetime partners (Morris, 1997). However multiple partner relationships may be very stable and one cannot assume that long-term married couples are not at risk as there may be stable extramarital partners.

Condoms

"Condom promotion for family planning or for AIDS prevention should present condom use as a responsible expression of love and as part of modern life. Such a positive approach often changes minds better than citing frightening health statistics." (Population Report) The female condom allows women more control in the decision to use protection and should also be explained and encouraged if available. Some suggestions to help people negotiate the use of condoms with their partner are shown in Table 5.3. The motivational tension that may arise for women when speaking about condoms with their partner is illustrated in Figure 5.6 (Mash, 2010).

Table 5.3 Tips for counselling about condoms

Encourage the person to consider the cost-benefit ratio. Pose the question: "Is more feeling and spontaneity worth dying for?"

Suggest experimentation with different brands of condom and lubricant.

Ensure that the patient knows how to use condoms correctly.

The patient should have condoms readily available when the need may arise.

The patient or partner should practise with condoms alone first to gain confidence in their use.

Suggest that negotiation over condom use should occur before things get hot and heavy.

Alcohol and drugs make it more difficult to stick to safe sex.

Encourage eroticisation of condoms. For example, if the patient's partner complains about prior experience with condoms, suggest that they respond by saying "'But you've never tried them with me".

If a new partner will not use condoms, the patient should consider whether the relationship is worth pursuing.

Figure 5.6 Motivational tension in the mind of a woman who is asked to negotiate condom use

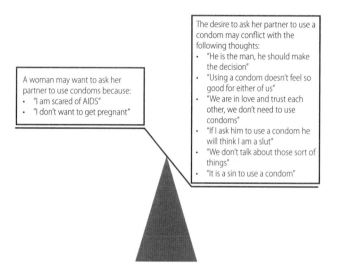

Circumcision

A Cochrane review found that medical circumcision of heterosexual men reduced HIV transmission by between 38% and 66% over one year (Siegfried, 2010). Given the safety of the procedure when performed by trained staff, it is recommended for the prevention of HIV transmission (WHO, 2009). However the prevalence of HIV is not lower in communities that practise traditional circumcision, which suggests the age of circumcision is an issue as well as the relationship between medical and traditional circumcision practices. There are also concerns that people who are circumcised may practise more unsafe sex if they believe they are protected. Nevertheless several countries such as Zimbabwe, Botswana and South Africa have embarked on male circumcision campaigns. Promising results have also been shown with tenofovir-containing microbicidal gel and further research will hopefully lead to a new form of prevention in the next few years.

The role of medication

The role of antiretrovirals and other medication in the prevention of the transmission, progression, and complications of HIV/AIDS is well established. Antiretroviral drugs, taken during pregnancy and labour, do markedly reduce the transmission of HIV from mother to child (McIntyre and Gray, 2000). After birth the avoidance of mixed feeding is recommended and the lowest risk of transmission is associated with exclusive formula-feeding. Exclusive breastfeeding is an option if formula-feeding is not a safe or practical option.

In patients with HIV, various types of chemoprophylaxis against opportunistic infections have been recommended in addition to general nutritional and social support. Co-trimoxazole prophylaxis for patients in WHO stages three and four or with a CD4 ≤ 200, and the prompt treatment of secondary infections continue to be of crucial importance. Key recommendations for chemoprophylaxis are summarised in Table 5.4. The use of INH prophylaxis for tuberculosis requires a robust TB management infrastructure. There is little evidence to support the routine use of influenza and pneumococcal vaccinations, although private sector guidelines recommend the routine use of influenza vaccination yearly in patients with a CD4 count > 200. Multivitamin preparations have been shown to delay the progression of HIV disease (Wawzi et al., NEJM: 2004, M Baum *et al.*, AIDS 2010), but are not a substitute for antiretroviral therapy. The use of immune booster preparations is not recommended concurrently with antiretroviral therapy, as some commonly used compounds have been associated with bone marrow toxicity and hepatic enzyme induction.

Highly active antiretroviral therapy (HAART) has been used in the most economically advanced parts of the world since the mid-1990s, and has been increasingly available in sub-Saharan Africa through public and private sector disease management initiatives since the late 1990s. Antiretroviral therapy is highly effective, and current computer modelling of efficacy (Walensky, 2005) suggests long-term control of HIV infection. This translates to ten to 15 years life gained in the individual patient. This is predicted on long-term adherence to multi-drug regimens in excess of 80%.

Table 5.4 Key recommendations for chemoprophylaxis in HIV/AIDS

Indication for prophylaxis	Target group	Medication	Comments
Pneumocystis jiroveci (PCJP) prophylaxis	All HIV-positive children with advanced or symptomatic disease All children born to HIV-positive mothers until diagnosis can be excluded – start at four to six weeks of age	Co-trimoxazole administered according to weight, in a twice-daily dose	Apart from treating PCJP, it also gives some protection against toxoplasma, bacterial pneumonia, bacteraemia, and *Isospora belli* diarrhoea. Studies done on dosage x3/week but adherence may be better on daily dose
	In all adults with a CD4+ count <200/μL, or CD4 count ≤350 cells/mm^3 (in patients with PTB/HIV or pregnant women) or MDR/XDR-TB irrespective of CD4 or WHO stage IV irrespective of CD4 count	Co-trimoxazole – one double-strength (960 mg) or two single-strength tablets (480 mg) daily	
Measles and chickenpox in children	Following exposure to measles (<five days) or -chickenpox (<three days)	Immunoglobulin (0.5 ml/kg) or zoster immunoglobulin (0.15 ml/kg)	
Tuberculosis (TB)	Patients with evidence of previous TB infection as assessed by a positive tuberculin skin test (Mantoux >= 5 mm) at any stage of HIV infection Certain high-risk groups, including those in contact with TB sufferers, health care workers, miners, and others living in dormitory conditions	Isoniazid for six to nine months – dosage 5 mg/kg/day (maximum 300 mg/day) or 15 mg/kg/dose (maximum 900 mg) given twice weekly	Secondary prophylaxis after treating TB is not recommended. Active TB must first be excluded. Medication use must be closely supervised and pyridoxine added to prevent peripheral neuropathy. Monitor for hepatitis.

Indication for prophylaxis	Target group	Medication	Comments
Diarrhoea in children	All children may be given vitamin A	Vitamin A – start dose every six months according to age: < six months 50 000 IU Six to 12 months 100 000 IU > 12 months 200 000 IU	An overdose of vitamin A can be dangerous. Vitamin A can reduce all cause mortality as well as that from diarrhoea

SOURCE: Harley (1999): Southern African HIV Clinicians Society (2000)

Tuberculosis (TB)

It is quite clear from epidemiological studies in the United Kingdom and the United States that addressing issues of poverty, hunger, malnutrition, and sanitation prevents or drastically reduces morbidity and mortality from tuberculosis. In the United Kingdom, "most of the decline from infectious disease appears to have occurred before effective immunisation, antibiotics, and chemotherapy became available" (McKeown, 1979). Unemployment, poor housing, overcrowding, poor education, and inadequate food supply are all relevant issues in South Africa. The HIV/AIDS epidemic is also an important factor. A person who has been exposed to tuberculosis as assessed by a positive tuberculin skin test, but who is not HIV-positive, has a 10% lifetime risk of developing tuberculosis. If this same person has HIV, they have a 10% risk every year of developing tuberculosis (Department of Health, 1998).

However, this does not mean that the National Tuberculosis Control Programme has no part to play in the prevention of tuberculosis. Important aspects of prevention include the following (Department of Health, 2009):

- *BCG immunisation* at birth can protect up to 80% of young children, especially against miliary tuberculosis and tuberculosis meningitis. If there is no record of BCG, or no BCG scar, it must be given up to the age of one year.
- BCG vaccination can lead to disseminated infection in HIV-infected children. However, due to the high TB burden in South Africa and the difficulty of determining HIV status at birth, it is recommended that routine BCG vaccination continues to be given at birth (Department of Health, 2009).
- The full immunisation programme is important as measles and whooping cough predispose to tuberculosis.
- A well child, under the age of five years, who is in intimate contact with a smear-positive tuberculosis family member or caregiver should receive INH prophylactic treatment. If the child is sick, appropriate investigations should be offered before treatment. This is often a missed opportunity to prevent TB disease in children.
- The prompt identification and treatment of smear-positive tuberculosis patients is also important in breaking the chain of transmission. This is why the programme focuses on smear-positive tuberculosis cases.

Malaria

The prevention of malaria in visitors to at-risk areas in southern Africa remains an important topic. No drug is totally effective in preventing malaria and visitors must take effective precautions to reduce their exposure to infected mosquitoes:

- Visit malaria areas during the lowest risk period (in winter).
- Avoid outdoor activities between dusk and dawn where possible. If you must go outside during the evening or night, cover the skin surface with clothing (long trousers and long-sleeved shirts) and wear closed shoes.
- Apply insect repellent to exposed skin between dusk and dawn. Repeated applications may be necessary as the action may only last four to six hours. Apply insect repellent sparingly to children and avoid using it on babies.
- Ensure that windows and doors have effective screens.
- Sleep under mosquito netting, preferably impregnated with pyrethroid insecticides.
- Use knock-down insecticides in dwellings.
- Burn mosquito coils or use vaporising mats.

The choice of chemoprophylaxis may be individualised depending on the patient's age, pregnancy status, medical history (such as immune status and allergies), length of stay, and degree of exposure. The pregnant backpacker camping in the bush for three weeks, for example, is obviously at higher risk than the company director staying overnight in a five-star screened hotel. The most widely used regimes are compared in Table 5.5.

High-risk patients, such as pregnant women, children under the age of two years and the immunocompromised, are more likely to get complicated malaria. Pregnant women and small children should avoid visiting a malaria area unless it is essential. In malaria endemic areas, prevention is an important component of malaria control. It is achieved through vector control (DDT spray of dwellings), personal protection measures such as insecticide-treated bed nets and preventive treatment with antimalarial drugs of vulnerable groups such as pregnant women, who receive intermittent preventive treatment.

Table 5.5 Chemoprophylaxis agents used in malaria

Regime	Adult dosage	Child dosage	Pregnancy	Side-effects	Contra-indications	Drug Interactions
Mefloquine	250 mg weekly starting one to two weeks before entry, then weekly for four weeks after leaving a malarious area	Not recommended < 5 kg weight 5–19 kg: 62.5 mg 20–30 kg: 125 mg 31–45 kg: 187.5 mg > 45 kg: 250 mg	Not recommended in first trimester or in three months before conception	Mild transient dizziness and gastro-intestinal upset Rarely neurological and psychiatric disorders	History of neuropsychiatric or cardiac disease Need for fine co-ordination, pilots, divers, etc.	Beta blockers and calcium-antagonists. Monitor effects on anticoagulants and anti-diabetic agents
Doxycycline	100 mg daily, starting 24–48 hours prior to entry, then daily and four weeks after leaving a malarious area	Not for use in children under the age of eight years	Contra-indicated	Gastro-intestinal upset, photo-sensitisation, *Candida* (thrush)		Decreased absorption with antacids containing calcium, magnesium, zinc and iron. May reduce efficacy of oral contraceptives

Regime	Adult dosage	Child dosage	Pregnancy	Side-effects	Contra-indications	Drug Interactions
Atovaquone 250 mg plus proguanil 100 mg	One tablet daily starting 24 hours prior to entry and for seven days after departure	Safe for all ages. Paediatric formulation available in SA One paediatric tablet = 62.5 mg atovaquone plus 25 mg proguanil 11–20 kg: one paediatric tablet daily 21–30 kg: two paediatric tablets daily 31–40 kg: three paediatric tablets daily > 40 kg: one adult tablet daily	Not recommended in pregnant women	Usually mild: Abdominal pain, nausea, headache		Limited data relating to drug interactions, but check effect on warfarin

The family physician's personal health

Doctors of all specialties tend to look after themselves badly. Many abuse alcohol and other substances and do not exercise enough. The reasons for this are complex and may relate to the fact that the profession is demanding and that it is often difficult to find or make time for relaxation and family. In order to care for patients appropriately, it is important for health professionals to ensure that they take good care of their own health.

A family physician should identify a colleague whom they can consult when s/he is unwell. This person should ideally also be a family physician and not be in the same practice or health care facility as this could lead to a conflict of interests. It is unwise for family physicians to self-medicate with medicines that normally cannot be obtained over the counter by members of the public. It is very difficult to be objective and self-diagnose. For example, if you have a fever, is it malaria or acute bronchitis, or is the symptom self-limiting, or is it the beginning of something serious? Sharing your health concerns with a trusted colleague is an appropriate method of personal preventive medicine.

Recommended reading

Department of Health. HIV/AIDS treatment guidelines. Pretoria: Department of Health. 2010.

Department of Health. Guidelines for the Prevention of Malaria in South Africa. Pretoria: Department of Health. 2009.

Department of Health. EPI (SA). Immunisation schedule. Pretoria: Department of Health. 2009.

Fomundam H, Mathews C (eds). Department of Health pocket guide on antiretroviral therapy in South Africa. 2nd edition. 2009.

Appendices

Immunisation schedule

Age of child	Vaccine needed
At birth	BCG, OPV (0)
six weeks	OPV (1), RV (1), DTaP-IPV//Hib (1), Hep B (1), PCV (1)
ten weeks	DTaP-IPV//Hib (2), Hep B (2)
14 weeks	RV (2), DTaP-IPV//Hib (3), Hep B (3), PCV (2)
nine months	Measles vaccine (1), PCV (3)
18 months	DTaP-IPV//Hib (4), Measles vaccine (2)
six years (both boys and girls)	Td vaccine
12 years (both boys and girls)	Td vaccine

Key:		
	BCG:	Bacilles Calmette Guerin;
	OPV:	Oral Polio Vaccine;
	RV:	Rotavirus Vaccine;
	DTaP-IPV//Hib:	Diphtheria, Tetanus, acellular Pertussis, Inactivated Polio Vaccine and *Haemophilus influenza* type b;
	Hep B:	Hepatitis B Vaccine;
	PCV 7:	Pneumococcal Conjugated Vaccine;
	Td vaccine:	Tetanus and reduced strength of diphtheria Vaccine

SOURCE: National Department of Health: EPI (SA)

AUDIT screening questionnaire

Question	Score				
	0	1	2	3	4
How often do you have a drink containing alcohol?	Never	Monthly or less	2–4 times/ month	2–3/week	4 or more times/ week
How many drinks do you have on a typical day when you are drinking?	None	One or two	Three or four	Five or six	Seven to nine*
How often do you have six or more drinks on one occasion?	Never	Less than monthly	Monthly	Weekly	Daily or almost daily
How often during the last year have you found that you were unable to stop drinking once you had started?	Never	Less than monthly	Monthly	Weekly	Daily or almost daily
How often during the last year have you failed to do what was normally expected from you because of drinking?	Never	Less than monthly	Monthly	Weekly	Daily or almost daily
How often during the last year have you needed a first drink in the morning to get yourself going after a heavy drinking session?	Never	Less than monthly	Monthly	Weekly	Daily or almost daily
How often during the last year have you had a feeling of guilt or remorse after drinking?	Never	Less than monthly	Monthly	Weekly	Daily or almost daily

Question	Score				
	0	**1**	**2**	**3**	**4**
How often during the last year have you been unable to remember what happened the night before because you had been drinking?	Never	Less than monthly	Monthly	Weekly	Daily or almost daily
Have you or someone else been injured as a result of your drinking?	Never	Yes, but not in last year (two points)		Yes, during the last year (four points)	
Has a relative, doctor or other health worker been concerned about your drinking or suggested you cut down?	Never	Yes, but not in last year (two points)		Yes, during the last year (four points)	

NOTE: Score of greater than eight (out of 41) is suggestive of problem drinking and indicates a need for more in-depth assessment. Cut off of ten points recommended by some to provide greater specificity.
*five points if response is ten or more drinks on a typical day.

CAGE screening tool

C   Have you ever felt you should **C**ut down on your drinking?

A   Have people **A**nnoyed you by criticising your drinking?

G   Have you ever felt bad or **G**uilty about your drinking?

E   Have you ever had a drink first thing in the morning to steady your nerves or to get rid of a hangover (**E**ye-opener)?

NOTE: If the person answers yes to two or more questions, you should consider harmful alcohol use, and if the answers to three or more of the questions are positive, the patient is likely to be dependent on alcohol (MayWeld *et al.*, 1974).

6 Management skills in the consultation

Bev Schweitzer
Division of Family Medicine
School of Public Health and Family Medicine
University of Cape Town

Ian Couper
Division of Rural Health
Department of Family Medicine
University of the Witwatersrand

Introduction

This chapter describes generic skills that are part of managing patients in most consultations. We start with an overview of the inner process of clinical decision-making and then look at how the consultation should be documented in the medical record. Many patients attend regularly with ongoing problems and chronic care requires a different approach to organisation and the consultation from that needed for acute episodic illness. We then consider prescribing medication, issuing of medical certificates and how to refer a patient.

Decision-making in family medicine

Traditional medical training teaches students to take a full history and then examine all the systems of the body before considering the diagnosis. This is known as inductive reasoning. In practice, however, clinicians usually have an idea of the diagnosis early on and then test it out as they progress with the consultation. This process is known as hypothetic-deductive reasoning.

Hypothesis formation and testing

From the moment the patient enters the room, the family physician starts to formulate hypotheses (Neighbour, 1987). As noted in Chapter 3, it is important not to settle on a diagnosis too early and ignore evidence that does not fit. Allow the patient to tell their story. Family physicians do not collect all the information from a systematic history, full examination, and side-room tests, and then sit down to decide on a diagnosis. It is instead a continuous process of hypothesis formulation and testing from the start of the consultation. During a single consultation, a number of working hypotheses may be created, tested, and discarded. Consider the following example:

THE INFORMATION	THE HYPOTHESIS
The patient complains of shortness of breath.	Asthma? The family physician asks about a history of asthma, wheeze, cough, and so on.
The patient's answers are not consistent with asthma, but she does seem nervous.	Hyperventilation due to anxiety? The family physician asks about stress and feelings of anxiety.
The patient has not experienced more stress than usual lately and her anxiety is related to her fear of hearing a bad diagnosis.	Cardiac failure? The family physician asks about change in effort tolerance, orthopnoea, nocturnal dyspnoea, and swollen ankles.
The patient confirms these symptoms.	Cardiac failure? The family physician looks for signs of and causes of cardiac failure.

If you attach too much value to the initial hypothesis, you might form a conclusion too soon and deny contradictory evidence. In the above example, the family physician would have done well to start with more open-ended questions, such as "Tell me more about your shortness of breath?" The patient might then have given more information from which to form the initial hypothesis.

Hypotheses should relate to the most probable cause, but bear in mind the possibility of uncommon, serious, or urgent problems. A patient with lower back pain, for example, is more likely to have mechanical backache than TB spine. However, the family physician must be aware of red flag symptoms that alert them to the possibility of a more serious disease, a concept that is especially useful in primary health care when the family physician is seeing many patients with the same complaint. He/she needs to distinguish between the common benign, but troubling, symptoms and the occasional symptoms that require urgent intervention. Examples include distinguishing tension headaches from headaches associated with subarachnoid haemorrhage (see page 192), distinguishing the dyspepsia of reflux from cancer of the stomach (see page 206) or distinguishing lower back pain from more serious spinal pathology (see page 214).

You will not have time to make a complete examination of every system in every patient. The examination is selective and should target signs that will increase or decrease the probability of your hypothesis being correct. The examination should also identify any complications. You are more likely to find signs if you are actively looking for them. Similarly, any special investigations should serve the same purpose. Throughout the process, you should have a clear idea of why you are asking a question, performing an examination or ordering a test.

Management decision-making is based on the hypotheses you have formulated and the likelihood that they are leading to the correct diagnosis. There is often more than one likely hypothesis to explain the symptoms and management decisions need to be made on the basis of probability. The risks of not intervening with respect to certain hypotheses also need to be considered. Every management decision, or element of treatment, must have a clear clinical reasoning process to justify it.

Hypotheses may be reformulated and tested between consultations. Observation over time and the patient's response to medication may form part of hypothesis testing.

While many problems are vague and most probably self-limiting, there are other problems that persist, which need to be investigated more fully at follow-up visits. Using time and ongoing consultations in this way relies on the continuity of care provided by seeing the same family physician or at least continuity of information in the medical records. This means that hypotheses – and the rationale for them – must be clearly documented in the patient record.

In primary care, medical students and newly qualified doctors tend to generate hypotheses based on their patho-physiological knowledge, whereas more experienced family physicians also use their knowledge of the patient's context to generate more accurate initial hypotheses. This includes knowledge of the patient's family, how diseases present locally, and what the most common problems are in the practice population (Hobus *et al*, 1987). In Khayelitsha, for example, a woman who complains that her "womb is dirty" is often concerned about infertility. A more experienced family physician would hypothesise that the problem is infertility early on, whereas a less experienced doctor might start with questions relating to the patho-physiology of the genital tract.

Pattern recognition

Some conditions in primary care are common and you can easily recognise them at a glance. Many skin problems, such as shingles, impetigo, or tinea capitis, are immediately recognised and diagnosed. Pattern recognition may also refer to behavioural patterns, such as the patient with an alcohol problem who frequently asks for a sick certificate after the weekend.

Algorithms

For many symptoms in primary care, the family physician develops an algorithmic approach to decision-making. There are many published guidelines with algorithms that the family physician can use to aid decision-making. Syndromic management approaches, such as for sexually transmitted infections or integrated management of childhood illness, follow established algorithmns.

The medical record

The functions of a medical record system in primary care have been defined as follows (Palmer, 1988):
- To improve patient care
- To make diagnosis clearer
- To make management decisions clearer
- To make follow-up systematic
- To avoid errors, such as repeating tests or drug interactions
- To aid communication between doctors, within the primary care team, and with outside agencies (for example, reports and referrals)
- As an *aide-mémoire* of the main events in the patient's life and family, and of previous consultations
- As a tool in research and quality assessment, teaching, and the planning of services
- As a medico-legal record
- As a means of charging appropriate fees for services.

Three types of information are required (Weed, 1969): a problem list, background information or a database, and ongoing progress notes at each consultation. The continuity of information between consultations is vital to the quality of care, especially if the patient does not see the same health care worker at each visit.

The ongoing notes

The SOAP format (subjective, objective, assessment, and plan) provides a problem-based system for writing notes (see Figure 6.1). Subjective information includes that derived from the patient, such as the history of symptoms and the illness experience. Objective information includes that derived from examining the patient and the results of investigations.

Figure 6.1 Patient notes for a 36-year-old woman using the SOAP format

S	*Chronic diarrhoea for two months with loss of weight. Watery diarrhoea, but no blood. No vomiting. Coming for HIV result. Attending with husband. Sore mouth with 'white stuff' inside.*
O	*HIV positive. Apyrexial. Oral candida. Loss of weight. Not dehydrated. Chest – clear. Abdomen – soft and non-tender. Crying ++*
A	<u>*Clinical:*</u> *HIV positive (stage three). Chronic diarrhoea. Oral candida.* <u>*Individual:*</u> *Feeling devastated at news – Worried about what will happen to her children. Fears loss of job if employer knows diagnosis.* <u>*Context:*</u> *Husband supportive – informed and agrees to be tested. Employed as a child care worker – loss of job?*
P	*Post-test counselling, including legal rights concerning employment. Loperamide two stat and one with each loose stool. Stool culture, microscopy and sensitivities.* *Mycostatin 2 ml four x daily to mouth after meals.* *Push oral fluids.* *Full blood count and differential, RPR and CD4 count.* *Husband informed – to be tested.*
Safety netting:	*See again in four days with husband.* *Give results. Do genogram? Disability grant?* *Not suicidal – has support.*

The assessment can be made in three stages. The clinical assessment includes the medical diagnoses, or hypotheses, and risk factors. Some clinical problems may be expressed as diagnoses and others at the highest level of certainty, depending in how sure you are about your hypotheses. You may speculate on possible differential diagnoses that you should consider. The level of certainty should be honestly reflected here. The individual assessment includes aspects of the patient's perspective and the contextual assessment aspects of the family, work or other environmental factors that are relevant to the illness. (See the notes on the three-stage assessment in Chapter 2.)

The plan should be based on the three-stage assessment. It may include medication as well as advice, information, or counselling. The latter should be documented as specifically as prescriptions! In a patient with insomnia, for example, you may indicate that you discussed sleep hygiene or coping with stress. It also includes any necessary further investigations or referral.

Remember to finish by recording your safety netting as described in Chapter 3 and any notes to yourself, to act as prompts in future consultations. An example is making a note to discuss smoking at a future visit.

The problem list

A problem list provides readily accessible information on current and past problems (see Figure 6.2) and should be in somewhere where it can be read at a glance, such as on the inside cover of the patient's folder. The list can be amended as old problems resolve or new ones occur or become better defined. The list can include medical, surgical, and psychosocial problems. Examples are dates of bereavements or episodes of domestic violence. Hospital admissions and other referrals can be noted. Include a record of the patient's hospital folder number to facilitate requests for further appointments or information.

Figure 6.2 A problem list for a woman with diabetes

Problem	Date
Diabetes type two	Diagnosed Sept. 1994
Hysterectomy	Nov. 2000
Smoker	Stopped Nov. 2000
Husband died	Jan. 2009

The database

Important information should be easily accessible, so the best place to record it would be either on the cover of the patient's folder or in a special section of the record. Make a place to file any correspondence relating to the patient.

- Record the patient's name, address, date of birth, and folder number.

- Include information about the family and context for patients whom you see regularly. A genogram is the most useful way to do this (see Chapter 4). Further notes can be added if necessary.
- Make a note of any preventive and health promotion measures. This will include information on blood pressure checks, smoking, alcohol abuse, vaccinations, cervical smears, family planning, and so on.
- Make a note of any drug allergies.
- Include the results of investigations.
- Billing and financial information should be recorded.
- Flow charts or annual summary charts (see Figure 6.3) should be included for chronic diseases.

Q How well does the primary care medical record or information system in your clinic or health centre fulfill the requirements as listed here? How could you modify or adapt the record to make it more practically useful?

Patient-held records

Patient-held records are a means of communicating information between different health care providers wherever the patient may seek help. In South Africa, the Road to Health card that records birth information, immunisations, childhood growth, and developmental milestones is a good example.

Computerised records

In more resource-rich settings, computerised patient records have been introduced. The family physician can access all the elements of the primary care record via a computer terminal on their desk. The computer can prompt the family physician with information regarding preventive tasks or drug interactions and can print out prescriptions as well as information leaflets. Coding diagnoses for billing or audit is also much easier.

Figure 6.3 Summary chart for non-communicable chronic diseases

WC CHRONIC DISEASE RECORD SHEET

USE THIS SHEET WITH THE DISEASE MANAGEMENT GUIDELINES

NAME
DOB: PATIENT STICKER
FOLDER NUMBER:
SEX:

HEIGHT ....m BMI .... Kg / m squared

WAIST CIRCUMFERENCE ....cm

☐ OTHER ______ ☐ DIABETES ☐ HYPERTENSION ☐ ASTHMA ☐ COPD ☐ EPILEPSY ______

DATE (DDMMYY)	WEIGHT (kg) OR WAIST (cm)	URINE DIPSTIX (PCR)*	BLOOD GLUCOSE (mmol / l)	DONE ON AN ANNUAL BASIS					70 80 90 100 110 120 130 140 150 160 170 180 190 / 100 150 200 250 300 350 400 450 500 550 600 PFR (o)	MDI TECHNIQ	ASTHMA CONTROL	MEDIC. EDUC	LIFESTYLE COUNSELLING				NO. OF SEIZURES / NO. OF MONTHS
				CHOL (mmol / l)	H bA1c (%)	CREAT mmol / l	EYE EXAM	FOOT EXAM					SMOKE	DIET	EXCER	ETOH	
EXAMPLE - BP 125/80 AND PEFR 450				6,7	7,8	56	✓	✓	X----------------------X O	POOR	PC	✓	NON SMOKER	–	✓	✓	2 / 6

SOURCE: District Health Services, Western Cape

Care of patients with chronic illness

Health systems have historically evolved around acute and infectious diseases more suited to episodic, reactive models of health care delivery (Swartz, 2002; Wagner, 2002). There is growing concern at the failure of such models to acknowledge the need for a sustained partnership between patient and doctor – especially in the management of chronic illness (Rundall, 2002). Chronic conditions have been defined by the WHO (2002) as health problems that require ongoing management over a period of years or decades. They include:

- Non-communicable conditions, for example heart disease, hypertension, diabetes, asthma, COPD, epilepsy, cancer
- Persistent communicable conditions, for example HIV/AIDS, TB
- Long-term mental disorders, for example depression, schizophrenia
- Ongoing physical/structural impairments, for example blindness, amputation, persistent pain problems.

Globally the burden of chronic illnesses is rising, and South Africa is no exception (Mayosi *et al.*, 2009). Yet all over the world patients with chronic illness are often poorly managed (Wagner *et al.*, 2001). This is partly because in primary care, acute problems often crowd out the less urgent need to manage chronic illness optimally (Bodenheimer *et al.*, 2002).

Chronic conditions have a number of features in common: they place great demands on patients and families over time, as well as on the health care system and often the socio-economic system. They require comparable management strategies, they challenge the efficiency and effectiveness of the health care system, and they demand a preventive focus as part of management.

The family

In the words of McDaniel *et al.* (2002), "Families, not health care providers, are the primary caretakers for patients with chronic illnesses." The family requires information and support from family physicians. Chronic illness places many demands on the family, who may develop unhealthy coping mechanisms. Attention may be so focused on the person with the illness that other members of the family are neglected. The demands of the illness may be so consuming that the family isolates themselves and miss out on sources of support. A balance needs to be achieved between the needs of the person with the illness and the needs of the rest of the family (see page 113).

Adherence

The term adherence is used rather than compliance to avoid the implication that the patient passively complies with the orders of the family physician. Instead, the family physician and the patient negotiate a plan together. Adherence depends on many factors that may need to be addressed. Low adherence to prescribed treatments is very common. On average, about 50% of patients adhere to prescribed chronic medication (WHO, 2003).

Reasons for non-adherence can be thought of under the following areas (WHO, 2003):

- Socioeconomic factors, for example the ability to pay for medication and the accessibility of the clinic
- Health care provider and system, for example knowledge about medication, poor communication skills, and doctor–patient relationship
- Condition-related factors, for example incapacity due to the illness or poor understanding of the disease
- Therapy-related factors, for example complex regime, frequent dosing, bad taste, side-effects or poor instructions
- Patient-related factors, for example particular beliefs, concerns or fears regarding the disease or therapy.

Certain interventions have been found to increase adherence to medication and improve outcome. However, these interventions were complex and included combinations of more convenient care, providing information, counselling, reminders, self-monitoring, reinforcement, family therapy, and other forms of additional supervision or attention. However, even with these interventions the increased adherence and improved outcomes was at best modest. Telling patients about possible side-effects did not worsen adherence (Haynes *et al.*, 1999).

Attendance

Even when the patient attends a state-run primary health care facility, where there is no charge for the consultation, there are other costs and difficulties. These include the cost of transport, distance from the facility and difficulties related to taking time off work or household responsibilities. Competing needs for the family's limited income means that other needs may take priority. At state clinics, the long waiting times and poor relationships with the staff at some facilities are further deterrents to frequent attendance.

General management principles

Seven principles (the seven Cs) are important in ensuring an optimal approach to the management of patients with chronic illness (Couper, 2007):

1. Commitment

Commitment to the patient as a person (see Chapter 2), rather than to the disease, underlies everything. There also needs to be a commitment to an ongoing relationship with the patient, rather than to a once-off encounter, and to enabling self-care. The patient in turn also needs to make a commitment to the relationship, to getting involved in their own care, and to returning for scheduled follow-up.

2. Continuity of care

Researchers predict that health expenditure will continue to escalate. They also warn of serious consequences if sufficient attention is not given to personal aspects of care such as continuity (Swartz and Dick, 2002). Poor adherence to chronic disease treatment, such as hypertension, has been noted as one such result (Epping-Jordan *et al.*, 2001; Levenstein, 1988). Research examining the relationship between continuity and the quality of care has shown that continuity is associated with increased patient satisfaction, fewer hospitalisations and emergency department visits, and lower health care costs (Cabana, 2004; Starfield, 1994). These findings are especially important in the care of chronic conditions where continuity has also been shown to improve adherence to treatment (Kerse *et al.*, 2004; Gill *et al.*, 2003). Continuity also saves time and money, for example by avoiding the need to repeat detailed history-taking or special investigations. Continuity is a key element in increasing the level of patient involvement and confidence in the management of chronic disease (Wagner, 2001). In this context successful interventions are complex and multifaceted with objectives such as improving patients' self-management and better patient–clinician interactions.

Such interventions demand a partnership between patient, family and provider that cannot be achieved without a continuing relationship. Continuity of care will ensure active sustained follow up, ongoing support and regular assessment. While continuity of care is often difficult to implement in the public health care context in South Africa, it is worth striving for; where it is achieved it makes a major difference to quality of care. Three dimensions to continuity have been defined by Kringos *et al.* (2010):

1. Longitudinal continuity of care: A long-term relationship between primary care providers and the patients in their practice beyond specific episodes of illness or disease is stressed. In many settings the relationship will not be with a specific carer but with a defined team of people.

2. Informational continuity of care: An organised collection of each patient's medical information readily available to any health care provider caring for the patient. This can be reached through medical record keeping, clinical support and referral systems.

3. Relational continuity of care: The quality of the longitudinal relationship between primary care providers and patients, in terms of accommodation of patient's needs and preferences, such as communication and respect for patients.

3. Collaboration

Health professionals and patients set goals and plan together. The patient is seen as a partner in their care rather than as a passive recipient of treatment. Patients achieve better outcomes when a patient-centred approach is used and they are actively involved in the consultation. Diabetic patients who ask more questions in the consultation have been found to achieve better glycaemic control. The patient develops knowledge and skills for self-care. While the health professional may advise and motivate, it is ultimately up to the patient to decide to take the treatment, eat appropriately, exercise and adapt to other lifestyle changes. When discussing lifestyle or behaviour change brief motivational interviewing is congruent with this collaborative approach (see page 130).

Collaboration is also needed with other members of the health care team, who can assist the patient towards better outcomes. Thus a patient with chronic osteoarthritis may be helped to lose weight by seeing a dietician, to strengthen muscles around the affected joints by seeing a physiotherapist, or to adapt their home or work circumstances by seeing an occupational therapist.

Collaboration of family and friends can play a major role in the management of the patient's illness. A person with diabetes whose family eats healthily and who respects the limitations of the patient's diet will face fewer temptations than a diabetic whose family and friends may be well-meaning but do not understand the disease.

Collaboration may be with other people who have the same or similar chronic condition. Associations such as the Arthritis Foundation, HIV support groups and the Diabetic Association of South Africa are examples of useful resources.

4. Comprehension

The patient's understanding of their illness and its management is central to self-care. Clear explanations by health professionals will facilitate this and could include drawings or models to enhance explanations. In addition, it is useful to give the patient and family written material to take home that they can go over at their own pace, and have available as a reference.

Comprehension also refers to the doctor's need to understand the patient. How does the patient understand their illness? What options will best suit the particular patient given their worldview and lifestyle? What are the barriers to adherence with medication or lifestyle changes?

5. Change

Every person living with a chronic condition will face significant changes in their life as a result of the illness and/or its management. This lifestyle modification is needed to promote optimal health, to prevent complications and/or to adapt to impairment. Many of these changes signify losses. Change may relate to a change in diet, change in habits, change in self-image, change in one's abilities or change in one's hope for the future. Change in help-seeking behaviour may also be required.

6. Clinical guidelines

Clinical guidelines are standard treatment approaches that offer a step-by-step approach to chronic conditions. Many of these exist for chronic diseases. For example, there are Standard Treatment Guidelines for primary care and district hospital level, as part of the Essential Drugs Programme of the National Department of Health. These are often supplemented by national and/or local protocols. Check that guidelines in use are up to date and based on good evidence (Sackett, 2000). It is important that these are used and followed by doctors who can often create difficulties by ignoring them in favour of personal experience or training. However, guidelines must be individualised to the particular patient.

7. Capture of information

Problem-orientated records will allow efficient care. Summary charts are useful to record patterns and trends, for example blood pressure, glucose, and peak flows (see Figure 6.3). Follow-up plans should also be documented, including specific dates for return visits or referral to other levels of care.

Each consultation

In applying the above principles in practice, the following five areas (the five As) should be considered in each consultation (WHO, 2004; Couper, 2007).

<u>Assess</u>:

- Complaints (concerns): Assess how the patient has been doing. How are they feeling? What symptoms have they experienced? Do they have any other concerns about the illness or management?
- Control (clinical status): Assess indicators of control, for example the frequency of need for reliever metered-dose inhaler, frequency of panic attacks and blood glucose levels.
- Compliance (adherence): Ask how the person is doing with the management of, for example diet, exercise, smoking reduction and medication. Ask about difficulties encountered.
- Complications (and risks): Ask if the patient has encountered any complications, for example hypoglycaemia in a patient with diabetes, bruising or sore throat in a patient on methotrexate for rheumatoid arthritis or infections in a patient with HIV.

<u>Advise</u>.

- Give information using neutral and non-judgemental language: "Your glucose level is high today. What do you think might be causing that?"
- Correct any misconceptions: "Even dark chocolate, although it is bitter, contains sugar."
- Management options: "You could eat diabetic chocolate, but the fat content is still high. Another option would be a cup of cocoa with skim milk and a sweetener to satisfy your chocolate craving. How do you feel about that?"
- Self-care: "Dry your feet carefully, especially between the toes".

<u>Agree</u>

- Goals of management: "Would you like to decrease or limit the amount of fits you have per year?"
- Treatment plan: "Are you willing to increase your dose of anti-epileptics to try and cut down on your seizures, despite the risk of increased drowsiness?"

Assist

- Health care team: Link patient to a dietician or chiropodist, for example.
- Community networking: Advise patients on local exercise group or Weigh-less, for example.
- Encourage the patient: "I'm delighted that you can feel the benefit from your regular walking. It will help you to lose weight and keep the sugar down and is also good for your circulation and general fitness."
- Problem-solving: For example, try to brainstorm options around the cost of a healthy eating plan.

Arrange

- Follow up.
- Referral if needed.

Appropriate prescribing

How do patients feel about the prescriptions family physicians give them? Here are some comments:
- An exasperated daughter: "Doctor, my mother's cupboard is full of pills but she never takes any."
- A reproachful patient: "But Doctor, aren't you going to give me anything?"
- The disgruntled patient: "I went to the doctor and all I got was pills!"

Rules for rational prescribing

The following list of rules for rational prescribing provides comprehensive guidelines for the family physician (adapted from Henbest, 1982):
- In the absence of a clear problem definition, be slow to prescribe.
- Choose a drug of first choice.
- Know the medication well. Develop your own personal formulary. Be wary of newer drugs that closely resemble less expensive, older drugs in the same class. They might increase costs without additional benefit (Morgan, 2005).
- Do not prescribe medication for which there is no reliable evidence of effectiveness.
- Use generic names so that you are aware of what you are prescribing.
- Use single agents (unless there is a particular indication for combination drugs). In this way, you can help avoid drug interactions.

- Keep dosage regimes as simple as possible. Once or twice-daily dosages are preferable if there is a choice.
- Use reliable sources of information about medicines, such as the South African Medicines Formulary.
- Consider risks, such as pregnancy and lactation, the age of the patient (especially children and the elderly), compromised renal or hepatic function, allergy, other disease, and interaction with other medication.

Unnecessary medication

Consider whether medication is necessary or whether the patient's health would be better served by any of the following:
- A clear explanation of the problem
- Reassurance about the prognosis
- Contact with a concerned family physician who listens and understands the problem
- Simple home remedies such as ginger in hot water to soothe a cough, or rest, ice packs and elevation for pain and swelling
- Treating the cause of the problem (for example, the treatment for insomnia may not always be a sleeping tablet)
- Lifestyle modification (for example, a patient with dyspepsia may be more in need of treatment for alcohol abuse than cimetidine)
- Relaxation techniques such as breathing exercises, deep muscular relaxation, hot baths, yoga and massage, which are all helpful for tension-related problems.

Some patients have high expectations of medication, while others are reluctant to use medication. The family physician needs to understand the patient's feelings, beliefs, and expectations about medication. This enables the family physician to make more informed management decisions and gives them the opportunity to correct misconceptions. For example, patients sometimes believe that metered-dose inhalers for asthma weaken the heart. This may be because they have experienced palpitations caused by beta-2 agonists, or perhaps they know people who have used inhalers for chronic obstructive pulmonary disease and later developed cor pulmonale. Understanding the patient's expectations does not mean that the family physician should go against their medical judgment and prescribe whatever the patient requests. Family physicians remain responsible for what they prescribe.

Consider the following example:

Mrs R has an upper respiratory tract infection. She asks for antibiotics as she says her colds go on to sinusitis and then she becomes very ill and requires antibiotics anyway. She cannot afford time away from work. The family physician explains that as her infection is viral, antibiotics will be of no benefit. Mrs R remains unconvinced even when the risks of unnecessary antibiotics are explained to her.

This consultation may move in one of two ways. A power struggle may develop between the family physician and the patient, with each demanding that the other agree with their own point of view and ending with one of them feeling dissatisfied. Alternatively, they may focus on their mutual aim, which is the best possible health for Mrs R, and come up with solutions, such as the use of a decongestant to prevent stasis in the sinuses. The solution should satisfy both the family physician and the patient.

Placebos

A placebo can be defined as a substance containing no effective medication, which is prescribed or given to reinforce a patient's expectation to get well. Placebos will have an effect in up to 30% of patients. Occasionally it may be appropriate to give a patient a placebo. However, there are dangers in doing this:
- Patients will come to expect a pill for every illness.
- Placebos encourage dependence on health services.
- Placebos discourage self-reliance.
- Giving a patient a placebo may affect the relationship of trust between the family physician and the patient.
- They may be used to avoid giving what the patient really needs, such as the need to be heard or the need for lifestyle changes.
- They may be used to treat the family physician's feeling of helplessness or to end the consultation.
- They may be used to give the impression that the patient is getting value for money by increasing the number of pills prescribed.

Information for the patient

The following guidelines for what the patient should know about their medication are from the Rational Drug Prescribing training course (Health Systems Trust, 1997):

- Explain the effects of the drug. It is important that patients understand the reason for taking the medication and what they can expect.
- Explain the side-effects. It has been found that explaining the side-effects of medication does not adversely affect adherence. Simple advice can help to avoid side-effects, for example patients should take iron tablets with food to prevent gastric irritation.
- Give instructions. Patients need to know how to use the medication, especially when specific techniques are required. An example is the use of metered-dose inhalers, where the family physician should observe the patient's correct use of an inhaler in the consultation and be able to demonstrate the technique themselves with a placebo inhaler.
- Warnings should be given where appropriate. Describe possible risks, such as the risk of drowsiness with some antihistamines and the effect of drinking alcohol with metronidazole.
- Follow-up is important. When should the patient consult again and what symptoms warrant immediate care?
- Ask if everything is clear. Check that the patient has understood and encourage them to ask questions. Written instructions can be helpful in complicated prescriptions. It is also useful to ask patients to reverse summarise their understanding.

The effectiveness of medications depends on more than just the chemical component of the medication. Once the family physician has decided that a prescription is necessary and has given the patient all the required information, they should prescribe with confidence and a positive attitude. Adherence to medication is discussed above on page 169.

The Essential Drugs Programme

The Essential Drugs List (EDL) is part of the Essential Drugs Programme, a World Health Organisation initiative. There are separate lists for primary and hospital care. The lists contain drugs that meet the needs of the majority of the population. By focusing on a limited number of essential drugs, the costs of drugs are reduced, and they are made more accessible and available. Health care professionals can have a better knowledge of fewer drugs and there is less unnecessary prescribing.

The books should be readily available in any primary care facility or district hospital. However, you can obtain the books that include standard treatment guidelines from the Department of Health (The Directorate: Pharmaceutical Programmes and Planning, Private Bag X828, Pretoria 0001) or at http://www.doh.gov.za/docs/factsheets/index.html.

Adverse drug reactions

It is important that all suspected adverse drug reactions are reported centrally so that the safety of medicines can be monitored. Reports in South Africa are made to the Department of Health (Medicines Control Council, Private Bag X828, Pretoria 0001).

Dispensing medication

Doctors and nurse practitioners need to complete a dispensing course in order to be licensed to dispense medication (see Medicines and Related Substances Control Amendment Act of 1997, and the Medicines and Related Substances Control Amendment Act 59 of 2002). This licence, if granted, needs to be renewed every three years.

All applications for a dispensing licence must be accompanied by a well-motivated reason as to why the practitioner wants to dispense. A notice needs to also be placed in the legal section of a local newspaper indicating the intention of the practitioner to apply for a dispensing licence.

It is illegal to buy or sell medications without a valid dispensing licence. This does not apply to medication given as a single dose during the course of the consultation such as an injection.

Legal requirements on a prescription

The following information must appear on all prescriptions:

- The name, qualifications, contact details, practice number and address of the prescriber.
- The name, age, sex and address of the patient.
- The prescription must be dated. All prescriptions are valid for thirty days from the date of issue, unless the prescriber wants the prescription to be repeated. The number of repeats must be clearly stated and not all schedules of medications can be repeated.
- The approved trade name or generic name of the product with clear instructions on dosage and duration of treatment.
- The diagnosis may only appear on the prescription if the patient has consented to this.

Generic substitution

Pharmacists who dispense medication are required by law to inform customers of generic equivalents of the medications on their script unless the prescriber has written "no substitution" or if the medication in listed as non-substitutable by the Medicine Control Council.

Medical certificates (Certificate of Illness)

Issuing a medical certificate is an important intervention that allows the patient appropriate time to rest and recover from illness. The employer may insist on knowing the nature of the illness for which the employee requires time off work. However, the patient is entitled to confidentiality and must give informed consent for any information given to their employer. A medical certificate therefore should be drawn up after discussion with the patient.

A medical certificate is a statement by a family physician of the patient's diagnosis and an approximation of the duration of the patient's incapacity to work. The family physician does not grant the sick leave as such.

A medical certificate recommending sick leave is different from a certificate of attendance that only confirms that the patient took time off work to visit the doctor.

Consider what you would do in the following cases:

Mr K works as a labourer for the city council. He presents with mild backache. He says that he has taken no leave for the past two years and would now like to use up the sick leave owed to him. He asks for a medical certificate recommending that he needs three weeks sick leave. Your examination findings show muscular tenderness but no limitation of movement or signs of nerve compression. Mr K insists that he has paid you and is entitled to his certificate of illness.

Mrs D is not ill but is grieving the recent loss of her aunt. She asks for a certificate of illness as she wants to attend the funeral in KwaZulu-Natal. Her employers only grant leave for funerals of the immediate family (as defined in Western culture). Her job will be at risk if she stays away and does not produce a medical certificate.

Mr M comes to see you with a urethral discharge which you treat using the syndromic approach for sexually transmitted infections. At the end of the consultation, he asks you for a certificate of attendance stating the reason for the consultation as back pain.

Do not write down anything that is untrue on a medical certificate. If you feel that the person does not have a medical diagnosis but a social problem, they should take ordinary leave to sort it out. If this is not possible then the doctor can advocate for time off with the employer if the patient is not able to. Encourage patients who have work-related issues to work with their trade unions (The South African Medical Association Committee for Human Rights (Ransome and Barker, 1999).

Referring patients

It is important to acknowledge the limits of one's ability and refer a patient who needs more specialised investigation and/or management.

If it is not an emergency, one can look at alternatives that may be more cost effective and convenient for the patient. The following are examples:

- A telephonic, telemedicine or faxed consultation: ECGs can be faxed for comments and digital x-rays or photographs can be emailed.
- Advice from a colleague at your health facility: Family physicians and other health professionals working in the facility have special interests and expertise, and are a valuable resource. Sometimes merely discussing the patient with a colleague helps you to solve problems.
- An alternative delivery of treatment may be appropriate: Patients with mild cellulitis or uncomplicated pneumonia do not always need to be admitted for intravenous antibiotics. Oral or intramuscular antibiotics and follow-up are appropriate if home circumstances are adequate. Where available, the district nurse can follow up on patients at home, if necessary.

Involve the patient in the decision-making

Explain to patients what they can expect from the referral. When patients do not turn up for their appointments, other patients have their appointments unnecessarily delayed. This may be prevented by involving the patient in the decision-making process (see Chapter 2). Sometimes patients are reluctant to be referred even for urgent conditions and negotiation is required.

Q How would you handle the following scenario?

A middle-aged woman with diabetes is helped into the consulting room by her husband and another patient. She is confused and unable to give a clear history or informed consent. As she has a delirium the family physician decides that referral for further investigation and treatment is essential. On explaining this, however, the husband is adamant that his wife's usual medication should be issued and she should be allowed to go home where she will be seen by a traditional healer.

If a patient requires secondary care, do not refer them to a tertiary hospital. Similarly, do not refer a patient to a hospital where the required skills or resources are not available. Telephone first if you are unsure. Do not refer patients to an emergency service when they have a non-urgent problem. They will not be able to obtain the care they require and will need to return at another time. This wastes time and resources.

In an emergency, make sure you review the patient continually until the ambulance comes; initial management interventions to stabilise the patient must be instituted until they can be safely transported.

The referral letter

The person to whom you are referring the patient should be given sufficient information so that they can provide efficient and effective care. The aim of the referral letter is to provide such information:

- *Identifying data for the patient*; that is, name, age, and folder number.
- *Identifying data for the family physician* (yourself); that is, name, facility (clinic or practice), address, telephone number, and fax number if available.
- *Date.*
- Statement of the *problem*. Remember that referral letters need to be read speedily in busy emergency or outpatient departments. Start your letter by clearly and concisely defining the problem and what you expect from the referral. Examples are:
    - *Cardiac failure, secondary to severe anaemia – history of malaena*
    - *Fell – fractured clavicle? For x-ray*
    - *Primary infertility – for investigation.*
- Give a *history* relevant to the problem. Include risk factors and other relevant information.
- Give the relevant *past medical and surgical history*.
- List *medications* that the patient is currently using.
- Note any *allergies* and other *adverse reactions to medication*.
- Include *examination findings*.
- Include the *results of special investigations*.
- Describe the *treatment* initiated and the effect of it.
- Give an *assessment*.
- State your *reason for referral*.
- State what *information* you have given to the patient regarding the referral.
- Indicate your willingness to be involved in *ongoing care*.

An example of a referral letter is given on the following pages.

Recommended reading

South African Medicines Formulary (2010) (9e). Cape Town: Health and
 Medical Publishing Group.

Dr S Gold
Mountain View Health Centre
Berg Road
Mountain View
Telephone: 26506
5 October 1999

The Doctor
Neurology OPD
St James Hospital

Re: Mrs J Garland
        14 Rose Terrace
        Mountain View
        Folder: 633924

Dear Doctor,

Thanks for seeing Mrs Garland (aged 62 years).

Problem:
Severe headaches
Symptoms of raised intracranial pressure and behaviour changes
Possible space-occupying lesion?

She has had severe, worsening, occipital headaches for the past six
weeks. They wake her at night. She has nausea, but no vomiting. Her
husband has noted that she has undergone mild personality changes —
she is more forgetful than usual, and no longer feels like socialising.

There is no history of head injury, and no changes in vision or hearing.
She has had tension headaches in the past but these are worse.
Symptoms of depression started about three weeks ago when her son
was arrested for dealing in drugs.

Past medical history:
Hypertension
Medications — Hydrochlorthiazide 12,5 mg daily, Paracetamol eight per
day for past ten days.
Allergies — Disprin causes gastritis.

Examination findings:
BP 136/86
Pulse 72/min
Temp. 36,8 degrees
Weight 65 kg
Heart, lungs and abdomen normal
Affect – blunted
Mood – depressed
Memory – was able to remember three named objects
Cognitive function – slow to answer but intact
PEARL
No papilloedema
Ears – normal drums
No neck stiffness
Cranial nerves normal
No cerebellar signs
Bulk, tone, power, reflexes equal bilaterally
No Parkinsonism.

Investigations:
TSH normal
Hb 12,5g%
Dextrostix 4,8 mmol/l
Trial of low-dose antidepressants was stopped by patient due to drowsiness.

Assessment:
Space-occupying lesion?
Worsening tension headaches?
Depression related to son's arrest?

I know the family well and would be willing to break bad news if necessary. I have told her that referral is to rule out the possibility of a brain tumour and that you will do a CT scan if necessary.

Yours sincerely
Stephen Gold

7 An approach to assessing common symptoms

Introduction

Primary care providers must be able to assess undifferentiated symptoms. Even if a specific diagnosis cannot be made at the first consultation, management will be based on the likelihood of serious pathology, need for urgent investigation and referral, or the opportunity for further assessment over time. By the time patients arrive at hospital there is usually a provisional diagnosis that guides further investigation and treatment. Primary care providers, however, need evidence-based, efficient and effective approaches to assessing common symptoms. This is in addition to understanding how to manage common diagnoses. Teaching has traditionally been structured around specific diseases and their accompanying signs and symptoms, rather than common symptoms and groups of symptoms and an integrated approach to assessing them.

This chapter looks at some of the most common symptoms that present in South African primary care (see Table 1.2 in Chapter 1) and provides a pathway for their assessment. The symptoms are presented in order of their frequency in primary care practice. The chapter finishes with a section on medically unexplained symptoms, as this remains an area that challenges and frustrates primary care providers.

Cough

History

Important features of the history are listed in Table 7.1. The two most useful diagnostic issues are the duration of the cough and whether it is productive or not.

Acute cough lasting less than three weeks: This is the most common cough and is often associated with a viral upper respiratory tract infection (URTI). Viruses cause hypersecretion of mucus by goblet cells and vasodilatation with nasal congestion, sneezing, nasal discharge and postnasal drip, which leads to throat clearing and cough. In South

Africa any cough lasting more than two weeks must be investigated for pulmonary tuberculosis (PTB), especially if associated with symptoms of weight loss, night sweats, tiredness or loss of appetite. Acute cough may also be due to pneumonia, acute bronchitis or lower respiratory tract infections.

Sub-acute cough lasting three to eight weeks: All of the causes of chronic cough can be considered, but there is also a prolonged post-infectious cough that may follow pneumonia, pertussis, or bronchitis.

Chronic cough lasting more than eight weeks: The following should be considered:

- Tuberculosis (TB)
- Chronic bronchitis and chronic obstructive pulmonary disease (COPD), which is typically associated with tobacco smoking or following TB
- Chronic uncontrolled asthma
- Lung cancer and other neoplastic conditions
- Cardiac failure
- Gastro-oesophageal reflux disease (GORD) and aspiration
- Interstitial lung disease and sarcoidosis
- Exposure to environmental pollution/irritants
- Psychogeneses (anxiety, habitual).

Examination

In addition to examination of the respiratory system, a general examination should record the vital signs (pulse, respiratory rate and temperature). Note any abnormal sounds (wheeze, stridor, voice) and look for nicotine-stained fingers, cyanosis, pallor, finger clubbing, lymphadenopathy, signs of heart failure (peripheral oedema, raised JVP) or polycythaemia.

Investigations

The commonest diagnosis is an upper respiratory tract infection which does not usually require any investigations. The most common investigations are to exclude TB by sputum microscopy and/or culture (see p. 256). A chest radiograph can help to diagnose the cause of a sub-acute/chronic cough or a serious acute condition (for example pneumonia). Other investigations in primary care will be guided by the diagnostic possibilities, for example:

- White cell count, C-reactive protein or erythrocyte sedimentation rate for suspected infection

- Peak expiratory flow tests or spirometry for asthma or COPD
- Sputum cytology for malignancy
- ECG for heart disease.

Other investigations are available at referral hospitals such as lung biopsy, oesophagoscopy or pH testing for gastro-oesophageal reflux.

Referral

Consider referral for further investigation or treatment if:
- Diagnostic uncertainty
- Severe disease such as pneumonia
- Haemoptysis
- Suspected lung cancer or other neoplasm.

Children

In children with chronic cough you may also need to consider the likelihood of other diagnostic possibilities, for example:
- Early months of life – milk inhalation/reflux, viral-induced wheeze, bronchiolitis, PTB, HIV and lymphoid interstitial pneumonitis
- Toddler/preschool – asthma, bronchitis, whooping cough, cystic fibrosis, croup, foreign body inhalation, TB, chronic HIV-associated lung disease including bronchiectasis
- Early school years – asthma, bronchitis, mycoplasma pneumonia, PTB
- Adolescence – asthma, PTB, smoking, psychogeneses.

Don't forget the possibility of passive exposure to tobacco smoke.

HIV and cough

The list of diagnostic possibilities should be expanded, depending on the state of the immune system and the likelihood of opportunistic infection or stage IV diseases. Patients with HIV have a greatly increased risk of developing TB and of having recurrent pneumonia. Recurrent TB and pneumonia may also lead to chronic lung disease and bronchiectasis. Patients with a CD4 count < 200 cells/µl are particularly at risk of opportunistic infections or unusual disease, for example:
- Pneumocystis pneumonia
- Pulmonary Kaposi's sarcoma
- Pulmonary cryptococcus

- Bacterial empyema
- Cytomegalovirus infection
- Disseminated histoplasmosis.

Table 7.1 Specific questions to ask a patient with a cough

History	Relevance
Duration of cough	· Acute causes < three weeks · Sub-acute causes three to eight weeks · Chronic causes > eight weeks
Nature of the cough	· Productive, for example URTI, TB, pneumonia, COPD · Non productive, for example laryngitis, asthma, GORD, croup · How the cough sounds, for example barking cough in croup, whooping cough
Age of patient	· Differential diagnosis is influenced by age. For example lung cancer is more likely in the older adult, croup in the pre-school child
Onset of cough	When the cough starts or what precipitates it may be helpful. For example: · A cough worse in the morning suggests postnasal drip, bronchiectasis or chronic bronchitis · If a child has a non productive cough at night it suggests asthma · Exercise induced cough suggests asthma
Amount of sputum	· How much sputum is coughed up each day – a spoonful, an egg cupful or a tea cup?
Sputum colour/blood	· Yellow/green/brown sputum suggests a viral or bacterial infection · Haemoptysis/altered blood suggests more serious pathology (for example TB, lung cancer, bronchiectasis, lung abscess, mitral stenosis) and often needs investigation or referral
Nature of sputum	· Thin, frothy, pink tinge suggests left ventricular failure · Offensive foul-smelling sputum suggests bronchiectasis or lung abscess
Periodicity	· Consistent dyspnoea and early morning cough suggests COPD · Intermittent cough and variable dyspnoea with atopy suggest asthma
Associated symptoms	· Fever in acute infections · Weight loss and night sweats in PTB · Wheeze in asthma and COPD · Ankle swelling in cardiac failure

History	Relevance
Smoking history	· Tobacco smoking is linked to an increased likelihood of infection, chronic bronchitis, COPD, PTB, lung cancer and uncontrolled asthma · Marijuana smoking may also be linked to the development of COPD · Indoor air pollution and the burning of biomass may also be linked to COPD and asthma
Past medical history and medication	· Diagnosis of HIV will increase chance of TB and opportunistic infections · Atopic conditions will increase the chance of asthma · Hypertension will increase the chance of cardiac failure · Adverse drug reactions should be considered · Response of cough to previous treatments should be considered
Occupational history	· Pneumoconiosis is relatively common in South Africa due to the large mining industry · Asthma is linked to certain occupational exposures, for example bakeries, spray painters.

SOURCE: Truter I. A therapeutic approach to coughing

Headache

History

When asking about a headache you should consider the following factors:

Time issues:
• Why has the patient consulted now?
• When did it start?
• How frequent is it and what is the pattern (episodic, daily, or unremitting)?
• How long does it last (minutes, hours, days)?

Character of the pain:
• How severe is the pain?
• What is the quality of the pain (dull, pressure, tight, pulsating, stabbing)?
• What is the site and spread of the pain (unilateral or bilateral)?
• What are the associated symptoms (for example aura, nausea, vomiting, photophobia, phonophobia, fever)?

Cause questions:
- What is the patient's perspective ("What do you think is causing your headache?" – this question often reveals psychosocial or mental issues)?
- Are there predisposing or trigger factors (for example stress, foods, analgesic use)?
- Are there aggravating or relieving factors (for example exercise, rest)?
- Is there a family history of similar headaches?

Response questions:
- What does the patient do during the headache?
- How much is normal activity limited or prevented?
- What medication have they used?

State of health between attacks:
- Are they completely well or do they have residual or persisting symptoms?
- Are there concerns, anxieties, or fears about recurrent attacks or their cause?

Classification of headaches

A simplified classification of headaches is shown in Table 7.2 and the features of some common primary headaches are outlined below. Despite popular belief hypertension is not a common cause of headaches. A headache diary may help with diagnosis in some patients. The history is almost always the most useful diagnostic tool.

Table 7.2 Classification of headache disorders, cranial neuralgias and facial pain

Primary	1. Migraine, including:
	1.1 Migraine without aura
	1.2 Migraine with aura
	2. Tension-type headache, including:
	2.1 Episodic tension-type headache
	2.2 Chronic tension-type headache
	3. Cluster headache and chronic paroxysmal hemicrania
	4. Miscellaneous headaches unassociated with structural lesion

Secondary	5. Headache associated with head trauma, including: 5.1 Acute post-traumatic headache 5.2 Chronic post-traumatic headache
	6. Headache associated with vascular disorders, including: 6.1 Subarachnoid haemorrhage 6.2 Giant cell arteritis
	7. Headache associated with non-vascular intracranial disorders, including: 7.1 Benign intracranial hypertension 7.2 Intracranial infection 7.3 Intracranial neoplasm
	8. Headache associated with substances or their withdrawal, including: 8.1 Acute alcohol induced headache 8.2 Chronic ergotamine induced headache 8.3 Chronic analgesics abuse headache 8.4 Alcohol withdrawal headache (hangover)
	9. Headache associated with infection, including: 9.1 Intracranial infection
	10. Headache associated with metabolic disorder
	11. Headache or facial pain associated with disorder of cranium, neck, eyes, ears, nose, sinuses, teeth, mouth or other facial or cranial structures, including: 11.1 Cervical spine 11.2 Acute glaucoma 11.3 Acute sinus headache
	12. Headache attributed to a psychiatric disorder
Neuralgias and other headaches	13. Cranial neuralgias, including: 13.1 Herpes zoster 13.2 Trigeminal neuralgia

SOURCE: Adapted from The International Classification of Headache Disorders. 2004

Primary headaches

Tension-type headache (TTH):
- Bilateral
- Band of pain, tight or pressure-like in nature
- Can last from several hours to several days
- Tends to worsen during the course of the day
- Tightening of scalp and pericranial tenderness
- Normal neurological examination
- Associated with psycho-social stress.

Migraine:
- Unilateral and severe pain
- Pulsating/throbbing in nature
- Associated nausea and sensitivity to light and sound
- Physical activity exacerbates it
- Aura present in 15-33%
- Recurrent and lasts four to 72 hours
- Made worse by psycho-social stress
- More common in women
- Positive family history
- Uncommon, but often missed in children. Children may have bilateral headache and gastrointestinal complaints.

Cluster headache:
- Unilateral in trigeminal area, over the eye and forehead
- Severe and stabbing in nature
- Rapid onset, shorter duration than migraine (one to three hours)
- Restless, may wake the person from sleep
- Lacrimation from one eye, nasal congestion, eyelid oedema, temporary ptosis
- Episodic, every one to two years, then recurrent daily for 6 to 12 weeks, often in the same season
- More common in men.

Medication overuse headache:
- May have features like migraine or tension headache, but is caused by patients using analgesics too often.

Secondary headaches

Headaches may be secondary to an underlying medical condition (see Table 7.2). Think about the possibility of a secondary headache when taking a thorough history and performing the examination.

Red flags

Headaches are common in primary care and most are due to benign conditions. It can therefore be easy to miss serious and even life-threatening causes of headaches. An awareness of red flag symptoms and signs should alert one to the possibility of a medical emergency.

1. **Sudden-onset headache:** Most patients with a benign headache have a history of the same headache occurring previously. Any patient presenting with a severe headache for the first time needs further assessment. A subarachnoid bleed, for example presents as a headache that starts suddenly and is very severe.

2. **Worsening-pattern headache:** This is a headache that progresses over weeks or months, but is characterised by continually getting worse and without periods of remission. A space occupying lesion or cancer may present in this way.

3. **Headache with systemic illness:** A headache in an acutely ill patient, with symptoms such as fever, rash, sweating, neck stiffness. Meningitis may present in this way.

4. **Focal neurological signs or symptoms:** For example, motor or sensory signs or symptoms (excluding the typical visual or sensory aura in some migraines).

5. **Papilloedema:** Raised intracranial pressure affects the appearance of the optic disc that can be seen during fundoscopy. The disc becomes pinker, retinal veins more dilated and the sharp margin of the disc is blurred and indistinct.

6. **Headache triggered by cough, exercise or Valsalva's manoeuvre:** These activities raise intracranial pressure and if they precipitate headache suggest that pressure is already raised. Headaches due to raised intracranial pressure may also wake the patient from sleep.

7. **Headache during pregnancy or post-partum:** Headache may be difficult to treat or indicate a more serious underlying pathology. May be associated with imminent eclampsia.

8. **New headache with history of cancer or HIV:** A headache developing for the first time is more likely to be due to pathology such as a metastasis in cancer or infection in HIV (for example cryptococcal meningitis).

9. **Headache following trauma:** May indicate intracranial pathology.

10. **Headache with jaw claudication:** May be due to temporal arteritis.

Focused examination

The following should usually be assessed and recorded in the medical record:

- Blood pressure, pulse and temperature
- Examine head and neck for tenderness, neck stiffness or sinus pain
- Neurological examination, including fundi.

Investigations

No investigations are useful in primary care for primary headaches. Investigations may be considered in specific patients with suspected secondary headache. For example:

- ESR in suspected inflammation (temporal arteritis)
- Skull radiograph in trauma
- Sinus radiograph or ultrasound in suspected sinusitis
- Tonometry in suspected glaucoma
- Urine test for illicit substances.

Some investigations, such as lumbar puncture, CAT scan or MRI scan, would only be performed in hospital after referral.

Fever

Fever is defined as a temperature of 37.8 °C or more, without the use of fever-reducing medications.

Causes of fever

Fever is usually seen as a sign of infection, but can also be caused by a variety of non-infectious conditions:

- Infections
  - Bacterial
  - Viral
  - Spirochaetal
  - Protozoal
  - Fungal
  - Ricketssial
- Neoplasms
- Allergic reactions
- Collagen disorders
- Drugs
- Granulomatous disorders or sarcoidosis
- Heat stroke
- Factitious fever.

Gathering information

Fever is often a diagnostic clue accompanying a more specific symptom such as sore throat, cough or diarrhoea. Occasionally, however, and more frequently in infants and small children, the main presenting problem is fever and the family physician needs an approach to investigating the cause. The following mnemonic may be helpful:

- **P** – precipitating/palliating/provoking factors, for example recent travel, underlying HIV
- **Q** – quality of fever, for example pattern of fever over time
- **R** – related symptoms, for example sore throat, earache, dysuria, cough
- **S** – severity of fever, for example measurement of temperature
- **T** – time course/treatment, for example duration and response to medication.

In the case of an unexplained fever a full examination will be required:

1. General impression: Toxic, sick or well looking
2. Vital signs: Temperature, respiratory rate, pulse and blood pressure
3. General: Jaundice, anaemia, cyanosis, lymphadenopathy, petechiae, oedema
4. Look for a focus of infection:
   - Ear, nose and throat infections - otitis media, tonsillitis, pharyngitis
   - Chest infection - pneumonia, bronchitis, pleural effusion
   - Skin infection and rashes - impetigo, tick bite fever, measles, chickenpox, rubella
   - Abdominal infection – appendicitis, gastro-enteritis, cholecystitis
   - Genito-urinary infection – pyelonephritis, cystitis, pelvic inflammatory disease
   - Neurological infection – meningitis.
5. Look for associated clinical signs such as:
   - Hepatomegaly - malaria, enteric fever, hepatitis
   - Splenomegaly - malaria, enteric fever, infectious mononeuclosis, lymphoma, infective endocarditis
   - Meningeal signs - neck stiffness, Kernig and Brudzinski signs
   - Lymphadenopathy – TB, HIV, lymphoma, toxoplasmosis, infectious mononucleosis, brucellosis
   - Jaundice – hepatitis.
6. Side room investigations
   - Urinalysis, for example evidence of urinary tract infection.

Special investigations

Special investigations should be focused and assist with management.
- Total and differential white blood cell count

- Urine culture and sensitivity only if urinary tract infection is suspected
- Chest radiograph if there are signs of pneumonia, empyema, pleural effusion or tuberculosis
- Rapid malaria test if in a malaria zone (or patient has recently visited one in the last four weeks)
- Special immunological tests like ANA (anti-nuclear antibody) and DsDNA (double-stranded DNA) should be done if one suspects disorders like systemic lupus erthyematosis, polyarteritis nodosa or other connective tissue disorders
- Polymerase chain reaction tests if indicated, for example HIV infection, swine flu
- IgM and IgG antibodies against tick bite fever, rubella, measles, herpes, and so on
- Lumber puncture for meningitis if raised intracranial pressure was excluded
- Blood cultures per indication.

Further assessment

Divide into a category:
- Children < three months: Treat as a severe bacterial infection. Give an immediate dose of systemic antibiotic (for example IM ceftriaxone), admit to hospital, and investigate fully for infection.
- Serious infection indicated by meningeal irritation, respiratory distress, purpura, surgical abdomen or shock: Resuscitate, give an immediate dose of intravenous antibiotic and refer as an emergency.
- Acute infection with focus of infection identified: Manage according to normal guidelines.
- Fever > one week and not responding to treatment: Repeat history, examination and consider more specialised investigations or referral.

Treatment of fever:
- Paracetamol and ibuprofen are safe in children.
- Paracetamol, aspirin and non-steroid anti-inflammatory drugs are safe in adults.
- As fever has an antimicrobial action, only treat if causing discomfort.
- Don't let the use of antipyretics distract from the cause of the infection.
- Fever does not always require an antibiotic and if more than two sites are affected, for example runny nose, coughing, sore throat and earache, the infection is usually caused by a virus.

Sore throat

Pharyngitis (URTI)

There is usually history of a painful throat, runny nose, malaise, fever and difficulty swallowing. On examination the throat is diffusely red. Pharyngitis is usually viral, but can also be bacterial. It may be impossible to exclude a bacterial infection clinically. To prevent complications from infection with beta-haemolytic streptococcus, such as rheumatic fever and acute glomerular nephritis, all children between three to 15 years with sore throat, pain on swallowing and/or pyrexia should be treated as having a streptococcal infection; unless they have clear evidence of a viral infection such as hoarseness, watery rhinitis and conjunctivitis.

Tonsillitis

Complaints may be similar with a sore throat, difficulty swallowing, fever and malaise. On examination the tonsils will be inflamed and swollen and may have pus visible. There is often cervical lymphadenopathy and a raised temperature. Tonsillitis may be viral (rhinovirus, adeno-virus, enterovirus) or bacterial (*Streptococcus* spp., pneumococcal, Staphylococcal, *H. influenzae*) Complications of rheumatic fever and acute glomerular nephritis are also possible and therefore tonsillitis is also treated as a streptococcal infection.

Indications for tonsillectomy include:

- Recurrent tonsillitis. Recurrent tonsillitis is usually viral and is defined as more than six episodes a year or more than four episodes a year for two years
- Peritonsillar abscess – unilateral swelling in front of the tonsil that pushes the uvula over to the other side
- Obstructive sleep apnoea syndrome
- Unilateral enlarged tonsil in an adult.

Acute laryngitis

Acute laryngitis is usually viral and may present like pharyngitis, but inflammatory changes extend to the mucosa of the epiglottis and whole of the supraglottis. It results in the loss of voice or a hoarse voice with an irritating dry cough that may last for seven to ten days.

A hoarse voice from acute laryngitis usually recovers within two weeks, but if it persists will require examination by indirect laryngoscopy to exclude other pathology. In older adults with a smoking history, largyngeal cancer may present in this way.

Diarrhoea

Diarrhoea is the passage of three or more loose or liquid stools per day, or more frequently than is normal for the individual. Diarrhoea in infants and small children is a major contributor to mortality and therefore most of this section refers to their assessment and management. The approach is largely based on the Integrated Management of Childhood Illness. Acute diarrhoea is usually infective from a viral (for example rotavirus or adenovirus) or bacterial cause (for example shigella, campylobacter, salmonella or *E. coli*). However chronic diarrhoea may also be caused by parasites (for example giardiasis), malabsorption (for example lactose intolerance), inflammatory bowel disease, and irritable bowel syndrome. HIV has also led to an increased incidence of acute and chronic diarrhoea and, in those with more advanced disease, a number of opportunistic infections.

Gathering information

The mnemonic PQRST can help recall key information in the history:
- **P** – precipitating/palliating/provoking factors, for example what fluids are being given at home?
- **Q** – quality of diarrhoea, for example the presence of blood or mucus
- **R** – related factors, for example vomiting, fever, abdominal pain
- **S** – severity, for example frequency, amount, ability to drink
- **T** – time course/treatment, for example duration and any self-medication.

On examination assess the degree of dehydration. The assessment of a child is shown in Table 7.3. Vital signs should be recorded – weight, temperature, pulse and blood pressure. Abdominal examination should also be performed.

Table 7.3 Assessing dehydration

Shock (one sign)	Severe dehydration (two signs)	Some dehydration (two signs)	No visible dehydration
Decreased level of consciousness	Lethargic	Restless or irritable	Alert
Decreased blood pressure and rapid thready pulse	Drinks poorly, unable to drink	Thirsty	Drinks normally
Capillary filling time of > three seconds	Sunken eyes	Sunken eyes	Wet mucous membranes
	Decreased skin turgor; skin pinch > two seconds	Decreased skin turgor; skin pinch < two seconds	Normal skin turgor

All this information will help categorise acute diarrhoea as:

- Diarrhoea with either no, some or severe dehydration/shock
- Dysentery (bloody diarrhoea)
- Severe dysentery due to associated dehydration or age under 12 months
- Persistent diarrhoea (lasts longer than 14 days)
- Severe persistent diarrhoea due to associated dehydration.

Management of dehydration

Those classified as severe dehydration or shock as well as those with severe dysentery or severe persistent diarrhoea should be referred to hospital.

Shock or severe dehydration:

- Rehydrate as per Figure 7.1 (Plan C).
- Refer to hospital.
- Give frequent sips of oral rehydration solution.
- Continue breastfeeding when possible.

Some dehydration:

- Rehydrate as per Table 7.4 at the health centre initially (Plan B).
- Continue breastfeeding/feeding.
- Give zinc for two weeks.
- Follow up in two days.
- Advise mother on when to return immediately.

No dehydration:
- Give fluids and food at home as per Table 7.5 (Plan A).
- Give zinc for two weeks.
- Follow up in five days if not better.
- Advise mother on when to return immediately.

The use of side room and special investigations

- Blood glucose if child is not fully awake and drinking well
- Urinalysis
- Consider the need for HIV testing
- Other investigations per indication.

Information to patients

- Diarrhoea causes dehydration and therefore the main treatment is rehydration.
- Continue to feed the patient during episodes of diarrhoea.
- Teach the patient or caregiver how to mix homemade sugar and salt solution (SSS): Half a level teaspoon of table salt + eight level teaspoons of sugar mixed with one litre of clean water.
- Advise the patient to return immediately if patient vomits everything, drinks poorly or has blood in the diarrhoea.
- Advise to return for an appointment to monitor malnutrition, anaemia and growth.

Medication

- No routine antibiotics unless specifically indicated as in dysentery (for example ciprofloxacin for three days)
- No anti-emetics in children
- No anti-diarrhoeal medication in children
- Give vitamin A supplementation in persistent diarrhoea in children
- In adults consider the use of anti-emetics or anti-diarrhoeal drugs such as loperamide.

Table 7.4 Plan B: Treatment for some dehydration

Task	Key points				
Determine amount of ORS to give during first 4 hours	Age	Up to 4 months	4 to 12 months	1 up to 2 years	2 up to 5 years
	Weight	< 6 kg	6–< 10 kg	10–< 12 kg	12–25 kg
	For 4 hours	200–450 ml	450–800 ml	800–960 ml	960–1600 ml
	Use weight rather than age as a guide when possible. 1 teacup = 200 ml				
Show the mother how to give ORS	• Give frequent sips from a cup • If the child vomits, wait 10 minutes. Then continue, but more slowly. • Continue breastfeeding whenever the child wants • If the child wants more ORS than shown, give more				
After 4 hours	• Reassess and classify the child • Select the appropriate plan for ongoing treatment • Begin feeding the child				

If the mother must leave or the clinic is closing	• Refer if possible. Otherwise:
	  – Show her how to prepare ORS at home
	  – Show her how much ORS to give over 4 hours
	  – Show her how to prepare SSS at home
	  – Emphasis the 3 rules: Give extra fluids, continue feeding, when to return.				

Table 7.5 Plan A: Treatment if no dehydration

Task	Key points
Counsel the mother	• Breastfeed frequently and for longer at each feed • If the child is exclusively breastfed then give sugar-salt solution (SSS) or oral rehydration solution (ORS) in addition to breastmilk • If the child is not receiving breastmilk or is not exclusively breastfed, give one or more of the following food-based fluids such as soft porridge, amasi (maas) or SSS or ORS • It is especially important to give ORS at home when the child has been treated for dehydration (Figure 7.1 and Table 7.4) or when the child cannot easily return to the clinic if the diarrhoea gets worse
Teach the mother how to mix and give SSS or ORS	• To make SSS: 1 litre boiled water (now cooled) + 8 level teaspoons sugar + half a level teaspoon of salt. SSS is used at home to prevent dehydration. • The ORS sachet is mixed with clean water and given to correct dehydration
Show the mother how much fluid to give in addition to the usual fluid intake	• Up to 2 years: 50 to 100 ml after each loose stool • Over 2 years: 100 to 200 ml after each loose stool Give frequent sips from a cup If the child vomits, wait 10 minutes. Then continue, but more slowly. Continue giving extra fluid until the diarrhoea stops

Figure 7.1: Plan C: Treatment of severe dehydration

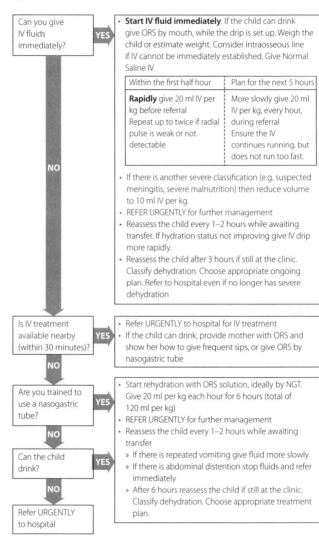

Abdominal pain

Introduction

The identification and management of patients who are severely ill or have an emergency should be the first priority. These patients may be recognised by any of the following red flags:

- Peritonitis suggested by rebound tenderness, guarding or rigidity of the abdomen
- Jaundice – bilary or hepatic disease
- Temperature $\geq 38\,°C$ – infective pathology
- No stool or wind for the last 24 hours and vomiting – possibility of intestinal obstruction
- On antiretroviral medication – possibility of lactic acidosis
- No urine passed for past 12 hours and swelling of the abdomen – possibility of urinary retention and obstruction
- Pregnant women with lower abdominal pain – complication of pregnancy or in labour.

Gathering information

Location

The location of acute abdominal pain may be associated with specific causes as shown in Table 7.6 (Kontoyannis, 2008).

Table 7.6 Likely pathology with abdominal pain at different locations

Location	Likely pathology
Right upper quadrant	Gallbladder disease, lower lobe pneumonia, hepatic disease
Epigastrium	Dyspepsia, peptic ulcer, peptic perforation, pancreatitis
Left upper quadrant and umbilical area	Small bowel obstruction, early appendicitis, mesenteric ischaemia, mesenteric adenitis (TB), gastro-enteritis, lower lobe pneumonia
Right or left flank	Ureteric colic, pyelonephritis, leaking abdominal aortic aneurysm
Suprapubic	Cystitis, acute urinary retention, pelvic appendicitis

Location	Likely pathology
Right iliac fossa	Appendicitis, carcinoma of caecum, mesenteric adenitis (TB), Crohn's disease of terminal ileum, ovarian cyst, salpingitis, ectopic pregnancy
Left iliac fossa	Diverticulitis, carcinoma of sigmoid colon, ulcerative colitis, constipation, ovarian cyst, salpingitis, ectopic pregnancy
Groin	Irreducible hernia

Some medical conditions may also be associated with abdominal pain such as diabetic keto-acidosis (hyperglycaemia) and hypercalcaemia. The widespread use of antiretroviral medication has made abdominal pain associated with hyperlactaemia and lactic acidosis a possibility.

Onset

Inflammatory pain tends to have a slower onset that is progressive as inflammation increases. A perforation typically has sudden onset and colicky pain that comes and goes rapidly.

Severity

Ask the patient to rate the severity on a scale of one to ten and watch how they react during the consultation and examination.

Nature

Pain may be described as aching, burning (for example dyspepsia or colic), stabbing (for example ureteric colic) or gripping (for example intestinal obstruction).

Progression

Abdominal pain may change over time. For example, appendicitis starts as a colicky central pain that later localises to the right iliac fossa with the onset of peritonitis. Colic may last seconds (intestinal), minutes (ureteric) or 20 minutes (gallbladder).

Radiation

The pain may appear to radiate to another place. For example, pain in retroperitoneal structures such as the pancreas or aorta may be experienced as back pain. Pain from the diaphragm may radiate to the shoulder tip and from the gallbladder to the tip of the scapula. Ovarian pain may radiate to the sacro-iliac region.

Exacerbating and relieving factors

Peritonitis is worse with movement so the patient lies still. Ureteric colic is unaffected by movement and the patient may move about trying to relieve the pain. Food may relieve a duodenal ulcer, but worsen a gastric ulcer. Fatty foods may worsen bilary colic, hot and spicy foods may worsen dyspepsia and peptic ulcers, milk may relive dyspepsia, but worsen bilary colic due to the fat content.

Associated symptoms

In a women with lower abdominal pain, ask about vaginal discharge (see page 223) and possibility of pregnancy (last menstrual period, abnormal menses, family planning, vaginal bleeding).

Ask about bowel movements to assess constipation or the total absence of stool in a patient with intestinal obstruction. Diarrhoea (see page 197) is commonly associated with colicky pain. Ask about the presence of worms in the stool and treat accordingly. Ask about blood and mucus in the stool.

Ask about urinary symptoms such as dysuria (see page 207) that may suggest urinary tract infection.

Ask about nausea and vomiting (see page 216).

Ask about HIV and consider the possibility of abdominal TB in those at stage three or four, with > five percent weight loss, cough > two weeks, fever or night sweats.

Examination

Examination includes attention to the patient's general appearance (sweating, pallor, position, behaviour), vital signs (temperature, pulse, blood pressure, respiratory rate), abdomen, and may include a rectal and vaginal examination.

Investigations

Investigations will depend on the hypothesis being considered but may include:

- Full blood count – anaemia, dehydration, infection
- Urea and electrolytes – renal function, dehydration
- Liver function tests – gallbladder, bilary or hepatic problems
- Amylase – pancreatitis
- Urinalysis – haematuria in ureteric colic and infection, leucocytes and nitrites in infection
- Pregnancy test
- Erect chest X-ray to look for free gas under the diaphragm or lower lobe pneumonia. Note that 30% of acute perforations are not visible on the erect chest X-ray
- Abdominal X-ray for signs of obstruction, free gas, calculi or gas in the bilary tree
- Abdominal ultrasound can examine most organs
- CAT scanning, barium or gastrografin studies, laparotomy and laparoscopy may have a place at the referral hospital.

Dyspepsia

Epigastric pain or discomfort is one of the commonest presentations of abdominal pain in primary care. Although no specific diagnosis is made in a large number of patients the following pathology should be considered:

- Duodenal ulcer
- Gastric ulcer or gastritis
- Gastric cancer
- Hiatus hernia, oesophagitis and gastro-oesophageal reflux
- Gall bladder disease
- Irritable bowel syndrome (colicky pain, abdominal bloating and alternating bowel hait).

The majority of patients with dyspepsia will recover spontaneously or with a course of antacids or acid suppression. A number of red flag signs and symptoms suggest the need for further investigation:

- Objective weight loss
- Anaemia or evidence of bleeding (malaena or haematemesis)
- Lymphadenopathy (Virchow's node)
- Age > 40 years when cancer becomes more likely
- Persistent vomiting – gastric outflow obstruction due to duodenal ulcer or gastric cancer

- Jaundice
- Poor response or recurrence after a course of empirical treatment.

In a patient with dyspepsia it is always important to enquire about medication and lifestyle factors that may be causing or worsening it:
- Non-steroidal anti-inflammatory drugs and corticosteroids
- Cigarette smoking
- Excessive alcohol intake
- Psychosocial stress.

The best investigation is endoscopy to exclude peptic ulcer disease, cancer, oesophagitis and hiatus hernia. Gallbladder disease will require liver function tests and ultrasound. Reflux may require manometry and pH testing to confirm. If peptic ulcer disease is suspected, tests for *Helicobacter pylori* should be considered. Tests include histology, urease testing of biopsies at endoscopy, antibodies in the blood and breath tests.

Dysuria

Dysuria is defined as pain, burning, or discomfort on urination, often accompanied by frequency or urgency and usually presents more commonly in women than in men. Dysuria results from irritation of the bladder trigone or urethral area. Inflammation or stricture of the urethra causes difficulty in starting urination, thereby causing a burning sensation on urination, while irritation of the trigone causes bladder contraction, leading to frequent and painful urination.

Urinary tract infection is the most frequent cause of dysuria, but empiric treatment without a sensible diagnostic approach is not always appropriate or advisable.

A good history and a sound diagnostic approach using inexpensive laboratory testing are often sufficient to determine the cause of dysuria (see Figure 7.2).

Figure 7.2 Diagnostic algorithm for dysuria

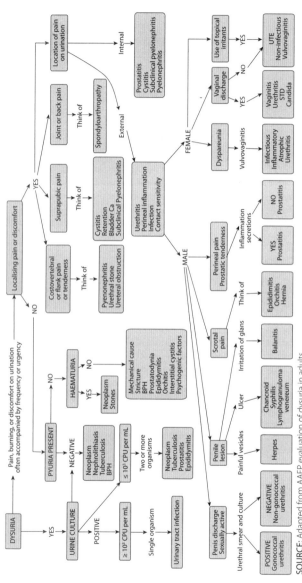

SOURCE: Adapted from AAFP evaluation of dysuria in adults

Red flags

Dysuria with any of the following findings should be further investigated:
- Fever
- Loin pain or tenderness in the renal angle
- Recent instrumentation involving the urethra
- Immuno-compromised patients with HIV, diabetes, or on corticosteroids
- Recurrent episodes (including frequent childhood infections)
- Known urinary tract abnormality.

Causes

Dysuria can be caused by any of the following:
- Infections: pyelonephritis, cystitis, prostatitis, urethritis, cervicitis, epididymo-orchitis, vulvovaginitis. Sexually transmitted infections that present with vaginal discharge and male urethritis syndrome are discussed on page 224. Urinary tract infection is also more common in pregnancy and this should be remembered in women of child-bearing age. Patients with possible immune suppression (with HIV or diabetes mellitus) or on immune-suppressing medication may present with vulvovaginitis and dysuria due to candidiasis
- Hormonal conditions: hypo-estrogenism (postmenopausal), endometriosis
- Malformations: bladder neck obstruction (with additional symptoms such as a weak stream, dribbling, hesitancy, intermittent stream or nocturia; especially in older men with benign prostatic hyperplasia (BPH)), urethral strictures or diverticula
- Neoplasms: renal cell tumour; bladder, prostate, vaginal/vulvar and penile cancers
- Inflammatory conditions: spondyloarthropathies (associated with backache, joint pain or eye irritation) and reactive arthritis (associated with joint pain, skin rash and mucosal lesions), drug side effects, auto-immune disorders
- Trauma: catheter placement, honeymoon cystitis after sexual intercourse
- Psychogenic conditions: somatisation disorder, major depression, stress disorders or anxiety, hysteria.

History taking

History taking should be aimed at discovering:

- Duration, timing, frequency, severity, and location of dysuria. Dysuria at the start of urination points to urethral pathology. Suprapubic pain after voiding is usually of bladder origin. Longer duration and more gradual onset of symptoms should prompt investigation for *C. trachomatis* or *M. tuberculosis* infection. A sudden onset of dysuria with haematuria usually suggests a bacterial infection.
- If the urine is bloody, cloudy, or malodorous
- The presence of any red flags
- Any urethral or vaginal discharge (amount, colour, and consistency). Urethral discharge has a high association with urethritis and, in men, is the most common symptom of a sexually transmitted infection. In sexually active patients, urethritis or vulvovaginitis is a likely cause of dysuria. A history of sexually transmitted infection can point to urethral scarring causing outflow obstruction with stream abnormalities and a predisposition to repeated infections, especially in patients with high-risk sexual behaviour
- The use of medications, herbal remedies and topical hygiene products. Dysuria may be caused by medications such as penicillin G, pyrazinamide, Rifater, amlodipine, hydrochlorothiazide, Cardura Xl, isosorbide-5-Mononitrate and some combination common cold/ allergy medications. Dysuria can also occur with the use of, among others, saw palmetto, pumpkin seeds, dopamine, or cantharidin, and with the use of a number of topical hygiene products, including vaginal sprays, vaginal douches, and bubble baths.

Physical examination

When doing the physical examination pay attention to the following:

- Temperature
- Tenderness over the kidneys (renal angles) or bladder
- A vaginal examination may be needed to identify discharge, trauma, sexually transmitted infections or vaginal atrophy
- Male genitalia should be examined for lesions, discharge, tenderness or swelling
- Other signs associated with suspected underlying causes such as skin rash, mucosal lesions and reactive arthritis; rectal examination to evaluate the size, consistency, and tenderness of the prostate in suspected obstruction.

Laboratory testing

Laboratory testing is directed at the most probable diagnosis and may include:

- Urine dipstick tests for identifying haematuria and pyuria. Leukocyte esterase is a marker for white blood cells and has a sensitivity of 75% for the detection of infection. Pyuria has a sensitivity of 96% for urinary infection. Positive testing for nitrites suggests a probable infection; however, it is not ruled out by a negative test.
- Microscopic examination of a spun, clean-catch, midstream urine sample. Pyuria is diagnosed by the presence of three to five white blood cells per high-power field and haematuria is diagnosed by the presence of three to five red blood cells per high-power field. Pyuria detected on urinalysis is associated not only with bacterial UTI, but also with *T. vaginalis*, *C. trachomatis* and other infections. Sterile pyuria may be present in patients with prostatitis, nephrolithiasis, urologic neoplasms and fungal or mycobacterial infections (TB).
- Urine cultures are not essential in young women when clear-cut signs and symptoms of acute dysuria indicate a high probability of uncomplicated cystitis.
- Vaginal and urethral smears with gram staining (although in primary care STIs will be dealt with syndromically and without specific tests (see page 228)).
- Radiologic studies and other diagnostic tests are indicated when the diagnosis is in doubt, when patients are severely ill or immunocompromised or do not respond to antibiotic therapy, and when complications are suspected.

Low back pain

Low back pain (LBP) is defined as pain that occurs posteriorly in the area between the bottom of the rib cage and the buttock creases (NICE, 2009). The initial evaluation should (Mash and Blitz-Lindeque, 2006):

- Attempt to place patients with LBP into one of the following categories
  - Non-specific LBP
  - LBP associated with radiculopathy or spinal stenosis
  - LBP associated with serious spinal pathology
  - LBP referred from a non-spinal source.
- Assess if there is social or psychological distress that may amplify or prolong the pain (Chou R *et al.*, 2007).

Natural history and aetiology

Table 7.6 lists the causes of LBP and the natural history is described below:

- Most LBP (80%) is non-specific and derives from the structural components of the lower back: bones, muscles, joints, discs, tendons, ligaments or nerves associated with lumbar vertebrae or pelvis. The exact structure causing the pain cannot be determined for most patients. It affects men and women equally, with onset usually between the ages of 30 and 50 years. The prognosis is favourable, as two thirds of patients with acute LBP substantially improve within six weeks (Deyo, 2001).

- The prognosis of LBP with radiculopathy (4%) caused by herniated discs is also favourable. More than 90% of symptomatic lumbar disc herniations occur at the L4/L5 and L5/S1 levels. Only about 10% of patients have so much pain after six weeks that surgery is considered.

- In contrast, spinal stenosis (3%) caused by hypertrophic degenerative changes of the facets and thickening of the ligamentum flavum, usually remains stable or gradually worsens.

- LBP is due to a specific spinal pathology in a minority of cases. They are important to detect because they often require aggressive evaluation and management (Deyo, 2001). In South Africa, spinal tuberculosis is more common due to the HIV epidemic (Oluruntoba, 2009).

- Back pain referred from a non-spinal source, such as abdominal or pelvic pathology, comprises about two percent of low back pain causes.

Table 7.6 Causes of low back pain (Speed, 2004)

Classification of cause	Examples
Structural	Non-specific
	Facet joint arthritis or dysfunction
	Prolapsed intervertebral disc
	Annular tear
	Midline disc herniation (Cauda equina syndrome)
	Spondylolysis or spondylolisthesis
	Spinal stenosis

Classification of cause	Examples
Infection	Discitis
	Osteomyelitis, for example staphylococcal
	Tuberculosis of the spine
	Paraspinal abscess
Inflammatory	Spondylo-arthropathies (for example, ankylosing spondylitis, psoriatic and reactive arthritis)
	Sacro-ilitis or sacro-iliac dysfunction
Neoplasm	Primary (for example multiple myeloma) or secondary (for example prostate and breast)
Metabolic	Osteoporosis and vertebral collapse
	Paget's disease
	Osteomalacia
	Hyperparathyroidism
Referred/non-spinal	Major viscera, for example kidneys and pancreas
	Retroperitoneal structures, for example dissecting aorta
	Urogenital system, for example pelvic inflammatory disease
	Hip, for example osteoarthritis

History

The onset and characteristics of the pain are important in differentiating non-specific from other categories of LBP. It is important to inquire about:

- Impact on physical function (sleep, work, dressing, sexual activity, recreation) and factors that improve or worsen the pain
- The tasks the patient performs at work and their level of physical activity off the job
- Radiating leg pain (sciatica) is suggestive of radiculopathy and disc prolapse and may be exacerbated by coughing, sneezing or straining during the Valsalva manoeuvre
- Spinal stenosis occurs usually in older patients and is characterised by pain in the legs on walking, which mimics ischaemic claudication. The pain is relieved by sitting down or bending forward
- Any red flag or non-spinal symptoms as described in Table 7.7.

Table 7.7 Red flags for low back pain

Possible cause	Key features on history or physical examination
Cancer	History of cancer with new onset of LBP
	Pain is progressive
	Unexplained weight loss
	Failure to improve after one month
	Age < 18 years or > 50 years
Vertebral infection	Fever and systemic upset such as night sweats and weight loss
	HIV
	Intravenous drug abuse
	Recent infection
Cauda equina syndrome	Urinary retention
	Motor deficits at multiple levels
	Faecal incontinence
	Saddle anaesthesia
Vertebral compression fracture	History of significant trauma
	History of osteoporosis
	Use of corticosteroids
	Older age
Severe/progressive neurological deficits	Progressive motor weakness
Inflammation (ankylosing spondylitis)	Early morning stiffness
	Improvement with exercise
	Alternating buttock pain
	Nocturnal awakening in early hours
	Younger age
Referred pain from abdomen or pelvis	Dysuria, fever, nausea/vomiting, abdominal pain, abdominal mass, localised tenderness on examination, genito-urinary symptoms

SOURCE: Adapted from: Kinkade S. 2007 and Chou R, Qaseem A, Snow V, *et al.* 2008

Assess psychosocial factors and emotional distress because they are stronger predictors of chronic disabling non-specific LBP than either physical examination findings or severity and duration of pain:

- Patient's perspective – beliefs, concerns, expectations, feelings
- Psychosocial stress – relational, financial, health, living situation, work related

- Mental health –depression, anxiety, substance abuse
- Secondary gain from potential compensation or disability grant.

Examination

A focused examination is adequate in patients with LBP whose history does not suggest serious spinal pathology or non-spinal causes, with particular emphasis on the following (Mash and Blitz-Lindeque, 2006):

- Palpate spine: Vertebral tenderness has sensitivity for infection, but not specificity. Tenderness may also indicate neoplasia or osteoporotic vertebral collapse.
- Movements: Limited spinal motion is not strongly associated with any specific diagnosis but suggests the degree of functional limitation.
- A positive result on the straight-leg-raising test (defined as reproduction of the patient's sciatica between 30 and 70 degrees of leg elevation) has a relatively high sensitivity but modest specificity for diagnosing herniated disc.
- The crossed straight-leg-raising test is more specific for a herniated disc but less sensitive.

Tests for sensation (light touch or pin prick), motor strength and reflexes are useful in localising the level of a disc herniation (See Table 7.8).

Table 7.8 Physical examination findings in nerve root impingements

Level of disc herniation	Nerve root impinged	Sensory loss	Motor weakness	Screening examination	Reflex
L3-L4	L4	Medial foot	Knee extension	Squat and rise	Knee/patellar
L4-L5	L5	Dorsal foot	Dorsiflexion ankle/great toe	Heel walking	None
L5-S1	S1	Lateral foot	Plantar flexion ankle and toes	Walking on toes	Ankle/Achilles

When to investigate or refer?

Because non-specific acute LBP typically does not have a serious aetiology and resolves with conservative treatment, most patients do not need investigations (Chou R *et al.*, 2009).

Patients with radiculopathy and suspected spinal stenosis should be investigated and referred if symptoms do not resolve in four to six weeks. Typical investigations in primary care include a full blood count, ESR and plain radiograph. CAT scans and MRI scans are often required at the referral hospital. Cauda equina syndrome and severe progressive neurological deficits must be referred as an emergency.

Vomiting

Vomiting is usually associated with nausea. In a child significant vomiting may be a general danger sign of underlying infection or severe illness.

Causes

- Gastro-enteritis or other infections, for example otitis media, urinary tract infection or hepatitis
- Gastro-intestinal conditions such as obstruction, appendicitis, pancreatitis or cholecystitis
- Physiological in pregnancy or motion sickness
- Metabolic and endocrine conditions causing hypoglycaemia, ketosis, uraemia or porphyria
- Neurological conditions such as head trauma, raised intracranial pressure or infections of the central nervous system
- Adverse drug reactions, for example to antibiotics, analgesics, digoxin, antivirals or chemotherapy
- Psychological issues such as attention-seeking behaviour or bulimia.

Gathering information

Explore the different causes listed above and specifically ask about:
- Appearance of the vomit and particularly any blood
- Duration, amount and frequency of vomiting
- Ability to keep down fluids and drink
- Associated symptoms such as nausea, diarrhoea, abdominal pain
- Use of medication
- Possibility of pregnancy.

If a gastro-intestinal cause is likely, then examination will focus on vital signs, dehydration and the abdomen. When the cause is less certain, a broader examination will be needed that includes a neurological assessment.

Side room and special investigations

- Blood glucose
- Urinalysis
- Pregnancy test.

Other special investigations will be done as indicated, for example amylase for suspected pancreatitis.

Management

Manage dehydration (see diarrhoea page 197).

Anti-emetics in adults are useful in self-limiting conditions such as gastro-enteritis, but should not delay identification and treatment of the underlying cause.

Medication should treat the underlying cause such as antibiotics for infections, or dexamethasone for raised intracranial pressure.

Joint pain

The two most common chronic joint conditions seen in the family physician's office are osteoarthritis (OA) and rheumatoid arthritis (RA). Consider the following six concepts when evaluating joint pain:

Is the joint pain really arthritis?

There are a variety of painful structures that can be interpreted as pain in the joint by patients.

Periarticular causes of pain can originate from a bursitis (for example, in the case of knee pain, an anserine bursitis could be the cause); tendonitis (for example, inflammation of some tendons of the anatomical snuff-box may cause wrist pain) and perceived regional joint pains may be caused by myofacial pain/fibromyalgia syndrome.

Nonarticular causes of pain may come from adjacent tumours of the bone; vascular pathology; osteomyelitis; or radiculopathy.

Articular pain arises from involvement of the joint itself. The signs of articular inflammation are swelling, tenderness, warmth and redness.

Is the condition acute or chronic?

Chronic refers to conditions lasting for more than eight weeks. Acute may mean a recent onset of a new condition or in other instances it may refer to a flare up of a chronic condition. With acute joint pain, one should first exclude a history of trauma before exploring other causes. The differentiation of acute from chronic joint pain is essential for making an appropriate management plan as shown in Table 7.9.

Is the problem inflammatory or non-inflammatory?

Differentiating between inflammatory or non-inflammatory conditions (see Table 7.9) helps in narrowing the differential diagnoses.

Table 7.9 Differences between inflammatory and non-inflammatory joint pain

	Inflammatory	Non-inflammatory
Early morning stiffness	> 30 minutes	< 15 minutes
Stiffness and pain	Increase with rest and are relieved by exercise	Increase with use and relieved by rest
Swelling	Often present	Not present
Microscopy of synovial fluid	Translucent, white cell count > 75 000 with polymorphonuclear cells > 50%	Translucent, white cell count < 2 000 with polymorphonuclear cells < 25%

It is critical to identify an inflammatory arthritis as, when present, disease-modifying anti-rheumatic drugs should be prescribed early. These drugs alter the progression and the course of the disease. If one is not trained in rheumatology, one should refer the patient to a rheumatologist immediately. On the other hand, all family physicians should be skilled in managing common rheumatological conditions such as gout.

What is the pattern of joint involvement?

Monoarthritis and oligo-/polyarthritis have differing diagnostic probabilities as shown in Table 7.10. Inflammatory pain with symmetrical small joint involvement is suggestive of RA. RA is the commonest inflammatory condition and it has a prevalence of 1% in the adult population. Inflammatory back pain may be a spondyloarthritis (ankylosing spondylitis).

Table 7.10 Pattern of joint involvement and diagnosis

Acute		Chronic	
Monoarthritis	**Oligo-/ polyarthritis**	**Monoarthritis**	**Oligo-/ polyarthritis**
Infective (septic)	Systemic illness	Osteoarthritis	Autoimmune (for
Gout (crystals)	Gout (crystals)	Gout (crystals)	example RA)
Reactive	Reactive	Infective (TB)	Osteoarthritis
Trauma	Post-streptococcal	Tumour	Gout (crystals)
			Reactive
			Psoriatic

Are there associated systemic features?

Most of the rheumatic conditions are systemic illnesses. It is therefore important to review all the systems when seeing a patient. Symptoms could include loss of weight, unexplained fevers, rash, chills and new disabilities. Psoriatic arthritis may have the typical skin rash and nail abnormalities. Reactive arthritis may follow urogenital or enteric infections. Rheumatic fever may follow a streptococcal infection.

What is the patient's profile?

Age, gender, family history and past medical history may provide clues. For example, fibromyalgia is typical in younger women; polymyalgia rheumatica mainly occurs in those over 60 years and is usually accompanied by a strikingly raised ESR. A family history of auto-immune diseases makes rheumatoid diseases such as RA more likely. Unexplained paediatric arthralgias have been found to be associated with psychosocial stress, school absenteeism and vitamin D deficiency. HIV commonly predisposes to a number of rheumatological problems.

Investigations

Targeted investigations are only useful if there is a high suspicion of a specific condition. Erythrocyte sedimentation rate and a C-reactive protein are commonly elevated in inflammatory conditions.

Arthrocentesis and investigation of synovial fluid can confirm infection and help differentiate inflammatory from non-inflammatory causes. Negative birefringent needle-like crystals in synovial fluid can clinche the diagnosis of gout. However, gout can be diagnosed on history, examination and elevated uric acid. The uric acid however is not always elevated in acute gout and may be mildly elevated in those without gout. Anti-CCP antibodies are used to diagnose RA (sensitivity 74%, specificity 94%) and IgM rheumatoid factor (sensitivity 75%, specificity 74%) is a predictor of disease severity. The rheumatoid factor must be highly elevated to support the diagnosis of RA.

Diagnostic imaging in the public sector health facilities in South Africa is usually confined to plain X-rays. X-rays can reveal the features of certain rheumatic diseases like OA and RA. It is also good in showing most fractures. In tertiary institutions, ultrasound and radionuclear bone scans can be used to detect early synovitis when there is a clinical doubt of arthritis. MRI and CAT scans provide information on soft tissue abnormalities.

Skin complaints and rash

In assessing skin complaints it may be more practical to take a brief history and then move immediately to examine the patient. The examination may provide an immediate diagnosis (by pattern recognition) or provide useful information, which will guide further history taking.

History

- The duration and temporal sequence of the rash is important:
  - Date of initial onset and duration
  - How the skin lesions have evolved and changed over time. For example they may have started as painful vesicles that then develop into pustules or ulcers. The lesion may have started in one part of the body and spread elsewhere
  - The speed of onset, that is did the lesions develop suddenly or slowly
  - A history of previous episodes at the same or different sites.
- Consider any associated symptoms or features:
  - Pruritus (for example papular pruritic eruption or drugs), pain (for example herpes)
  - Presence of systemic illness or high fever
  - Any medication, topical or systemic, prescribed or over the counter.
  - Relationship to recent travel, stress, work or activities
  - Recent exposure to someone with a similar skin condition.
- Associated diseases: Diabetes mellitus, HIV, tuberculosis, atopic conditions such as allergic rhinitis or asthma
- Previous treatment: strengths of medication (be aware of the four

groups of steroid potency), duration of treatment (often too short), and whether it worked or not

- Type of work: hands in water and detergents all of the time, exposure to other chemicals or irritants
- Lifestyle and habits: washing with antiseptics soaps will irritate already sensitive skin, exposure to chemicals such as cosmetics, hair products, perfumes, plants.

It is important to note the individual patient's expectations. It is not uncommon to find a patient who has been to several different health practitioners, and who has had various combinations of steroids, antihistamines, antifungals, antibiotics, and advice. The patient is often very anxious to know what the definitive diagnosis is, whether there is definitive treatment that will cure the rash, and why they have this problem.

Examination

- Take a look at the patient. Make sure the patient undresses enough to ensure adequate examination. Note the morphology of the lesions:
  - Circumscribed, flat, non-palpable, changes in skin colour: Macule, patch
  - Palpable elevated solid masses: Papule, nodule, plaque, wheal
  - Circumscribed superficial elevations of the skin formed by free fluid in a cavity between the skin layers: Vesicle, bulla, pustule, cyst
  - Loss of skin surface: Fissure, erosion, ulcer
  - Material on the skin surface: Crust, scale, peel
  - Vascular: Petechiae, purpura, telangectasia
  - Other: Lichenification, atrophy, excoriation, scarring.
  - Eczema is a complex morphology, but is very common and may be:
    - Acute: Wet, red, vesicles, erosions, crusting
    - Chronic: Dry, lichenified, excoriations.
- Note the distribution of the lesions: Scalp, face, lips, mouth, trunk, body folds, limbs, hands and feet, nails. Some lesions also occur in particular arrangements such as:
  - Ring shaped (annular), for example tinea infection (ringworm), syphilis, urticaria
  - Clustered together, for example herpes simplex, shingles, insect bites
  - Linear (in a line), for example scars, warts, insect bites
  - Reticulate (in a network), for example erythema ab igne, lichen planus.

- If a diagnosis is not immediately apparent then the combination of history, morphological appearance, distribution and particular arrangements should enable a differential diagnosis to be made. For example:
  - Tender, reddish nodules on the anterior surface of the lower legs suggests erythema nodosum, of which the two most common causes to exclude are tuberculosis and streptococcal infection.
  - Involvement of the palms of the hands and soles of the feet suggests syphilis, tick-bite fever, or psoriasis.

Investigation

Take a blood test. Only two are generally needed: VDRL and HIV. All the allergy tests, such as IgE, RAST, eosinophil counts, are expensive and generally do not help one clinch a diagnosis.

Take a skin scraping. If considering a fungus infection, especially in persistent skin rashes, it is best to confirm a diagnosis prior to treatment. Scraping some of the scales from the rash with a glass slide onto another slide, and sending it to the laboratory, for addition of potassium hydroxide and microscopy, may help in the diagnosis. If scabies is considered, especially in persistent cases, the scraping must be made of the deeper layers of the skin, for example until bleeding points appear.

Take a photograph. Any average cell phone or digital camera will do. Natural light is best, without a flash. Remember to get the patient's consent. Send it via MMS or email attachment to a dermatologist associated with your work place, accompanied by a short history.

Take a skin biopsy. This is not for every rash, but certainly in persistent cases, where everyone is guessing, lots of treatments have been tried, and the patient is losing hope and spending money, a simple skin biopsy aids tremendously in making a proper diagnosis. The easiest method is a punch biopsy.

Assessment

The clinical diagnosis can quite often be placed into one of five major areas:

1. Infectious: Bacterial, viral, fungal, parasitic, spirochetes
2. Eczema: Atopic, contact, nummular, photosensitive, seborrhoeic, stasis
3. Drug related: Drug hypersensitivity syndrome, urticaria, Stevens-Johnson syndrome, fixed drug eruption, lichenoid reaction

4. Psoriasis: Plaque, erythrodermic, pustular, guttate, flexural (inverse)
5. Other: Acne, erythema nodosum, erythema multiforme, lichen planus, lupus erythematosis, vitamin deficiencies, tumours such as Kaposi's sarcoma or melanoma.

This is not an exhaustive list, but from the history and examination it is very useful to think in big categories, and make sure one quickly sifts through these major areas, and then pursues a management plan according to the most likely diagnosis, while awaiting blood or biopsy results.

Management

1. Treat a specific diagnosis, not a rash.
2. Remove any offending agents (tight boots, perfume), deal with stress, reassure and discuss skin hygiene (use basic soaps).
3. Arrest pruritis. Use high enough dosages of antihistamines for a long enough time period. Sometimes a month of high dosages is needed.
4. Use steroids in sufficient amounts and adequate potency for short periods of time, expecting results and then taper down, as opposed to low potency 1% hydrocortisone for extensive periods of time.
5. Be kind to the skin. Use liberal amounts of emulsifying ointment or aqueous cream, even occlusive dressings, not rubbing too hard, not scratching, and remember sunscreen.

Vaginal discharge

History and examination

The following information is important:

- Colour, any blood, smell
- Duration
- Associated symptoms such as lower abdominal pain, pruritus, fever
- Last menstrual period, contraception and possibility of pregnancy
- Patients perspective on the possibility of a sexually transmitted infection or causation
- Sexual partners, for example, new partners, unfaithful partners, intimate partner violence, and use of condoms
- Previous cervical smears and results, previous treatment for vaginal discharge or diagnosis of HIV.

The patient should be examined to confirm the presence of a discharge and to observe it directly. A speculum and bimanual examination should be routine and focus on:

- The appearance and origin of the discharge
- Appearance of the cervix and opportunity for a cervical smear
- Any cervical excitation tenderness or adnexal tenderness and masses
- Any uterine abnormalities or pregnancy
- Any other pathology such as genital ulcers, carcinoma or foreign bodies.

Physiological discharge

The physiological discharge is due to normal secretions from the cervix and vagina mixed with bacteria from the normal flora and shed epithelial cells. Patients with a white physiological discharge are otherwise asymptomatic. The discharge normally has a pH of 3.8 to 4.5, a wet slide with normal saline solution would show a few white cells, no clue cells and a predominance of lactobacilli seen as long rod shaped bacteria.

Increased physiological discharge occurs in:

- Puberty
- Pregnancy
- Women who do little physical exercise
- Menopause
- Ovulation
- Sexual stimulation.

Pathological discharge

Causes of pathological discharge are listed below. The ability to reach a reliable diagnosis based on the appearance of the discharge is poor. Discharge may be due to an overgrowth of the normal flora as in:

- Bacterial vaginosis
- Candida infection.

Discharge may be due to a sexually transmitted infection as in:

- *Trichomonas vaginalis* infection
- *Neisseria gonorrhoea* infection
- *Chlamydia trichomatis.*

A foreign body, such as a forgotten tampon, may present with a foul-smelling infected discharge.

Discharge that is often blood-stained may be a sign of carcinoma of the cervix or other less common carcinomas.

Oestrogen deficiency at the menopause may lead to a discharge from atrophic vaginitis.

A discharge may complicate pregnancy in the case of a threatened or inevitable abortion, premature rupture of membranes and in the post-partum period as lochia gradually reduces.

The commonest of the above pathological causes are bacterial vaginosis, trichomonas vaginalis and candida infection.

Bacterial vaginosis

The process seems to start with a decrease in lactobacilli, resulting in reduced production of peroxidase in the vagina thus increasing the vaginal pH. This allows the overgrowth of facultative anaerobic bacteria such as *Gardenerella vaginalis*, *Mycoplasma homonis*, *Mobiluncus* species and other anaerobes. The diagnosis is confirmed if three of the following are present:

- A grey–white vaginal discharge, which is sometimes foamy
- A positive amine or Whiff test (the detection of a fishy smell when a drop of 10% of potassium hydroxide is added to a drop of vaginal fluid)
- A vaginal pH > five (with no contamination from cervical mucus, blood or semen as they can all raise the pH)
- Clue cells (epithelial cells with a stippled appearance from being covered with bacteria) in a normal saline wet smear.

Trichomonas vaginalis **infection**

This is normally sexually transmitted, but can also be transmitted in other ways. The organism can survive in chlorinated swimming pools, hot tubs and tap water. Perinatal transmission is also possible, but beyond infancy its presence is strongly suggestive of child sexual abuse.

The clinical features include a malodorous, frothy green-yellow discharge. The diagnosis is confirmed by microscopically examining a normal saline wet smear. The organism is recognised by its characteristic jerky movements in 50-70% of the trichomonads.

Candida **vaginitis**

This is caused by *Candida albicans* in more than 70% of all cases. The infection is often linked to a predisposing cause such as HIV infection, diabetes, steroid therapy, malnutrition, pregnancy, menstruation, oral contraceptives, prolonged broad spectrum antibiotic use, immuno-suppressive medications and coitus. Most of these suppress immunity or alter the local environment in the vagina allowing *Candida* to become pathological.

Clinical features include an itchy, curd-like, cheesy yellow or white discharge adherent to the vulvovaginal mucosa leaving a raw bleeding surface when detached. Superficial dyspareunia is sometimes present. The pH is 4.5 or less. Infection under the foreskin of the penis of the sexual partner may also occur.

The diagnosis is confirmed by making a wet smear of the discharge with 10% potassium hydroxide where hyphae and spores are seen micro-scopically. Any predisposing cause should be considered.

Pelvic inflammatory disease

Pelvic inflammatory disease results from ascending infection that causes inflammation of the uterus and adnexa. It is a sexually transmitted disease caused by a mixture of organisms of which *Neisseria gonorrhoea*, *Chlamydia trachomatis* and anaerobes such as *Bacteroides* are the most common.

Symptoms include lower abdominal pain, fever, and foul smelling yellow purulent vaginal discharge. Examination may reveal a sick or ill-looking patient with a raised temperature, lower abdominal tenderness (or generalised tenderness due to peritonitis if a tubo-ovarian abscess has burst), and vaginal discharge from the cervical os. There is positive cervical excitation tenderness and a pelvic mass may be palpable in the posterior fornix.

Diagnosis is usually made clinically, but can be confirmed by pelvic ultrasound or laparoscopic examination. A cervical swab should be taken for microscopy, culture and sensitivity. Blood should be taken for culture and sensitivity if the patient is febrile.

Syndromic management

In primary care it may be difficult to reliably make a specific diagnosis as infections are frequently mixed, clinical features non-specific, time is limited and laboratory services far away. A syndromic approach to the initial management has therefore been recommended, which ensures the most likely causes are all treated simultaneously at the one visit. In patients suspected of having a sexually transmitted infection it is impor-tant to manage the patient holistically and not just prescribe medication. The following issues should be considered:

- Condoms should be used during treatment
- Contact tracing is needed to also treat the sexual partner(s)
- Counselling on safer sex, condom use, testing for HIV and syphilis
- Contraception needs
- Cervical cancer screening
- Completing all the treatment even if the symptoms improve quickly.

The syndromic approach to vaginal discharge and lower abdominal pain is shown in Figures 7.3 and 7.4. A follow up visit may be needed to ensure treatment is successful, continue counselling and to give the results of any investigations.

Figure 7.3 Vaginal discharge syndrome

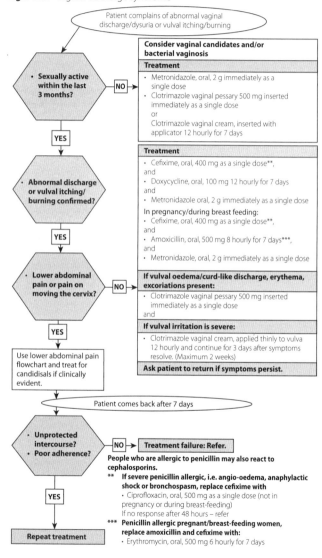

Patient complains of abnormal vaginal discharge/dysuria or vulval itching/burning

- **Sexually active within the last 3 months?** — NO →

Consider vaginal candidates and/or bacterial vaginosis

Treatment
- Metronidazole, oral, 2 g immediately as a single dose
- Clotrimazole vaginal pessary 500 mg inserted immediately as a single dose
  or
  Clotrimazole vaginal cream, inserted with applicator 12 hourly for 7 days

YES ↓

- **Abnormal discharge or vulval itching/burning confirmed?**

Treatment
- Cefixime, oral, 400 mg as a single dose**, and
- Doxycycline, oral, 100 mg 12 hourly for 7 days and
- Metronidazole oral, 2 g immediately as a single dose
In pregnancy/during breast feeding:
- Cefixime, oral, 400 mg as a single dose**, and
- Amoxicillin, oral, 500 mg 8 hourly for 7 days***, and
- Metronidazole, oral, 2 g immediately as a single dose

YES ↓

- **Lower abdominal pain or pain on moving the cervix?** — NO →

If vulval oedema/curd-like discharge, erythema, excoriations present:
- Clotrimazole vaginal pessary 500 mg inserted immediately as a single dose
and
If vulval irritation is severe:
- Clotrimazole vaginal cream, applied thinly to vulva 12 hourly and continue for 3 days after symptoms resolve. (Maximum 2 weeks)
Ask patient to return if symptoms persist.

YES ↓

Use lower abdominal pain flowchart and treat for candidisals if clinically evident.

↓

Patient comes back after 7 days

- **Unprotected intercourse?**
- **Poor adherence?** — NO → **Treatment failure: Refer.**

People who are allergic to penicillin may also react to cephalosporins.
** If severe penicillin allergic, i.e. angio-oedema, anaphylactic shock or bronchospasm, replace cefixime with
- Ciprofloxacin, oral, 500 mg as a single dose (not in pregnancy or during breast-feeding)
If no response after 48 hours – refer
*** Penicillin allergic pregnant/breast-feeding women, replace amoxicillin and cefixime with:
- Erythromycin, oral, 500 mg 6 hourly for 7 days

YES ↓

Repeat treatment

Figure 7.4 Lower abdominal pain

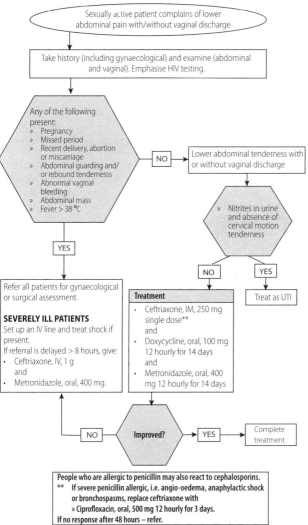

Dizziness

The history gives the most valuable information and it is helpful to initially categorise the patient into one of four possible diagnostic groups. History and examination can then proceed in a more focused way:

- Syncope: the patient feels as if they are going to faint
- Vertigo: the patient feels the world is spinning or rotating around them
- Disequilibrium: the patient feels as if they have lost balance in their legs
- Light-headedness: often ill-defined and cannot be clearly placed in one of the other categories.

Syncope

Typical symptoms usually precede a faint such as dizziness, unsteadiness, pallor, nausea, sweating, closing in of visual field or blurred vision. This leads to a collapse with brief loss of consciousness and then rapid spontaneous recovery. Syncope is due to insufficient cerebral blood flow. Occasionally syncope may lead to a brief tonic-clonic seizure that starts after the loss of consciousness.

Specific causes include:

- Simple faint due to a vasovagal reaction to some trigger such as pain, emotion, prolonged standing, heat and excess sweating, or insufficient fluid intake. The majority of people will experience a simple faint at some point and it does not indicate a serious disease. Some people also react to nausea and vomiting, micturition, defaecation or coughing. A few people may have oversensitive carotid sinuses that react strongly to pressure such as a tight collar when turning the head.
- Drug-induced syncope should always be considered. A wide variety of medication may induce syncope due to hypotension (for example antihypertensives), bradycardia (for example beta blockers) or predisposing to arrhythmia (for example erythromycin).
- Orthostatic syncope is due to loss of the reflex maintenance of blood pressure when standing up from a lying or sitting position. It can be due to prolonged bed rest, medication, diabetic autonomic neuropathy, or fever and dehydration. There is a more than 20 mmHg drop in systolic blood pressure on standing.
- Cardiac syncope is dangerous and typically presents during exercise with preceding palpitations or chest pain. It may be due to an arrhythmia (brady- and tachycardias), acute coronary syndrome, severe aortic stenosis, hypertrophic cardiomyopathy or cardiac

tamponade. Patients need urgent investigation and usually referral. Cardiac syncope is more common in the older adult or elderly.

- Hypovolaemia from any cause such as diarrhoea, diuretics or bleeding may present with syncope.

Vertigo

Vertigo presents with a strong sense of rotation, spinning and falling. Vertigo may be accompanied by ear-related symptoms such as tinnitus or deafness. Look for evidence of nystagmus and perform examination of the ear and neurological system:

- Vertigo arising from disease of the inner ear, for example benign positional vertigo, Meniere's disease and vestibular neuronitis fall into this category
- Vertigo arising from disease of the acoustic nerve, for example acoustic neuroma falls into this category
- Vertigo arising from disease of the brain stem or cerebellum, for example transient ischaemic attack or circulatory disturbance, multiple sclerosis and chronic alcohol abuse fall into this category
- Vertigo related to medication, for example toxicity from phenytoin or carbamazepine falls into this category.

Vertigo in the elderly is often multifactorial as degenerative disease of the vestibular system and other senses, circulatory disturbances and polypharmacy may co-exist.

Disequilibrium

Dizziness is actually experienced as a loss of balance and may be felt more in the legs than the head. Typical causes would be Parkinson's disease, peripheral neuropathy, following a stroke, loss of proprioception or cerebellar disease. A full neurological examination is required.

Light-headedness

Dizziness which is difficult to define is often related to psychological causes and is a common feature of anxiety disorders. Panic attacks may also include dizziness as an acute symptom. Look for hyperventilation, mental disorders and psychosocial stressors.

Ear pain

The main causes of a painful ear are:
- Local infection – pustule/furuncle
- Otitis externa – acute or chronic
- Acute otitis media
- Trauma, for example lacerations, barotrauma and perforation of the tympanic membrane
- Foreign body.

Otitis externa

Otitis externa is generalised inflammation involving the skin of the external auditory canal, including the surface of the tympanic membrane. The main contributing factors to acute otitis externa are trauma to the ear canal, for example by scratching with a finger or earbud, and moisture in the ear.

The diagnosis is usually fairly easy as the external canal is acutely inflamed, tender and weeping freely, it is extremely painful to handle and nothing can be seen of the interior of the canal without causing the patient pain. Glands in front and behind the ear may be inflamed.

Acute otitis media

Pain and hearing loss are the main symptoms of otitis media. The diagnosis is largely based on the red and inflamed appearance of the tympanic membrane. If the membrane perforates then pus may be discharged from the ear. Diagnosis of otitis media in infants and young children may be difficult because they are unable to articulate symptoms and a screaming child may also develop a red tympanic membrane. Infants may simply be unwell and pyrexial. Any child with an undiagnosed illness or pyrexia must have their ears examined.

Acute otitis media is an acute inflammation of the lining of the middle ear cleft and is usually preceded by an URTI. The most common organism cultured is *Streptococus pneumoniae*, followed by *Haemophilus influenzae* and *Moraxela (Branhamella) catarrhalis*. Viruses probably play an indirect role in the aetiology of acute otitis media. There are two peaks – one one at 6 to 12 months of age and another at school entry. Children with acute otitis media must be followed up to ensure there is no hearing loss. Success of treatment must be gauged by the degree to which the eardrum, tuning fork tests and hearing return to normal.

Children with acute OM should be referred if:
- There is no response to treatment after five days.
- A bulging drum is not responding to treatment after one day.

- There is incomplete resolution of acute otitis media.
- There is persistent middle ear effusion for three months after an attack of acute otitis media. Middle ear effusion: 70% of children will have an effusion present two weeks from the time of diagnosis, 40% at four weeks, with 10% having persistent effusions for three months or more.
- There is persistent apparent or proved deafness.
- There is evidence or suspicion of acute mastoiditis or other severe complications.
- Acute perforation of the tympanic membrane has not healed in six weeks.
- There is attic perforation and/or persistent discharge - suspected cholesteatoma.

Complications of acute OM include:
- Perforation of the tympanic membrane
- Serous otitis media (glue ear) may lead to impaired hearing and delayed speech and language development in pre-school children.
- Acute mastoiditis: Painful swelling and tenderness behind ear over the mastoid process. Urgent referral is needed.
- Chronic otitis media, usually with a persistent discharging ear and perforation. Cholesteatoma should be excluded.

Chest pain

Cardiac and respiratory problems are the focus of the initial diagnostic evaluation. After these problems are excluded, other conditions affecting structures in and around the thoracic cage enter into the differential diagnosis, for example, diseases of the oesophagus, upper abdomen, head, neck and chest wall.

Approach to assessment

Step 1: Emergency care

The initial step is to perform a focused history and physical examination, and consider doing an ECG, chest X-ray or cardiac biomarkers (serum troponin or if unavailable creatine kinase muscle brain isoenzyme (CK-MB)). The primary goal is to identify patients with potentially life-threatening causes for chest pain in whom **emergency care** is needed as shown in Figure 7.5. These patients need immediate hospitalisation and initiation of appropriate definitive treatment.

Figure 7.5 Categorisation of life threatening causes of chest pain

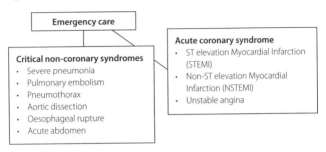

The pain's quality, location, radiation, temporal elements, provocative factors, palliative factors, severity and associated symptoms may assist in distinguishing ischaemic chest pain from non-ischaemic chest pain as shown in Table 7.10. It is important to remember that descriptions of chest discomfort due to myocardial ischaemia may differ depending on the patient's culture, gender, age and presence of co-morbid conditions such as diabetes.

Table 7.10 Characteristics of chest pain that increase/decrease likelihood of myocardial infarction (JAMA, 2005)

Descriptions increasing the likelihood of MI	Descriptions decreasing the likelihood of MI
Radiation to right/left/both arms or shoulders	Pleuritic
Exertional	Positional
Associated with sweating	Sharp
Associated with nausea or vomiting	Reproducible with palpation
Worse than previous angina or similar to previous MI	Inframammary location
Described as pressure	

Other important points in the history for emergency causes of chest pain include the following:

• Pain associated with a pneumothorax or a vascular event (aortic dissection/acute pulmonary embolism) classically has an abrupt onset with the greatest intensity of pain at the beginning. The onset of ischemic pain is more often gradual with an increasing intensity over time.

- Exertional dyspnoea is common when chest pain is due to myocardial ischaemia and may predate the sensation of angina.
- Syncope associated with chest pain should raise a concern for aortic dissection, pulmonary embolus, or critical aortic stenosis.
- Patients with chest pain who use cocaine are at increased risk of acute coronary syndromes.

Physical examination should be focused on the cardiac and respiratory systems, but the extent of the examination is primarily determined by the diagnoses that are being considered. The general appearance of the patient suggests the severity and possibly the seriousness of the symptoms. A full set of vital signs can provide valuable clues, for example a marked difference in blood pressure between the two arms suggests the presence of aortic dissection. A careful examination of the abdomen may be important, with particular attention to the right upper quadrant, epigastrium, and the abdominal aorta.

An ECG should always be performed when a diagnosis of acute coronary syndrome is suspected. A normal ECG markedly reduces the probability that chest pain is due to acute myocardial infarction, but it does not exclude a serious cardiac aetiology, particularly unstable angina. ECG findings must be considered in the context of the history and physical examination.

A chest X-ray is required when cardiac, pericardial, aortic, or pulmonary disease is considered.

Step 2: When emergency care is not needed

When the diagnosis of coronary heart disease (CHD) appears likely based on symptoms that are suggestive of angina and/or a history of cardiac risk factors (such as smoking, diabetes mellitus, hypertension, dyslipidaemia, family history of vascular disease, and obesity), the patient needs further evaluation. Consider performing additional investigations such as exercise stress testing, and starting outpatient treatment.

Step 3: When evaluation for CHD is negative

One also needs to consider alternative diagnoses for patients with chest pain who do not have CHD as reflected in Table 7.11.

If symptoms suggest a **respiratory aetiology** then evaluate the patient further for lower respiratory tract infection, tuberculosis, asthma, chronic obstructive pulmonary disease or bronchiectasis. More rarely lung cancer or other tumours may cause chest pain. HIV often underlies recurrent, severe or unusual respiratory infections.

If symptoms suggest a **musculoskeletal aetiology**, a trial of a NSAID is appropriate. Musculoskeletal chest pain is often insidious and persistent, lasting for hours to weeks. It is frequently sharp and localised to a specific area such as the xiphoid, lower rib tips, or midsternum, but may be diffuse and poorly localised. Pain may be reproducible on palpation or exacerbated by deep breathing, turning, or arm movement. Pain may also originate in the spine but radiate to the chest.

If symptoms suggest a **gastro-intestinal aetiology**, for example dyspepsia or heartburn, evaluate the patient for gastro-intestinal disease. This may initially involve a trial of acid suppression/and or endoscopic examination. Since the heart and oesophagus share a similar neurological innervation, it may be difficult to distinguish between chest pain due to myocardial ischaemia and that originating from the oesophagus. Oesophageal candidiasis is common in patients with HIV.

If symptoms suggest a **psychogenic aetiology**, evaluate the patient for psychosocial stress and mental problems such as an anxiety disorder or panic attacks.

Other **cardiovascular aetiologies** are possible and a recent history of infection, especially viral, may precede an episode of pericarditis or myocarditis.

Consider **chest anatomy** as a guide to other less common causes of non-life threatening chest pain including chest wall pain from herpes zoster or breast disease.

If **diagnostic evaluations are negative**, the patient probably has chronic idiopathic chest pain and you should consider referral to a pain management centre.

Table 7.11 Alternative diagnoses to CHD (JACC, 1999)

Non-ischaemic cardiovascular	Pulmonary	Gastro-intestinal
Aortic dissection	Pleuritis	Biliary
Myocarditis	Pneumonia and lower respiratory tract infections	Cholangitis
Pericarditis	Pulmonary embolus	Cholecystitis
	Tension pneumothorax	Choledocholithiasis
Chest wall	Acute asthma	Colic
Cervical disc disease	Exacerbation of COPD	Pancreatitis
Costochondritis	Lung cancer and other tumours	Peptic ulcer disease
Fibrositis		**Oesophageal**
Herpes zoster	**Psychiatric**	Oesophagitis
Neuropathic pain	Anxiety disorders (including panic attacks)	Spasm
Rib fracture	Depression	Reflux
Sternoclavicular arthritis	Unexplained somatic complaints	Rupture
Breast cancer		

Dyspnoea

Perform an immediate assessment and initiate emergency management

The assessment and management of the patient is based on a quick initial assessment and if necessary immediate emergency management.

Gather information

Once the patient is stable the family physician can pursue a definitive diagnosis and management. Shortness of breath has many different causes that can be related to the upper airways, lungs, heart and a variety of other problems. Specific information that may be useful includes:

- Duration and pattern of dyspnoea, for example asthma may be intermittent and recurrent, COPD persistent and progressive, or pneumonia of an acute onset

- Associated symptoms, for example cough, chest pain, wheeze, ankle swelling, fever, weight loss, night sweats, trauma, anxiety
- Severity of the dyspnoea, for example the New York classification of dyspnoea was developed to assess cardiac disease:
  - I – No dyspnoea from ordinary activity
  - II – Comfortable at rest, dyspnoea with ordinary activities
  - III – Less than ordinary activity causes dyspnoea, which is limiting
  - IV – Dyspnoea at rest, all activity causes discomfort.
- Past medical history such as respiratory (for example asthma, COPD, previous severe pneumonia and TB), cardiovascular (for example myocardial infarction, hypertension, cardiac failure or diabetes mellitus), HIV
- A history of smoking, substance use, medication and occupation may also be useful.

Clinical examination explores the differential diagnosis as shown in Figure 7.6. The presence of stridor, wheeze and crepitations can help categorise the possibilities.

Additional investigations may be performed depending on the differential diagnosis. These could include a chest radiograph, peak flow rate, electrocardiogram, sputum microscopy and culture, full blood count, urea and electrolytes, glucose, urinalysis, blood culture, pulse oximetry and arterial blood gases.

In South Africa causes of dyspnoea associated with HIV are common and are related to different stages of the diseases and CD4 counts. Causes include recurrent pneumonia and TB and with a CD4 count less than 200, *Pneumocystis* pneumonia, Kaposi's sarcoma as well as viral and fungal infections are all possible.

Figure 7.6 Algorithm for the differential diagnosis in shortness of breath

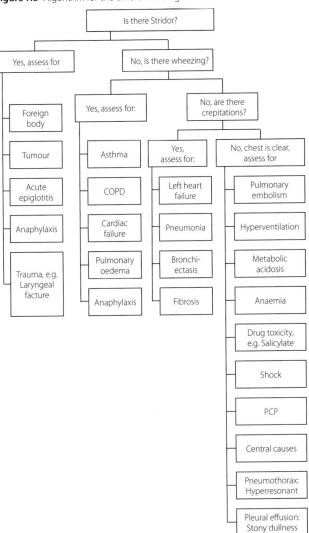

Does the patient need admission to hospital?

A patient presenting with any of the following signs should be referred to hospital:

- Temperature > 38 °C
- Systolic blood pressure < 90 mmHg or diastolic < 60 mmHg
- Pulse: > 110/minute or < 60/minute
- Respiratory rate > 30 breaths/minute
- Oxygen saturation < 90%/PaO_2 of 60 mmHg

The mnemonic CURB-65 has been used to identify patients with community-acquired pneumonia that requires admission and stands for:

- Confusion: Any altered mental state
- Urea > 7 mmol/l
- Respiratory rate > 30/min
- Blood pressure: Systolic < 90 mmHg and diastolic < 60 mmHg
- Age > 65 years

Make a specific diagnosis

Table 7.12 shows the typical features of specific conditions that may help you make a diagnosis. Once a specific diagnosis has been made then you can manage the patient accordingly.

Table 7.12 Key diagnostic symptoms and signs in a patient with shortness of breath

Clinical assessment	In favour: clinical symptoms and signs	
	Symptoms	Signs
1. Upper airway obstruction		
Foreign body/ choking	Occurred while eating History of foreign body inhalation Very sudden onset Grasping neck	Cyanosed Stridor
Anaphylaxis	History of previous anaphylaxis Exposure to food or medication prior to attack	Swollen neck/tongue Wheeze and stridor Urticaria Angio-oedema
Upper airway trauma	History of trauma to neck	Evidence of trauma

Clinical assessment	In favour: clinical symptoms and signs	
	Symptoms	Signs
Severe upper airway infection (pharyngeal abscess, diphtheria, peritonsillar abscess, epiglottitis)	· Sore throat · Barking cough	· Difficulty swallowing/ drooling · Stridor · Fever
Inhalation burns	· History of exposure to fire or smoke · Hoarseness, raspy cough	· Difficulty swallowing secretions · Burns around mouth and nose
2. Asthma	· Younger age group, · History of atopy (eczema, allergic rhinitis) · Family history of atopy · Intermittent dyspnoea, wheeze, cough (often nocturnal), sputum · Ask about triggers: cold air, exercise, emotions, allergens (house dust mite, pollen, animal fur), drugs (aspirin, NSAIDS), viral infection, acid reflux, occupation	· Reversible airway obstruction · Wheeze · Hyperinflated
3. COPD	· Older age group > 40 years often · History of prolonged smoking/TB · Persistent and progressive dyspnoea · Chronic productive cough	· Irreversible airway obstruction · Wheeze · Hyperinflated · Fever with exacerbation · Right-sided heart failure

Clinical assessment	In favour: clinical symptoms and signs	
	Symptoms	**Signs**
4. Cardiac failure	• Cough is non-productive or frothy • Orthopnoea, paroxysmal nocturnal dyspnoea, • Swollen ankles • History of hypertension, ischaemic heart disease, valvular heart disease, rheumatic fever or other underlying cause	• Signs depend on ventricle most affected: • RVF: Raised JVP, peripheral oedema, ascites, tender hepatomegaly • LVF: Bilateral basal fine crepitations, gallop rhythm, cool peripheries, hypotension, narrow pulse pressure, wheeze, displaced apex beat (LV dilatation), RV heave (pulmonary hypertension)
5. Pneumonia		
Bacterial/ viral	• Cough • Pleuritic chest pain • Rigors • Malaise • Purulent sputum • Haemoptysis • HIV positive	• Fever • Tachycardia • Bronchial breathing • Localised crackles • Consolidation • Pleural rub
***Pneumocystis jiroveci* pneumonia (PJP)**	• Dry cough • HIV positive	• Fever • Hypoxia • Chest mostly clear
Tuberculosis	• History of TB contact • Cough > two weeks duration • Weight loss, night sweats • HIV positive	• Signs of consolidation or cavitation, typically in upper lobes
Bronchiectasis	• Cough productive of copious yellow or green sputum • History of TB, recurrent infections • Worsening symptoms associated with infections	• Finger clubbing • Coarse crepitations

Clinical assessment	In favour: clinical symptoms and signs	
	Symptoms	Signs
6. Pulmonary embolism	· Abrupt onset · Pleuritic chest pain, haemoptysis, dizziness, syncope · Past or family history of thrombo-embolism · History of risk factors for thrombosis such as immobilisation and surgery	· Pyrexia, cyanosis, tachypnoea, tachycardia, hypotension · Increased JVP · Pleural rub or pleural effusion
7. Metabolic acidosis Diabetic ketoacidosis, lactic acidosis	· History of diabetes mellitus or renal failure · Prolonged use of anti-retroviral drugs especially stavudine (D4T) or ddI · Salicylate poisoning	· Rapid, deep and sighing respiration
8. Panic attack	· Sudden onset · No obvious underlying disease · Often young patient · Associated symptoms of anxiety such as numbness, tingling, light-headedness, nausea, palpitations, trembling, chest pain	· No localising signs
9. Pneumothorax	· Trauma, · Abrupt onset · Chest pain	· Unilateral increased resonance · Decreased breath sounds · Tracheal deviation · Displaced apex beat · Hypotension or weak pulse
10. Cardiac tamponade	· History of HIV/TB/malignancy	· Distant heart sounds · Distended neck veins · Tachycardia, weak pulse, pulsus paradoxis · Peripheral oedema (right heart failure)

Vaginal bleeding

A normal menstrual cycle takes 28 days, although some women may have a shorter cycle of 21 days. Bleeding may take five to seven days with total blood loss of approximately 40 ml. Deviation from normality is associated with the following terms:

a. Menorrhagia: excessive uterine bleeding in amount and duration that occurs at regular intervals
b. Metrorrhagia: uterine bleeding at irregular intervals
c. Menometrorrhagia: frequent irregular excessive bleeding
d. Oligomenorrhoea: infrequent irregular bleeding occurring at intervals of more than 45 days.
e. Post menopausal bleeding: any amount of vaginal bleed that occurs at least six months after the last normal menstrual period.

In their reproductive period, about 20% of women will present with problems related to abnormal uterine bleeding. Causes of abnormal bleeding are listed in Table 7.13.

Table 7.13 Cause of abnormal vaginal bleeding

Category	Specific examples
Pregnancy related	Spontaneous or threatened abortion Ectopic pregnancy Gestational trophoblastic disease
Hormonally related	Anovulation Excessive oestrogen intake / production
Vulvovaginal	Condylomata Cervical polyp Cervical cancer Cervicitis Trauma / sexual assault
Uterine	Fibroids Endometrial polyp Endometrial hyperplasia / carcinoma
Ovarian	Tumours
Systemic	Coagulopathy

History

Age: The probability of different conditions is age-related and should guide the diagnostic process. For example dysfunctional bleeding is more likely in younger patients and carcinoma more likely in older patients.

Pattern of bleeding: What is the normal menstrual pattern and when did it change? Is the bleeding regular (cyclical), irregular in anovulatory cycles or completely irregular (non-cyclical)? How much bleeding is there? For example is there only spotting or heavy bleeding with clots? How frequently must the patient change her sanitary wear?

Abdominal pain: Is there lower abdominal pain? Is the pain bilateral or unilateral? Is there usually dysmenorrhoea? Is there dyspareunia?

Family planning: What method of family planning is being used or when was it stopped?

Sexual history: Is the patient sexually active?

Infection: Are there any symptoms of infection? For example a temperature, vaginal discharge, dyspareunia or dysuria?

Past medical history: Previous pregnancies, previous pap-smears, other medical conditions or medication that could cause bleeding or interfere with family planning.

Stress: Is there a possible mental disorder or history of recent psychosocial stress?

Pregnancy: A pregnancy test should be performed. The question of whether the pregnancy is intrauterine or extrauterine (ectopic) should be considered.

General examination

Routine observations should include temperature, pulse and assessment of anaemia. A high temperature suggests infection, a tachycardia may suggest haemodynamic instability and severe blood loss, a blood pressure should then be taken, clinical signs of anaemia can be followed up by a finger prick haemoglobin determination (Hbg%) or full blood count. The abdomen should be examined.

Visualisation of the lower genital tract

A speculum examination of the lower genital tract should be performed. Confirm that the bleeding is really coming from the genital tract. Is the lower genital tract normal? The vulva, vagina and particularly the cervix should be inspected. A pap-smear should be taken. If bleeding excessively the blood can be gently cleaned from the cervix with a cotton swab. Macroscopic suspicion of a cervical cancer should lead to referral.

Bi-manual palpation

Is the upper genital tract normal? Consider:
- Pregnancy with enlarged uterus
- Ectopic pregnancy with unilateral tenderness, rigidity, mass and cervical excitation
- Inflammation with tenderness and cervical excitation
- Ovarian cysts or enlargement
- Fibroids with enlarged uterus.

If the upper and lower genital tracts are normal on examination then other causes should be considered. These can be considered as dysfunctional bleeding, side-effects of family planning (injectable progesterone, oral contraceptives, IUCDs) or more rarely endocrinopathies (polycystic ovaries with chronic anovulation, prolactinomas, thyroid disease, diabetes) and bleeding disorders (thrombocytopenia, liver disease, warfarin therapy).

Dysfunctional bleeding is common at the time of the menarche and menopause and occasional anovulatory bleeds can occur in all women. As a family physician don't forget the effects of psychosocial stress, weight loss and weight gain on the hypothalmic-pituitary-ovarian axis.

Assessment

Any identified specific cause should be treated. Patients with severe bleeding and anaemia may need to be referred immediately. If no cause is identified an empirical approach can be adopted. If three courses of empirical treatment are not successful then further investigation or referral should be made. The intra-uterine cavity should be explored, for example by pelvic ultrasound scan (intramural or subserosal fibroids, functional ovarium cysts, other ovarian tumours) or hysteroscopy (polyps, tumours, submucous fibroids) In older women an Endopap, Acurette or similar intra-uterine sampling device can be taken as an initial investigation of the intra-uterine cavity.

Medically unexplained problems

Many patients who present to primary health care services have no organic reason for their symptoms. Symptoms may include body pain, weakness or gastro-intestinal symptoms to mention but a few, for which no biological cause can be identified. The distress of these patients is often ignored and they are subjected to inappropriate and expensive investigations by doctors working from a purely biomedical perspective. Both the doctor and the patient can end up feeling frustrated and disillusioned.

Why do people develop unexplained symptoms?

Unexplained somatic symptoms are more common in those suffering from depression and anxiety or exposed to acute or chronic psychosocial stressors. The neuro-endocrine system mediates physical responses to emotions and psychological states and may help explain many of these symptoms. Psychosocial factors may also predispose people to disease, precipitate disease or perpetuate disease once it is established (Mayou, 2002).

Possible factors why specific people develop medically unexplained symptoms:
- Increased sensitivity to bodily sensations
- Being brought up in a family where physical, but not emotional problems, were given attention
- It may be easier to discuss physical rather than emotional symptoms
- Expectations that the doctor is interested in physical rather than emotional problems (which frequently is the case)
- Emotional strain may result in less tolerance of physical discomfort, so that sensations that are usually tolerated, take on more significance
- Defense mechanisms may result in a person focusing on a symptom in order to avoid focusing on another, more threatening issue.

Assessment

The following principles are adapted from McDaniel et al. (2002):
- **Explore both organic and psychosocial aspects in an integrated way from the beginning.** Ask about both physical and emotional factors in the initial history: "When did the headaches start to get worse?" "Do you remember what else was happening in your life around that time?" This communicates to the patient that equal respect will be given to them, no matter what the cause of the problem.

- **Screen for anxiety and depression.** Include questions to screen for depression and anxiety in your history. For example: "Do you feel sad or like crying for no reason?" "Are you thinking too much?"
- **Identify problems of living.** Be sensitive to cues, both verbal and non-verbal, and respond by giving the patient an opportunity to talk: "You look worried. Do you want to tell me what's on your mind?" The genogram can help you to identify stressors in the patient's life (see Chapter 4). It can also help you to identify supportive relationships. Common problems relate to alcohol, drugs, intimate partner violence, work, relationships, finances, fertility, fear of illness such as HIV, sexual problems or difficult living conditions.
- **Explore possible underlying trauma and hurt.** Patients with unexplained somatic complaints often have a history of abuse or other severe hurt in the past. One might gently ask "Is there anything that maybe you find difficult to talk about that might be affecting you?"
- **Acknowledge the physical symptoms.** Acknowledge the severity and the impact of the symptoms on the person's life. Once the patient feels that you have taken their physical symptoms seriously, they will be more open to ideas of causation.
- **Explain the symptom.** Explain the link between stress or emotions and physical symptoms: "The difficulties you have been facing in your life cause the muscles around your head to pull tight and that causes pain." Give other common examples of how the body expresses emotions, such as the heaviness on one's chest when one feels very sad.
- **Explore the meaning of the symptoms for the patient.** With some patients, one can move onto a metaphorical level by saying: "What do you think this headache is trying to tell you?" "You describe it as a heavy pain. Are there times when you feel that everything seems to be weighing down on you?"
- **Make use of the expertise of the patient.** "What do you think would have to happen in order for the headaches to get better?"
- **See the patient regularly.** This is necessary even when they are free of physical symptoms, if you feel that the symptoms are based on a need for contact. In this way, attention is independent of the patient's physical complaints.
- **Do not be discouraged by the persistence of symptoms or presentation of new ones.** Judge progress in terms of how the patient functions at work or in the home rather than in terms of the symptoms.

- **Avoid unnecessary investigations or referral, but do take symptoms seriously.** Remember that people with unexplained symptoms also get organic illnesses.
- **Advise on relaxation and recreation.** Deep-muscle relaxation, physical exercise, and planning pleasurable activities may all help. Anxiety can cause hyperventilation, which results in symptoms such as dizziness and tingling in the fingers. These symptoms then worsen the anxiety. Deep-breathing exercises are calming. They should be practised regularly to prevent tension and also when the patient is experiencing anxiety:
  - Breathe slowly through the nose for the count of three seconds.
  - Slowly breathe out through the mouth to the count of three seconds.
  - Pause for three seconds before breathing in again.

  Abdominal breathing is the most relaxed kind of breathing. Place a hand on the abdomen to feel it move as you breathe.
- **Cognitive techniques are helpful.** Refer for cognitive therapy if possible. You can also help the patient to replace negative thinking patterns and self-talk with a more positive approach to avoid the downward spiral of negative thoughts and feelings.

Further reading

Handbook of Dermatology for Primary Care, 2nd ed. Saxe, Jessop, Todd. A little pocket booklet produced by the Division of Dermatology, University of Cape Town (UCT). An excellent book to read through, just looking at many pictures of common skin conditions, with a short description of each.

8   Managing common conditions

This chapter outlines the management of common diagnoses in primary care. Diagnoses have been chosen in terms of the burden of disease and what actually presents in ambulatory primary care (see Chapter 1). In addition, a number of diagnoses have been included because they are common, but often missed, such as intimate partner violence, depression and alcohol use disorders. Finally two broader areas, disability and palliative care, that are common and require a slightly different approach to management are also described.

HIV and AIDS

The National Department of Health has written guidelines for the management of HIV/AIDS in adults and adolescents, children, and pregnant women (DOH, 2010). However, this handbook does not have the scope to cover all of the guidelines and, instead summarises the key issues of a three-stage management plan. A three-stage assessment is particularly relevant in gaining an understanding of the person living with HIV.

HIV testing

HIV is a manageable, chronic illness, which requires early diagnosis so that patients receive optimal care and so that transmission can be prevented. Early diagnosis requires testing large populations. Limited HIV testing was previously justified in the context of absence of treatment, and the huge stigma associated with the diagnosis. The trend now, however, is towards simpler, provider-initiated testing that can be incorporated into routine consultations and which might help to de-stigmatise the disease (Cameron, 2009). A more streamlined approach to testing, with the acronym ACTS (Advise, Consent, Test, and Support), is being promoted and is estimated to take five minutes or less. This allows HIV testing to be incorporated into routine consultations and provides more time for intensive counselling and support for HIV-positive patients. The four steps of ACTS are shown in Figure 8.1.

In children younger than 18 months, the HIV ELISA or HIV rapid test may be positive because of the presence of maternal antibodies and so the HIV DNA PCR test is instead used to confirm a diagnosis.

Figure 8.1 HIV testing using the ACTS approach

HIV TESTING IS FOR **EVERYONE**

A — ADVISE

- **Advise all clients to have an HIV test today**
  - If they decline, respond to concerns and motivate with benefits of testing
  - If HIV negative, client can learn how to stay negative
  - If HIV positive, client can get the care needed to stay healthy
- **If HIV positive, ensure that client is in care**
  Ask client about questions/concerns and if ready to get an HIV test

C — CONSENT

- **Explain consent:** they can only be tested for HIV if they give permission by signing the consent form
- **Explain confidentiality:** no one outside of the health team will be told about their HIV test or status without their permission
  Have client sign the consent form

T — TEST

- **Explain testing procedure:**
  - Finger prick to test a drop of blood for HIV
  - Results of test ready in approximately 15 minutes
- **If first test is positive, explain need for confirmatory test**
  Perform rapid test or take client to nurse for finger prick

S — SUPPORT

Give test result ▶ Allow time to react ▶ Respond to concerns and support

Client HIV negative	**Client HIV positive**
• You tested HIV negative today	• You tested HIV positive today, which means you have HIV infection
• What will you do to stay negative? **Discuss prevention options:**	• Coping
• Abstain; don't have sexual intercourse	• Ask about & respond to client's concerns
• Be faithful to one or reduce number of partners	• Reassure client; knowing status can save their life
• Condomise correctly **EVERY TIME** you have sex	• Living positively
• Encourage partner testing and condomising	• Explain importance of knowing CD4 & HIV Stage
• Get tested again every year or sooner	• Stress importance of returning for CD4 results to find out if they need ARVs
If you have: STI, new partner, unsafe sex, fall pregnant or if you become sick	• Protect your health & your partner
Ask client if they have any questions	• Avoid re-infection by HIV or new STIs
	• Use condoms **EVERY TIME** you have sex
	• Encourage partner testing & condomising
	• **Obtain blood for CD4 test and do HIV staging**
	• **Assess if client needs further counselling**
	• **Verify 2+ contacts for recall**

NURSES CAN FOLLOW THESE 4 STEPS DURING EVERY CLINICAL VISIT

1 Determine reason for client's visit ▶ **2** Start ACTS. If client consents, begin the testing process ▶ **3** Provide service per reason for visit ▶ **4** Give HIV result & support per above

SOURCE: SA ACTS   www.ACTSHIVTEST.org.za

Clinical assessment and plan

The following clinical issues should be considered when consulting with a patient who is newly diagnosed with HIV:

- What is the clinical stage of HIV infection (see Table 8.1)? What is the CD4 count? The following patients are eligible for ART (see Table 8.2):
  - CD4 count ≤ 200 cells/mm^3 irrespective of clinical stage
  - CD4 count ≤350 cells/mm^3 (in patients with PTB or pregnant women)
  - WHO stage IV irrespective of CD4 count
  - MDR/XDR-TB irrespective of CD4.
- Does the patient have any current opportunistic infections or diseases (see Table 8.1)? Check for signs and symptoms of TB at every consultation.
- What prophylaxis (such as co-trimoxazole or INH) should the patient be taking? Is nutritional support needed?
- What preventative interventions are recommended, such as cervical smears?
- Are lifestyle changes being made? This includes diet, exercise, avoidance of smoking, alcohol and other harmful substances, and safe sex to prevent re-infection.

The following issues should be considered in a patient taking ART:

- Is any routine monitoring required to evaluate treatment efficacy or potential adverse effects of treatment? Is treatment effective (for example clinical response, CD4 count and viral load)? Review results of routine safety monitoring (for example renal or liver function and anaemia).
- Is the patient experiencing any adverse effects of treatment, for example reduced renal function in patients taking tenofovir; hyperlactataemia, particularly in patients on regimens containing stavudine or didanosine (including unexplained weight loss, abdominal symptoms or dyspnoea); peripheral neuropathy; lipoatrophy; lipodystrophy; hepatitis; skin rash?
- Is the patient adhering to the treatment programme?.
- Are there any symptoms or signs suggestive of TB? Have they developed any new signs or symptoms of other opportunistic infections, including immune reconstitution syndromes?
- Can prophylaxis be stopped if the patient's immune system has improved sufficiently?

Table 8.1 WHO clinical staging of HIV disease in adults and adolescents

Clinical stage 1

1. Asymptomatic
2. Persistent generalised lymphadenopathy

Clinical stage 2

1. Moderate unexplained weight loss (under 10% of presumed or measured body weight)
2. Recurrent respiratory tract infections (sinusitis, tonsillitis, otitis media, pharyngitis)
3. Herpes zoster
4. Angular cheilitis
5. Recurrent oral ulcerations
6. Papular pruritic eruptions
7. Seborrhoeic dermatitis
8. Fungal nail infections

Clinical stage 3

1. Unexplained severe weight loss (over 10% of presumed or measured body weight)
2. Unexplained chronic diarrhoea for longer than one month
3. Unexplained persistent fever (intermittent or constant for longer than one month)
4. Persistent oral candidiasis
5. Oral hairy leukoplakia
6. Pulmonary tuberculosis
7. Severe bacterial infections (for example pneumonia, empyema, meningitis, pyomyositis, bone or joint infection, bacteraemia, severe pelvic inflammatory disease)
8. Acute necrotising ulcerative stomatitis, gingivitis or periodontitis
9. Unexplained anaemia (below 8 g/dl), neutropenia (below 0.5 x 109/l) and/or chronic thrombocytopenia (below 50 x 109/l)

Clinical stage 4

1. HIV wasting syndrome
2. *Pneumocystis jiroveci* pneumonia
3. Recurrent severe bacterial pneumonia
4. Chronic herpes simplex infection (orolabial, genital or anorectal of more than one month's duration or visceral at any site)
5. Oesophageal candidiasis (or candidiasis of trachea, bronchi or lungs)
6. Extrapulmonary tuberculosis
7. Kaposi's sarcoma
8. Cytomegalovirus disease (retinitis or infection of other organs, excluding liver, spleen and lymph nodes)
9. Central nervous system toxoplasmosis
10. HIV encephalopathy
11. Extrapulmonary cryptococcosis including meningitis

12. Disseminated non-tuberculous *Mycobacteria* infection
13. Progressive multifocal leukoencephalopathy
14. Chronic cryptosporidiosis
15. Chronic isosporiasis
16. Disseminated mycosis (histoplasmosis, coccidiomycosis)
17. Recurrent septicaemia (including non-typhoidal *Salmonella*)
18. Lymphoma (cerebral or B cell non-Hodgkin)
19. Invasive cervical carcinoma
20. Atypical disseminated leishmaniasis
21. Symptomatic HIV-associated nephropathy or HIV-associated cardiomyopathy.

SOURCE: Revised WHO clinical staging and immunological classification of HIV and case definition of HIV for surveillance. 2006.

Table 8.2 Standardised national ART regimens for adults and adolescents

1st line		
All new patients needing treatment, including pregnant women	TDF + 3TC/FTC + EFV/NVP	For TB co-infection EFV is preferred. For women of child bearing age, not on reliable contraception, NVP is preferred
Currently on d4T based regimen with no side-effects	D4T + 3TC + EFV	Remain on d4T if well tolerated. Early switch with any toxicity. Substitute TDF if at high risk of toxicity (high BMI, low Hb, older female)
Contraindication to TDF – renal failure	AZT + 3TC + EFV/NVP	
2nd line		
Failing on a d4T or AZT based 1st line regimen	TDF + 3TC/FTC + LPV/r	
Failing on a TDF based 1st line regimen	AZT + 3TC + LPV/r	
Salvage		
Failing any 2nd line regimen	Specialist referral	

Notes: 3TC Lamuvidine; AZT Zidovudine; d4T Stavudine; EFV Efavirenz; FTC Emtricitabine; LPV/r Lopinavir, Ritonavir; NVP Nevirapine

Individual assessment and plan

General principles for counselling patients with HIV are as follows (Baumann, 1998):

- Help the patient with HIV/AIDS to feel in control. Provide information so that the patient can make their own decisions.
- Encourage the patient to maintain a healthy self-esteem. Help the patient to build on the positive, to challenge comments and behaviour that erode self-efficacy, and to counter negative reactions from others.
- Encourage the patient to continue to find meaning in their experience.

The role of the counsellor is not to have all the answers, but rather to guide people to reach their own decisions with the provision of relevant and accurate information. Provide a collaborative, empathic, confidential, non-judgmental, and respectful environment in which patients can explore their feelings and make their own decisions. The goal is not just to make the person feel better, but rather to help the person to gain confidence and skills for assuming, rather than avoiding, responsibility.

With the initial diagnosis of HIV the patient may be asymptomatic, but experience stages of grief regarding loss of their healthy self. They face the challenge of accepting the diagnosis, and disclosing the diagnosis to others. They may fear the effects of disclosure - stigma, rejection and economic consequences. Emotions may include fear, guilt, anger, depression and anxiety. They may struggle with the meaning of the illness in terms of their spiritual beliefs.

The Health Profession's Council of South Africa (HPCSA, 2010) has ethical guidelines for good practice with regard to HIV and guidelines on how to approach ethical dilemmas are given in Chapter 12.

Contextual issues

Patients can apply for a temporary disability grant if they are too ill to work and they have not yet stabilised on ART. A person caring for a patient with HIV/AIDS can apply for a grant-in-aid. Patients with irreversible complications of HIV/AIDS, or concurrent disability, may need a permanent disability grant.

The Employment Equity Act (1998) prevents discrimination against employees on various grounds, including HIV status.

Include family and friends in your management plan wherever possible. Explore who else in the family needs to know about the HIV, assist with disclosure and testing of partners or children.

Consider referring the patient to support groups in the community which may offer social and practical support. Consider home-based care or referral for palliative care in advanced disease or if the family is having difficulty caring for the patient.

Pulmonary tuberculosis

In order to have an impact on the TB epidemic, an 85% cure rate for smear-positive patients and a 70% case detection rate needs to be achieved. Cure rates lower than 85% may worsen the epidemic, as patients who are not cured will remain infectious for longer.

TB testing

Obtain one sputum sample immediately and one sample the following morning. However, if the patient is unable to return the following day, take two sputa samples, one hour apart, on the same day. The sputa are tested for acid-fast bacilli on microscopy. If one sputum sample is positive for acid fast bacilli (AFB), treat the patient for TB.

In addition, culture and sensitivity of the sputa should be requested if the person has had TB previously, is a contact of a patient with MDR/XDR, is a health worker or is in prison.

If both sputa are negative, treat with antibiotics, encourage an HIV test and follow up until symptoms have resolved. If the patient is HIV positive or symptoms are not resolving, then send a third sputum sample for AFB and culture and do a chest X-ray. The decision to treat is then made based on the chest radiograph and clinical rationale, while awaiting the culture results.

Clinical assessment and plan

Medication: Prescribe medication according to the latest regimens as per the National TB programme (see Table 8.3). If the patient has HIV:

• Continue with routine HIV care
• Ensure that the patient is on co-trimoxazole prophylaxis
• Give pyridoxine 25 mg daily (protection against neuropathy)
• Consider if eligible for ART (see HIV on page 251).

Smoking: Counsel the patient to quit smoking as this worsens the TB outcome.
Nutrition: Encourage a healthy diet and if the BMI is 18.5 or less, refer for nutritional support.
Stopping excess alcohol will aid nutrition and adherence with medication.
Family planning: Combined oral contraceptive should contain at least 0.05 mg ethinyloestradiol. Shorten pill free interval to four days. Give injectable contraceptives at shorter intervals – medroxyprogesterone acetate 150 mg, eight weekly, norethisterone enanthate 200 mg, six weekly. If available, consider IUD.

HIV testing: All patients diagnosed with TB should be offered an HIV test.
Arrange follow up and safety netting: Ensure that the patient is warned to return if symptoms worsens or they develop side effects of medication (see Table 8.4).

Table 8.3. TB treatment for adults and children > 8 years (DOH, 2009)

	Intensive phase	Continuation phase
New patients	Isoniazid, rifampicin, pyrazinamide and ethambutol for 7 days a week for 2 months	Isoniazid and rifampicin for 7 days a week for 4 months
Retreatment patients	Isoniazid, rifampicin, pyrazinamide and ethambutol for 7 days a week for 3 months Streptomycin injections for 7 days a week for first 2 months.	Isoniazid, rifampicin and ethambutol for 7 days a week for 5 months

Table 8.4 Approach to the management of side effects of TB drugs (DOH, 2009)

Minor symptoms	Drug(s) responsible	Management
Anorexia, nausea, abdominal pain	Rifampicin	Continue TB drugs. Give tablets last thing at night
Joint pains	Pyrazinamide	Continue TB drugs. Aspirin.
Burning sensation in feet	Isoniazid	Continue TB drugs. Pyridoxine 25 mg daily
Orange / red urine	Rifampicin	Continue TB drugs. Reassurance
Major symptoms	**Drug(s) responsible**	**Management**
Skin itching / rash (anaphylactic reaction)	Streptomycin	Stop streptomycin. Treat as for hypersensitivity reaction
Deafness (no wax on examination)	Streptomycin	Stop streptomycin
Dizziness (vertigo and nystagmus)	Streptomycin	Stop streptomycin if severe
Jaundice (other causes excluded)	Most TB drugs	Stop TB drugs until jaundice resolves, then re-introduce one by one.
Vomiting and confusion (suspected drug induced pre-icteric hepatitis)	Most TB drugs	Stop TB drugs, urgent liver function tests
Visual impairment	Ethambutol	Stop ethambutol
Generalised reaction, shock, purpura	Rifampicin	Stop rifampicin

Individual assessment and plan

Ensure understanding of the illness, and the management and the importance of adherence for the full duration of treatment – even when the patient feels well. Elicit and discuss the patient's concerns about the illness and management.

• Hear the patient's concerns: "How do you feel about being told that you have TB?"
• Explore potential barriers to adherence: "What do you think will be most difficult about taking medications every day for the next six months?" Most patients are able to predict their own adherence accurately, taking their lifestyles, habits, and past experience into account (Hausler, 2000). Ask about the patient's plans for the next six months. If they plan to move or to be away for a significant time, they will need a letter to transfer to a different clinic. When patients don't take their medication, avoid judging and blaming. Rather explore the reasons and plan accordingly.
• Discuss options for Directly Observed Treatment (DOT). Patients should be allowed to choose who they would like to supervise their treatment. It could be the clinic nurse, an employer, a community health worker, a family member, or a teacher. Make plans together and ask questions such as: "Who would you like to help you with your tablets?" "How will you remember to take your tablets later, when you are feeling well?" DOT has been criticised for being paternalistic and undermining the patient's autonomy. To minimise this, introduce it in a way that focuses on the needs of the patient. Give patients information that allows them to feel more in control, rather than passive recipients of therapy. Listen to their experience of their disease and of treatment and be responsive to any difficulties.

Contextual assessment and plan

• Screen household contacts who are symptomatic, five years or younger, or HIV positive.
• Notify the diagnosis using the standard form.
• What are the family or community beliefs around TB and its treatment? Ask how people at home will react to the diagnosis.
• Patients with drug responsive TB are no longer infectious after two weeks of treatment, but may need more time off work to recover – this has employement and financial implications.
• Enquire about social support. If inadequate, you might suggest a support group for patients or identify people in the community who can assist. Patients who are destitute, who are unable to access the

clinic, or who have no- one to care for them at home may require admission to a TB ward or hospital.

- Ask about the availability of food at home. Treatment taken on an empty stomach causes more side-effects. Supplements or food parcels may be necessary.

Children

The following combination can be used to make the diagnosis of TB:

- A history of exposure to a patient with infectious TB or confirmed infection with a positive Mantoux
- Symptoms of TB such as persistent cough, fever, failure to thrive, fatigue, night sweats or swollen neck glands
- An abnormal chest radiograph suggestive of TB.

The diagnosis can be confirmed by collecting a gastric aspirate, fine needle aspiration or induced sputum for smear and culture.

Any child under the age of five years, who has a positive Mantoux test or close TB contact, without TB disease, needs prophylaxis with isoniazid.

Sexually transmitted infections (STIs)

The syndromic approach to STIs means that treatment is directed towards syndromes such as urethral discharge or genital ulcers rather than the specific causative organisms. It is advocated in primary care because:

- One cannot make a reliable bacteriological diagnosis based on clinical findings
- STIs are common and transmissible, and can result in serious complications
- Diagnostic tests are difficult to provide at the primary care level due to the fastidious nature of the organisms, distance from the laboratory and the need for special equipment
- Treatment can be provided at the same visit rather than delayed while waiting for test results
- Symptoms are often caused by multiple infections simultaneously.

Disadvantages of the syndromic approach are:

- Overtreatment of some patients
- Possible development of resistance from widespread use of antibiotic cocktails

- Misdiagnosis of STI in some patients with possible social consequences for relationships and families.

Clinical assessment and plan

Management protocols are available in "Standard Treatment Guidelines and Essential Drugs List" published by the National Department of Health, South Africa (2008). The treatment recommendations for lower abdominal pain, vaginal discharge are shown in Chapter 7, and for male urethritis syndrome and genital ulcer in Figures 8.2 and 8.3. It is important to explain that all the treatment should be taken even if symptoms rapidly improve. Pay attention to any issues which may have an impact on adherence, such as potential side-effects. All patients with an STI should be offered testing for HIV and syphilis.

Individual assessment and plan

The importance of treatment and the sensitive nature of the illness makes it especially important that people with STIs are treated with acceptance and respect. For many people the diagnosis of a STI is a traumatic experience, as it requires questioning the faithfulness of one's partner or having one's own faithfulness confronted. The patients' perspective in terms of their sexual behavior should be explored in order to reduce their future risk of STIs.

Abstaining from sex or being faithful to one partner who is uninfected and not at risk will prevent STIs (including HIV). Reducing the risk of STIs can focus on the following four 'Ps':

- Partners (reduce the number of partners, avoid concurrent partners, avoid high-risk partners who have multiple partners or other risky behavior such as IV drug abuse)
- Protected sex (use condoms correctly)
- Practices (avoid high-risk practices such as sex during menstruation, anal sex, dry sex, sex under the influence of alcohol or drugs, sex when there are sores or abrasions on the genitalia)
- Prompt treatment of STIs.

Common reasons for not using condoms (Myer, 2005, Mash, 2010):

- Condoms can be uncomfortable, awkward and result in decreased sensation, especially if not used skillfully
- Unequal power differentials between the sexes limit the ability of women to insist on condoms as men often make sexual decisions
- Younger women with older partners, on whom they depend for

material support or gifts, may be afraid that he will leave if she asks him to use a condom
- Women may also be afraid of a violent response if they ask men to use a condom
- Lack of negotiating skills or cultural ability to talk about sexual matters openly
- Use of or arguing for condoms implies that you are promiscuous or that you are dirty and infected
- Condoms are seen to signify a lack of trust and love in the relationship and therefore one should not use condoms if you are really in love
- Belief that the partner is monogamous or that you are not at risk – this concept of invulnerability is especially common with teenagers
- In some religions using condoms is seen as a sin
- Accessibility of condoms. Although condoms are available free in public sector clinics, they tend to be placed in public places and people feel embarrassed to be seen taking them. Young women asking for condoms at clinics feel intimidated by the disapproval of the staff. Despite findings that the availability of condoms at schools does not promote sexual activity, there are virtually no schools in South Africa where condoms are freely available.

Contextual issues

It is important to manage all sexual contacts in order to prevent re-infection of the patient and further spread of infections in the community. Contacts will often not attend for treatment spontaneously as their infection may be asymptomatic and active tracing is therefore required.

Figure 8.2 Male urethritis syndrome (MUS)

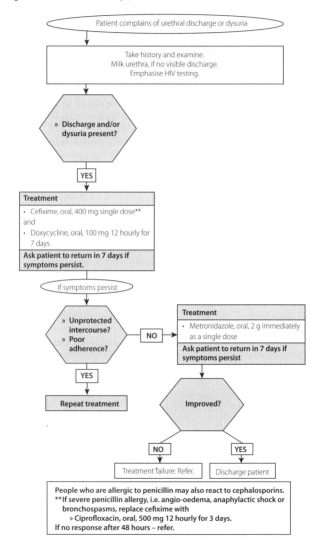

Figure 8.3 Genital ulcer syndrome (GUS)

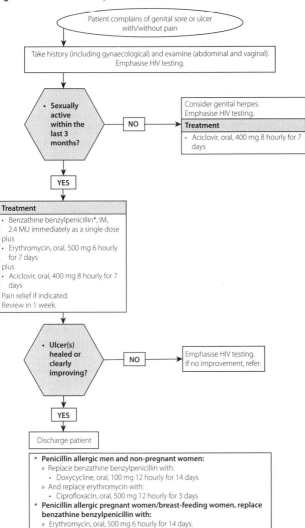

Intimate partner violence

Intimate partner violence (IPV) has been defined as a pattern of aggressive and coercive behaviour that involves a current or former intimate partner in a dating, married, or cohabiting relationship (Joyner and Mash, 2010). Abuse may be experienced in many forms including physical, emotional and psychological, verbal, environmental, social, financial, sexual, ritual, and religious/spiritual abuse (Cherniak, *et al.*, 2005: 368).

Identify the abuse

Abused women are often reluctant to disclose the problem to health workers spontaneously. The following cues should raise the index of suspicion (Joyner and Mash, 2010):

- Vague non-specific symptoms
- History of mental problems or psychiatric medication
- Fatigue, sleep problems, unexplained somatic complaints
- Symptoms of depression
- Feeling anxious/dizzy/thinking too much
- Chronic pain syndromes
- Repeated sexually transmitted infections
- Assault or trauma
- Suspected alcohol or substance abuse.

Direct questions can then be asked sensitively: "Are you unhappy in your relationship?" "Do you sometimes feel unsafe with your partner?" "Has your partner ever hurt you?"

Patients should feel that they will be believed and that the family physician will consider their problem important. The patient must feel safe so you should ensure confidentiality and privacy.

Clinical management and plan

- Check for sexually transmitted infections/HIV
- Care for injuries and ensure adequate forensic documentation (use J88)
- Check for pregnancy, offer contraception, termination and/or sterilisation as appropriate.

Individual assessment and plan

- Listen attentively to your patient's story.
- Screen for mental problems such as anxiety disorders, depression, substance abuse, or post-traumatic stress disorder.
- Offer follow-up counselling and support.
- Listen and believe their experience of abuse. If you are critical or uncomfortable about what the patient says, they will hold back. Having one's story heard, in itself, can be therapeutic.

Assure the patient that they are not alone and are not to blame. Abused women often feel alone and abandoned. Abusers often isolate their partners from friends and family. The abuser may blame the spouse for provoking them. The patient may believe this. It is important to be firm and stress that perpetrators are responsible for their actions. Point out that there are many abused people in similar situations.

Defend the patients' right to live without fear of violence. The abused person often has very poor self-esteem and believes that they have no rights. Remind them that they have a right to live without fear of violence. No one deserves to be beaten no matter what.

Contextual assessment and plan

Refer to any or all of the following legal resources:
1. Family court for a protection order
2. Victim Empowerment Unit at police station for support
3. NPO sector for legal aid.

The Domestic Violence Act (1998) requires police to find the abused person a safe place to stay and help them to access medical care if necessary. They must inform the abused person of their legal options of laying a charge and/or applying for a protection order. They should supply the person with an application form and explain that a temporary protection order will come into effect as soon as it has been served on the abuser. If the order is contravened, the abuser will be arrested.

Assess her current social situation and future options. A formal risk assessment can assess her imminent risk of harm. Consider the following risk factors for imminent injury and death:
- Increasing severity and frequency of abuse
- An available weapon
- Threats to kill the patient, the children, or the abuser
- Previous attempts to kill the patient, the children, or the abuser
- A suicide attempt by the patient.

Help the patient plan for their safety. If it is not safe for them to return home, organise accommodation where they will be safe. Discuss plans for the patient to leave the abuser. Consider also any children that are involved and who may also be suffering or require maintenance payments.

Encourage the patient to seek help and support. LifeLine has the telephone numbers of shelters in different provinces. Women's groups such as NICRO offer group and individual counselling. Social workers can help with practical advice and counselling. Spiritual leaders may sometimes be of help.

Support the patient's decisions. This may be difficult for the family physician. No matter what the patient decides, the family physician needs to respect their autonomy and their reasons for making the choices they make, even if they are apparently self-destructive. They may decide to stay with the abuser, or leave and then return to the abuser again and again.

Respiratory tract infections

The appropriate medication for respiratory tract infections, according to the National Treatment Guidelines (2008), is summarised in Table 8.5.

Table 8.5 Treatment of respiratory tract infections in primary care

Respiratory tract infection	Medication recommended
Common cold and influenza	Paracetamol, decongestants, cough syrup
Tonsillitis and pharyngitis	Benzathine benzylpenicillin* IM, as a single dose or Phenoxymethylpenicillin* oral for ten days
Acute sinusitis	Amoxycillin* oral and paracetamol and oxymetazoline nose drops for five days
Uncomplicated acute bronchitis	Paracetamol, decongestants, cough syrup
Acute bronchitis with HIV	Amoxycillin,* paracetamol
Pneumonia in children	Amoxycillin,* paracetamol Refer if < two months

Respiratory tract infection	Medication recommended
Severe pneumonia in children	Oxygen, ceftriaxone IM and co-trimoxazole as single doses, and refer to hospital
Pneumonia in adult	Benzylpenicillin* IM stat and amoxycil-lin* for five days* Add erythromycin 500 mg QID for five days if no response after 48 hours Consider need to refer
Mild pneumonia in adult > 65 years or with other medical condition	Amoxicillin/clavulanic acid Amoxycillin, oral, for five to ten days Consider need to refer
Severe pneumonia in adult	Oxygen, ceftriaxone IV/IM, as single dose and refer to hospital
Pneumocystis pneumonia	Cotrimoxazole according to weight for 14-21 days Consider need to refer

*Erythromycin if allergic to penicillin

Malnutrition

South Africa faces a double burden of malnutrition with being under-weight a problem mainly present in children and being overweight a problem in many adults. The focus here, however, is on childhood malnutrition, because malnutrition in the first two years of life makes a significant contribution to childhood mortality and morbidity and has serious effects on brain development that affect intelligence and behaviour in later life. The immediate causes of malnutrition will be a combination of decreased nutritional intake (for example lack of food or resources to store food, illness and neuro-developmental problems), increased nutritional losses (for example diarrhoea, vomiting and malabsorption) or increased requirements for nutrition (for example fever and infection).

Prevention and early intervention

1. Weigh and measure children at each contact with a health facility. Plot their growth on the Road to Health charts and address poor growth or weight loss immediately.
2. Take a proper feeding history including what they eat, how often they

eat, how their food is prepared, how their food is stored, how their milk is mixed, and whether they eat from their own plate.

3. Identify conditions that predispose children to malnutrition (for example HIV, fever, chronic diarrhoea, mouth ulcers and oral thrush) and address them appropriately. Increase daily food intake.

4. Give extra food during the recovery period after illness.

5. Treat for worms and give vitamin A if this is due.

Clinical assessment and plan

Severe malnutrition presents with very low weight, visible severe wasting or oedema of both feet and is initially treated in hospital. Management is a multi-professional effort and may include the physician, clinic nurse, social worker, dietician, occupational therapist, physiotherapist, psychologist (behaviour modification) and sometimes speech therapist to help with feeding disorders.

1. Resuscitate the child if necessary as they are very prone to hypothermia, hypoglycaemia and septicaemia. Be careful not to overestimate dehydration.

2. Plot weight, height and head circumference on age-appropriate tables.

3. Detect immediate causes of malnutrition such as medical conditions which cause loss of appetite or discomfort with eating (such as TB, oral candidiasis and mouth ulcers), increase nutrient losses (such as diarrhoea, vomiting and malabsorption) or increase nutrient requirements (such as fever and infection). Neuro-developmental conditions such as cerebral palsy and encephalopathy may also make eating difficult.

4. Keep the child warm.

5. Treat infection aggressively with IV antibiotics, covering for both gram positive and gram negative organisms.

6. Give extra dosage of vitamin A according to age.

7. Give folic acid at 5 mg/day for 14 days.

8. Give multivitamins and minerals, particularly zinc, potassium and magnesium to fill depleted stores. Don't give iron until oedema and infections have cleared.

9. Give high-calorie milk and increase daily. F-75 is the starter formula. Start immediately after resuscitation and continue for two to seven days. Start with 120 ml/kg per day and increase daily with 10 ml/kg per day. As soon as the child is stable switch to F-100. When switching to F-100 keep the same volume for one day and then increase to the maximum of 200 ml/kg per day.

10. Address the social circumstances or refer to social worker. Make sure about grants.
11. Refer the child to a feeding scheme.
12. Expect weight gain of 10–15 g/kg per day.
13. Follow up regularly, ensure immunisations are up to date, and weigh at every visit.

Individual assessment and plan

Understand the family's perspective on the problem and any specific beliefs, concerns or expectations that they may have regarding nutrition, food or the child. Take a proper feeding history and refer to a dietician or nutrition adviser. Be respectful and supportive. Even among poor families different beliefs and feeding behaviour can make a difference to the development of malnutrition.

Contextual assessment and plan

Assess immediate social causes of malnutrition such as a lack of food in the house or inability to prepare or store food. Underlying this may be poverty with inadequate access to food, family dysfunction affecting the child or mother, a lack of access to health services or a poor environment that causes unhygienic water or poor sanitation. This may lead the family physician to think more broadly about the social determinants of malnutrition in the community they are responsible for.

Hypertension

The clinical management should be based on the latest South African Guidelines which were last published in 2006 (Figure 8.4).

Figure 8.4 South African Hypertension guidelines on when to initiate treatment

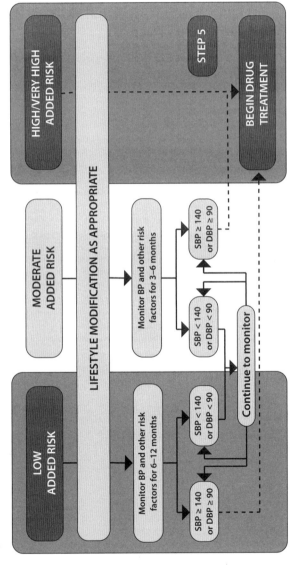

Check the blood pressure

Management decisions and lifelong treatment will be based on the blood pressure measurement. This measurement therefore needs to be as accurate as possible. A number of factors need to be taken into account:

- Is the BP machine accurate and recently calibrated?
- Are you using the correct size cuff? Using too small a cuff in an obese patient may produce an artificially high reading.
- Is the patient relaxed and sitting or lying down?
- Has the patient recently smoked tobacco, drunk caffeine or eaten a meal?
- Is there tight fitting clothing around the upper arm?
- Are you supporting the arm at the level of the heart?
- Have you considered the effect of white coat hypertension? Blood pressure increases when the patient sees the doctor and may decrease with repeated readings as they relax.

A diagnosis of hypertension is not made on the basis of one reading. A mildly raised blood pressure can be repeated at the next visit in a few weeks time, a moderately raised blood pressure can be repeated in a few days time and a severely raised blood pressure can be repeated in a few hours time.

Clinical assessment and plan

Look for other cardiovascular risk factors

In addition to the blood pressure reading, information on all cardiovascular risk factors should be obtained:

- Family history of premature cardiovascular disease (men < 55 years, women < 65 years)
- History of tobacco smoking
- Evidence of being overweight/obesity (BMI or waist circumference > 102 cm in men and > 88 cm in women)
- Dyslipidaemia (xanthoma, total cholesterol > 6.5 mmol/l or LDL-cholesterol > 4.0 mmol/l or HDL-cholesterol < 1 mmol/l in men and < 1.4 mmol/l in women)
- Diabetes mellitus (check blood glucose)
- Age (> 55 years in men and > 65 years in women).

Look for evidence of early target organ damage

If there is already evidence of early target organ damage then the cardiovascular risk is obviously increased:

- Heart: left ventricular hypertrophy on ECG
- Kidneys: microalbuminuria (if available)
- Kidneys: slightly elevated creatinine (115–133 µmol/l in men and
  07–124 µmol/l in women).

Look for evidence of associated clinical conditions

If there are cinical signs and symptoms of associated clinical conditions
then the need to treat is clear:

- Cardiac failure
- Ischaemic heart disease
- Peripheral vascular disease, for example bruits over carotid and renal
  arteries and poor peripheral pulses
- Chronic kidney disease, for example proteinuria, haematuria, raised
  creatinine and calculated glomerular filtration rate
- Stroke or transient ischaemic attack
- Advanced retinopathy, for example haemorrhages or exudates and
  papilloedema.

Assess the patient on overall cardiovascular risk

Table 8.6 shows how one can combine the information on risk factors,
target organ damage and associated clinical conditions with the blood
pressure to make an assessment of cardiovascular risk. The management
of the patient is based on this total risk assessment and not the isolated
blood pressure reading.

Table 8.6 Stratification of cardiovascular risk in four categories

	Blood pressure (mmHg)				
No other risk factors	Average risk	Average risk	Low added risk	Moderate added risk	High added risk
One to two risk factors	Low added risk	Low added risk	Moderate added risk	Moderate added risk	Very high added risk
Three or more risk factors, for example metabolic syndrome, subclinical organ damage or diabetes	Moderate added risk	High added risk	High added risk	High added risk	Very high added risk
Established cardiovascular or renal disease	Very high added risk	Very high added risk	Very high added risk	Very high added risk	Very high added risk

Low, moderate, high and very high risk refers to ten year risk of a cardiovascular fatal or non-fatal event. Added risk indicates that in all categories risk is greater than average. The dashed line indicates how the definition of hypertension may be variable, depending on the level of total cardiovascular risk.

Think about red flags for secondary causes

Most hypertension in primary care has no identifiable underlying disease – so-called essential hypertension, but in a small number of patients it is secondary to another diagnosis. The most common secondary cause is chronic kidney disease. Patients with secondary hypertension may be more refractory to treatment.

Look out for red flags that may indicate an underlying problem:
- Pre-existing renal disease (for example proteinuria, haematuria and raised creatinine)
- Co-arctation of the aorta (for example delayed brachial-femoral pulse and notching of ribs on chest radiograph)
- Conn's disease (for example unexplained low potassium)
- Phaechromocytoma (for example tachycardia, palpitations, anxiety and paroxysmal hypertension)
- Cushing's disease (for example central obesity, moon face, bruising and striae).

Treatment goals

Management of hypertension is individualised. The goals of treatment are as follows:

1. The primary goal of treatment is to achieve maximum reduction in the long-term total risk of cardiovascular disease.
2. This requires treatment of the raised BP *per se* as well as of all associated reversible risk factors.
3. BP should be reduced to at least below 140/90 mmHg and to lower values, if tolerated, in all hypertensive patients.
4. Target BP should be at least 130/80 mmHg in diabetics and in high or very high risk patients, such as those with associated clinical conditions (for example stroke, myocardial infarction, renal dysfunction and proteinuria).
5. In order to more easily achieve goal BP, antihypertensive treatment should be initiated before significant cardiovascular damage develops.

Medication

Drug therapy consists of using a step care approach by starting with a low dose thiazide diuretic and then adding drugs from other classes. The second and third steps include the addition of an ACE inhibitor and/or a CCB. However, there may be compelling reasons why one would use one class of drug in favour of these traditional steps as shown in Table 8.7. One would carry on adding drug therapy from other classes after increasing the drug dosage to the maximal tolerable dose until one gets good control.

Table 8.7 Compelling indications to start treatment with a specific class

Compelling indications	Drug class
Angina	Beta-blocker OR CCB (rate lowering preferred)
Prior myocardial infarct	Beta-blocker AND ACE (ARB if intolerant). Verapamil if beta-blockers contraindicated. If heart failure, see below.
Heart failure	ACE (ARB if intolerant) AND certain beta-blockers AND aldosterone antagonist For combination ARB and ACE Loop diuretics for volume overload
Left ventricular hypertrophy (confirmed by ECG)	ARB (preferred) OR ACE
Stroke: secondary prevention	Low-dose thiazide-like diuretic and ACE or ARB
Type-one or –two diabetes with or without evidence of microalbuminuria or proteinuria	ACE or ARB – usually in combination with a diuretic
Chronic kidney disease	ACE or ARB – usually in combination with a diuretic
Isolated systolic hypertension	Low-dose thiazide or thiazide-like diuretic or long-acting CCB

ACE = Angiotensin I converting enzyme inhibitor, ARB = Angiotensin II receptor blocker
CCB = Calcium channel blocker

Individual assessment and plan

Doctors frequently overestimate the adherence of patients to their treatment and do not spend enough time eliciting patient's ideas and beliefs on the seriousness of hypertension, risk of complications and effectiveness of treatment. Remember that patients with hypertension are often expected to take long-term medication when they do not feel ill, to prevent some theoretical future cardiovascular event. Time spent on understanding the patient's perspective and exchanging information will not be wasted.

Counselling should also address the following issues and a guiding style (see Chapter 5) is preferable:
- Weight reduction
- Dietary salt reduction
- Restricted alcohol consumption

- Limited total fat intake
- Increased fruit and vegetable consumption.
- Limited free sugars
- Increased physical activity (150 minutes per week of moderate intensity aerobic exercise)
- Smoking cessation
- Psychosocial stress.

Lifestyle modification is attempted first in those with mild added risk (for six to twelve months) and moderate added risk (for three to six months) before prescribing medication.

Contextual assessment and plan

Lifestyle issues may need involvement of the family. Reduction of psychosocial stress may also assist with adherence and reduction in blood pressure.

Refractory hypertension

It is not uncommon for patients on treatment to have uncontrolled hypertension. Before labelling the patient as refractory, increasing the dose or just adding another medication to the prescription consider the following:

- Did the patient take their medication today? Medication is often omitted when patients get up early to go to the clinic.
- Poor adherence to treatment is very common and may be due to many different factors. Try and have a respectful, curious, open and non-judgemental conversation about this. For example, the patient may not understand the importance of taking treatment, may have experienced side-effects, may not understand how to take the medication, may have concerns about the diagnosis or treatment, may have significant psychosocial problems, or may have not received all their treatment due to stock problems.
- Is the patient taking another medication that causes hypertension? For example patients are often prescribed NSAIDs. Prednisolone and hormonal medications may also interfere.

A patient not optimally controlled on three or more classes of antihypertensive drugs is classified as having refractory hypertension. In these patients one needs to exclude secondary causes of hypertension or refer the patient to a hypertensive expert.

Type-two diabetes

Patients with type-two diabetes typically suffer from a combination of high blood glucose, high cholesterol and hypertension which are associated with being overweight/obesity, unhealthy eating and physical inactivity (IDF Africa Region Task Group 2006).

Clinical assessment and plan

Medication

Biguanides (glucophage) reduce the production of glucose in the liver (gluconeogenesis) and allows glucose to enter muscle and fat cells more effectively (reduces insulin resistance). Glucophage is the first line treatment in most patients with type-two diabetes, especially those who are overweight. It should be used with caution in the elderly and the most serious potential side effect is lactic acidosis. Start at a low dose and increase three-monthly to the maximum dose of 2 g per day.

Sulphonylureas (for example glibenclamide and gliclazide) work mainly by stimulating the cells in the pancreas to make more insulin. Some may also help the insulin to work more effectively in the body. They can be first line treatment in those that are not overweight. Otherwise they are usually added when control remains poor on glucophage alone. They may cause hypoglycaemia and shorter-acting drugs such as gliclazide should be used in the elderly. Start at low dose and increase three-monthly to the maximum dose.

Failure to control the blood glucose on one type of medication should lead to combination oral therapy.

Insulin, however, is eventually needed in most type-two diabetes when the HbA1c remains above seven percent in patients taking maximal oral medication and attempting lifestyle modification. There are two options:

- Supplemental intermediate-acting insulin is given as a single injection at bedtime. Dose is (weight in kg) × 0.2 IU. This is added to combination oral therapy if control is poor. Glucophage can be continued and the sulphonylurea dose halved or stopped altogether.
- Substitution insulin treatment involves twice daily injections, before breakfast and before supper. A pre-mixed short/intermediate acting combination is usually used with the starting dose being 0.2 IU per kg split into two thirds in the morning and one third in the evening. Oral medications are usually stopped, but in the obese glucophage may be continued.

A variety of new medications are now available but due to cost are still not widely used in South Africa.

Control

Diabetic control should be monitored regularly at the clinic by:

- Measuring HbA1c, which is the best indicator of glucose control over the previous few weeks. The ideal target is less than seven percent. Fasting glucose is difficult to measure routinely and random glucose, although easy to measure, only gives information about control at the time it is measured. Random glucose should ideally be between four to eight mmol/l.
- Measuring blood pressure. The ideal target is < 130/80 mmHg.
- Measuring cholesterol and triglycerides. The ideal targets are total cholesterol less than 4 mmol/l, LDL-cholesterol less than 2 mmol/l, HDL-cholesterol greater than 1 mmol/l and triglycerides less than 2 mmol/l
- Waist circumference should ideally be less than 94 cm in men and less than 80 cm in women.

Ideal targets are often difficult to attain and individual targets should be set with the patient as even modest improvements in the measurements (such as a one percent drop in HbA1c) have substantial benefits in terms of the risk of complications.

Complications

The clinic should also regularly monitor the patient for signs of complications. If complications are detected early they can often be prevented or delayed. Table 8.8 summarises the routine activities that should be done (IDF Africa Region Task Group 2006). This requires a high level of organisation, teamwork and continuity of information.

Table 8.8 Guidelines for the routine care of diabetic patients

First visit (when diabetes is diagnosed)

Check the following:
- Weight, height and body mass index (BMI) (= weight in kg/height squared in m²)
- Waist circumference
- Urine for glucose, ketones, microalbuminuria/proteinuria
- Blood pressure
- Visual acuity and dilated fundoscopy (cataracts, retinopathy)
- Feet (pulses, peripheral neuropathy, infection, minor trauma)
- Mouth (gums and caries)

Do tests for:
- Fasting blood glucose
- HbA1c
- Cholesterol
- Creatinine (if proteinuria)

Management guidelines:
- Discuss lifestyle modification (diet, exercise, smoking); see dietician if possible
- Prescribe medication immediately if random blood glucose is higher than 15 mmol/l (if lower than this you may try lifestyle change alone before medication)
- Plan education programme; give educational material

Follow up visits (1- to 3-monthly or more frequently if necessary)
- *Assess, advise, assist and arrange*
- Assess concerns, problems or questions
- Assess clinical status and check blood glucose (fasting if possible)
- Assess adherence to medication and management plan
- Assess for any complications (e.g blood pressure, feet)
- Offer advice or share information (e.g. lifestyle choices)
- Review and agree on the management plan
- Assist patient to utilise health care team and community resources
- Think family
- Arrange further follow up

Annual check
- *Assess, advise, agree, assist and arrange*
- Review medical history

Check the following:
- Weight, BMI and waist circumference
- Urine for microalbuminuria/proteinuria
- Blood pressure
- Visual acuity and dilated fundoscopy (cataracts, retinopathy)
- Feet (pulses, peripheral neuropathy, infection, minor trauma)
- Mouth (gums, caries)
- Insulin injection sites

Do tests for:
- Blood glucose (fasting if possible)
- Cholesterol if previously high or if there is atherosclerosis
- HbA1c
- Creatinine (if proteinuria)

Management guidelines:
- Review medications and the need for other interventions (referral to dietician, chiropodist, opthalmologist, etc)

Individual assessment and plan

The management of diabetes requires a well-informed and motivated patient who is able to engage with a variety of individualised self-care activities. This requires a commitment to a structured, systematic and empowering education programme. Education may be offered to a group or individuals and may involve doctors, nurses, health promoters, dieticians or pharmacists. High quality educational materials in an appropriate language are also needed to reinforce the information at home. Changes in lifestyle often involve commitment from the whole family as discussed in Chapter 4.

Motivational interviewing or a guiding style is more appropriate than a directing or authoritarian style. Patients may have a variety of beliefs about what causes diabetes and how to treat it. Having a basic understanding of what diabetes is will be important in order to make sense of the benefits of self-care activities.

Healthy eating

The diabetic diet is a healthy diet for the whole family. It is important to discuss the diet with the patient and the person who shops and cooks at home. A useful starting point is to make use of the food-based dietary guidelines for South Africans. They are simple, positive messages that are intended to assist patients or any member of the community in making healthy food choices (see Table 8.9). The following issues are important:
- What is eaten from the different food groups
- Portion size and how much is eaten
- Frequency and timing of meals
- Cooking methods used to prepare food
- Dealing with special situation such as fasting.

Table 8.9 Dietary guidelines for South Africa (Food-based dietary guidelines, 2006)

1.	Enjoy a variety of foods
2.	Be active
3.	Make starchy foods the basis of most meals
4.	Eat plenty of fruits and vegetables every day
5.	Eat dried beans, peas and lentils regularly
6.	Meat, chicken, fish, eggs, milk and dairy can be eaten every day
7.	Use fat sparingly
8.	Use salt sparingly
9.	Drink lots of clean, safe water
10.	If you drink alcohol, drink sensibly

Physical activity

Increasing physical activity as part of a normal routine is an important goal. It is recommended that people with diabetes get at least 150 minutes of aerobic exercise each week (moderate intensity such as walking, jogging, dancing or cycling). It is also recommended that people with diabetes do resistance activities three times a week or more. Resistance activities are activities that use muscular strength to move a weight or work against a resistant load.

Adherence to medication

Most diabetic patients will have to take medications and it is important that they understand how these work, how to take them and what the side-effects are. Patients may have specific concerns regarding their medication, which should be addressed. Patients should all know how to recognise and manage hypoglycaemia.

Other lifestyle issues

Tobacco smoking increases the risk of cardiovascular disease. Psychosocial stress may impact on diabetic control. Alcohol abuse may affect glucose and lipid metabolism and adherence to medication and other self-care activities.

Foot care

Prevention of foot ulcers is far more effective than treatment. Diabetes can cause loss of sensation in the feet, causing injury to go unnoticed. It also decreases the patient's ability to fight infection and healing is slowed by the poor blood supply. Guidelines to give the patient are as follows:

- Wear well-fitting, closed shoes.
- Custom-made insoles may be necessary.
- Never walk barefoot. Your foot could be injured without you even feeling it.
- Keep your feet dry.
- Check your feet every day for redness or any skin changes. See your family physician immediately if there are any changes.
- Have your family physician examine your feet regularly.
- Do not smoke. This causes the blood vessels to constrict.
- Ensure good control of your sugar level.
- Exercise.
- Cut your nails flush with the end of the toes.
- Corns and calluses are a sign of tight-fitting footwear. See your family physician or chiropodist.
- Do not try to cut away calluses yourself.
- Do not use wart paint or corn preparations.
- Keep your feet clean.
- Never treat athlete's foot with creams containing steroids. This allows a more severe infection with invasion of the tissues.

Asthma

The diagnosis of asthma is difficult in young children. Parental identification of wheeze is not reliable (Russel, 2008). "Transient early wheezes" usually settle completely by the age of three years. "Non-atopic wheezes" persist longer, but also mostly settle by the age of five years. Wheezing is usually precipitated by a viral infection. They can be distinguished by pulmonary function tests, but they appear the same to the primary care provider. "IgE-associated wheezes" persist and a diagnosis of asthma can eventually be made. These children usually have evidence of atopy (family or personal history) (Russel, 2008).

In adults it is not uncommon to find a variety of diagnostic labels such as wheezy bronchitis or even asthma/chronic obstructive pulmonary disease (COPD). This uncertainty in diagnosis may translate into uncertainty in terms of treatment and overall management. This also implies that when patients labelled as asthmatic are seen for the first time, one should first ask whether it is asthma. See the section on COPD for how to distinguish between them.

Clinical assessment and plan

Control

Control is assessed by asking five simple questions about asthma over the previous four weeks and measuring the peak expiratory flow (PEF) (Lalloo, 2007). An exacerbation is defined as an asthma attack that required the attention of a health worker. Control is assessed over the last four weeks for all the features except exacerbations, which are counted over the previous year (see Table 8.10).

Table 8.10 Assessment of asthma control

Characteristic	Well controlled (All of the following)	Partly controlled (Any measure present in any week)	Uncontrolled
Daytime symptoms	$\leq$ two per week	> two per week	Three or more features of partly controlled asthma in any week
Night-time symptoms or awakening	None	Any	
Limitation of normal activities	None	Any	
Need for reliever/ rescue treatment	$\leq$ two per week	> two per week	
Peak expiratory flow	Normal	< 80% predicted or personal best (if known)	
Exacerbations	None	One or more per year	One in any week

Check inhaler technique

It is important to have the patient demonstrate their inhaler technique and for them to receive constructive feedback (see Figure xx]). It is also useful for the health worker to have a placebo inhaler and to show the correct technique. The most important step in use of the metered-dose inhaler (MDI) is the co-ordination of inspiration and actuation of the inhaler.

Although some patients will immediately improve once shown how to use the MDI, there are many who continue to struggle and for them a spacer must be prescribed. Providing a spacer will improve delivery of medication in all patients and, if easily available, can be recommended to all patients on inhaled steroids. The spacer technique should also be taught (Figure 8.5). When using the spacer, single actuations should

Figure 8.5 Assessment of good Inhaler technique

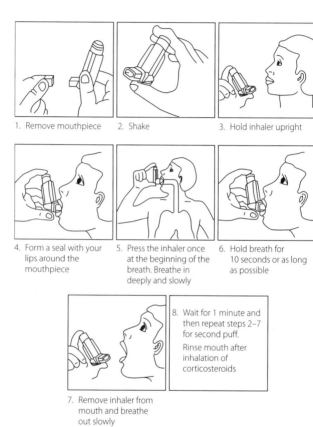

1. Remove mouthpiece

2. Shake

3. Hold inhaler upright

4. Form a seal with your lips around the mouthpiece

5. Press the inhaler once at the beginning of the breath. Breathe in deeply and slowly

6. Hold breath for 10 seconds or as long as possible

7. Remove inhaler from mouth and breathe out slowly

8. Wait for 1 minute and then repeat steps 2–7 for second puff.

Rinse mouth after inhalation of corticosteroids

For further details on using a spacer see Mash, B. Chapter 28: How to use inhalers and spacers. In: *South African Family Practice Manual*. Pretoria. Van Schaik, 2006.

be used at a time and normal tidal breathing with a valved-spacer is as effective as single deep breaths in drug delivery. Children younger than four years will always need a spacer with a face mask, between four to six years a spacer with a normal mouthpiece and older than six years children may also be able to use a dry powder device or breath-actuated MDI.

Teaching and checking inhaler technique is not a once-off activity, but should form part of the ongoing care.

Consider treatment options

In the new guidelines the appropriate steps and different options in treating asthma are well described (Figures 8.6 and 8.7).

For the partly or uncontrolled asthma patient it will also be necessary to consider if a short course of oral steroids is required. Short courses are indicated when symptoms and/or lung function progressively deteriorate or when the patient consults as an emergency. In adults prednisone can be given as 30–40 mg per day for 7–14 days as a once-daily dose in the morning and in children for 5–7 days at a dose of 1–2 mg per kg per dose. There is no need to tail off the course gradually and it can be stopped abruptly at the end. Short courses should not be given in isolation and attention should be given to the other management issues, appropriate safety netting and follow-up.

There may be co-morbid medical conditions such as gastro-oesophageal reflux, rhinitis, sinusitis or cardiac disease where better management will also improve control of asthma.

Figure 8.6 Treatment steps in adults with asthma

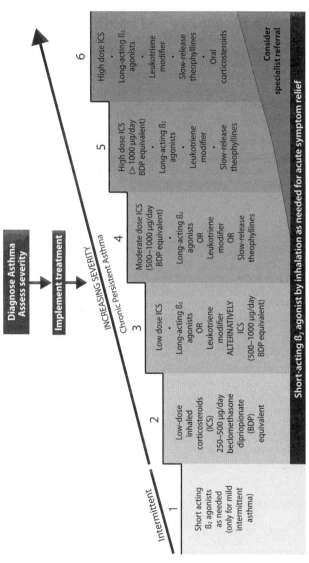

Figure 8.7 Use of controller medication in children (Motala, 2009)

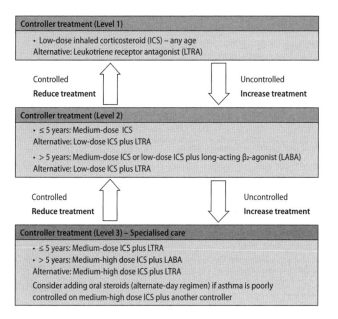

Individual assessment and plan

Check adherence and understanding of medication

The patient's ability to appreciate the difference between their controller and reliever medication is associated with better adherence (Nizami, 2008). Misunderstanding often leads patients to believe that the controller is ineffective, as it does not provide immediate relief, or that the controller should only be added to the reliever when they are really desperate. Evaluating patients' use of, ideas and concerns about their medication should therefore be a routine part of care.

Empower patient self-management

One of the goals of asthma management is to empower the patient to manage their own asthma between visits to the doctor. There is evidence to show that personalised action plans result in fewer days off work, fewer emergency visits, less hospitalisation and a better quality of life (Lalloo, 2007).

Self-management requires the patient to be well informed about asthma, have confidence in themselves and the necessary skills to implement their own decisions. Realistic goals for asthma care should be set with the patient. Key information includes:

- Knowledge regarding the classification (controller/reliever), name, strength, dose and frequency of each medication
- Knowledge on how to self-assess control of asthma. This can be done on the basis of symptoms and does not necessarily require a PEF meter
- Knowledge on what to do when control deteriorates and how to initiate a short course of oral prednisone. Options should be pre-determined, clearly defined and written down
- Knowledge of when and how to obtain emergency help.

Contextual assessment and plan

In the partly or uncontrolled patient there may be a host of aggravating factors that can be modified. Consider if the patient is being exposed to triggers or allergens at home or in the workplace:

- Personal or second-hand tobacco smoke
- Furry animals
- Pollen
- Burning of biofuels
- House dust mite

- Dust or fumes in the workplace
- Foods or beverages containing preservatives
- Drugs that aggravate asthma such as NSAIDs, aspirin or beta-blockers (including eye drops)
- Emotional upset or psychosocial stress.

Chronic obstructive pulmonary disease

In our context COPD may not only be due to prolonged smoking, but also to previous tuberculosis, heavy cannabis use or prolonged exposure to the burning of biomass in informal housing (Greenblatt, 2004).

The history is the most useful way to distinguish between asthma and COPD (Table 8.10). A chest radiograph may show features consistent with previous TB and help exclude other diagnoses, such as cardiac failure. Lung function testing with a PEF meter may help provide supporting evidence.

Reversibility of airway obstruction is helpful when demonstrated and supports the diagnosis of asthma. A lack of reversibility does not exclude asthma. The following tests can be used:

- Increase in PEF (> 20%) 15–30 minutes following inhalation of 200-400 µg beta agonist(salbutamol) via a spacer
- Increase in PEF (> 20%) after a two-week trial of prednisone 40 mg daily
- Decrease in PEF (> 20%) immediately after running for five minutes
- Variability of PEF (> 20%) over a one to two week period. A PEF meter is taken home and the PEF recorded morning and night. The daily variation (%) is calculated as (Maximum PEF-Minimum PEF) ÷ (Maximum PEF + Minimum PEF)/2 × 100.

In COPD there is little or no reversibility (no symptomatic improvement or < 20% increase in PEF) to inhaled beta agonists and/or a two-week trial of oral corticosteroids.

Table 8.10 Distinguishing asthma and COPD

Features of asthma	Features of COPD
• Symptoms started during childhood or early adulthood (usually before the age of 20 years) • History of hayfever, eczema and/or allergies • Family history of asthma or other allergic conditions • Symptoms are intermittent with periods of normal breathing in between • Symptoms are usually worse at night or in the early hours of the morning or during an upper respiratory tract infection • It may be precipitated by seasonal changes, airborne allergens, or pollutants, emotional factors or occupational hazards (consider occupational asthma) • Symptoms improve or disappear after using inhaler or oral steroids.	• Symptoms start later in life (usually after the age of forty years) • Symptoms slowly worsen over a long period of time • Long history of daily or frequent cough and sputum production (usually starts long before the onset of shortness of breath) • Symptoms are persistent rather than only at night or during the early hours of the morning • History of heavy smoking (more than 20 cigarettes per day for 15 years or more), previous tuberculosis, heavy cannabis use or prolonged exposure to the burning of biomass.

Clinical assessment and plan

How severe is the COPD?

The severity of a person's COPD can be classified as mild, moderate or severe using the factors described in Table 8.11. Unfortunately it is not usually possible to measure FEV1 in primary care.

Table 8.11 Assessing severity of COPD

	Mild	Moderate	Severe
Dyspnoea / functional impairment	Limits strenuous activity, for example running, climbing stairs	Limits activities performed at normal pace, for example walking	Impairs activities of daily living, for example washing, dressing Cannot walk more than 200 m
FEV1 (% predicted)	60–79%	40–59%	< 40%
Additional features			Repeated hospitalisation for exacerbations, right heart failure

Improvement of breathlessness

See the recommended treatment steps for different severity of disease on Table 8.12.

Table 8.12 Treatment steps for COPD

	Step 1	Step 2	Step 3	Step 4
Initiation of treatment according to severity	Mild	Moderate	Severe	
Option 1	Inhaled short- OR long-acting beta-agonist regularly	Inhaled short- OR long-acting beta-agonist regularly *plus* inhaled short- OR long-acting anticholinergic regularly	Inhaled short- OR long-acting beta-agonist regularly *plus* inhaled short- OR long-acting anticholinergic regularly *plus* SR theophyllines	Inhaled short- OR long-acting beta-agonist regularly *plus* inhaled short- OR long-acting anticholinergic regularly *plus* SR theophyllines *plus* ICS 800 µg/day in selected patients

	Step 1	Step 2	Step 3	Step 4
Initiation of treatment according to severity	Mild	Moderate	Severe	
Option 2	Inhaled short- OR long-acting anticholinergic regularly	Inhaled short- OR long- acting beta- agonist OR anticholinergic regularly *plus* SR theophyllines		

* Frequent exacerbations (> two per year) or rapid deterioration or where a two-week trial of responsiveness to oral corticosteroids shows >15% or 200 ml improvement in FEV$_1$

Improvement of quality of life

- Provide verbal and written information on COPD, smoking cessation and management options.
- Offer referral to an exercise programme to improve skeletal muscle fitness.
- Advise regarding optimal nutrition and weight.
- Consider long term domiciliary oxygen in patients with severe disease (Stage 3), persistent hypoxaemia (saturation < 90% at rest) when stable and who are non-smokers. Refer for specialist assessment only if all three criteria are met.

Prevention and treatment of exacerbations

- An exacerbation presents as increased breathlessness, often accompanied by wheezing, chest tightness and increased cough and sputum (sputum often changes in volume and colour). Exacerbations are usually precipitated by an infection.
- Exacerbations should be distinguished from other causes such as pneumonia, pneumothorax, congestive cardiac failure, arrhythmia and pulmonary embolism.
- Prevention involves annual vaccination for influenza and five-yearly pneumococcal vaccination
- Outpatient treatment involves four to six hourly use of inhaled

beta-agonists and/or anticholinergics via nebuliser or MDI/spacer, a seven-day course of 40 mg of oral prednisone and antibiotic therapy such as amoxycillin 500 mg tds or doxycycline 100 mg bd for ten days. Hospitalisation may be required if there is no improvement on treatment.

Treatment of complications

Right heart failure is the commonest complication (for example oedema, raised jugular venous pressure, ascites and hepatomegaly). Treat any precipitating causes (acute respiratory infection, worsening airflow obstruction) and reduce oedema with a diuretic such as furosemide 40 mg. Avoid over-diuresis, which may cause hypotension. Advise salt and water restriction.

Individual assessment and plan

Smoking cessation

Ask each patient about their smoking status. Provide or refer for brief counselling on smoking cessation in a guiding style. Consider use of nicotine replacement or bupropion. Refer to a support group if available and acceptable.

Patient's perspective and adherence

As with asthma, it is important to check for the patient's ability to use their inhaler and for their understanding of the different medications or other concerns, beliefs or expectations.

Contextual assessment and plan

It may be helpful to involve the family in supporting smoking cessation, lifestyle issues or reducing indoor air pollution.

Epilepsy

Epilepsy is a chronic condition characterised by recurrent, unprovoked seizure activity. In the majority of patients with epilepsy there is no identifiable cause.

Aetiology of seizures

Identifiable causes for seizures include:

- Children: Congenital brain malformation, inborn errors of metabolism, febrile seizure
- Adult: Intracranial infection, tumours, alcohol or drug withdrawal, trauma, eclampsia
- Elderly: Cerebral degeneration, cerebro-vascular accident, tumours, drug reactions
- All ages: Hyponatraemia, hypocalcaemia, hypoglycaemia, non-ketotic hyperglycaemia, uraemia, malignant hypertension, hypoxemia.

Seizures are sometimes confused with other conditions that cause collapse or altered consciousness such as vertigo, syncope, disequilibrium, cerebro-vascular accidents, panic attacks, hypoglycaemia, narcolepsy or alcoholic blackouts.

Classification of epilepsy

Partial (focal) seizures

- Simple partial – consciousness not impaired
  - With motor symptoms
  - With somato-sensory or special sensory symptoms
  - With autonomic symptoms/signs
  - With psychiatric signs.
- Complex partial – impairment of consciousness
- Partial (simple or complex) evolving to secondary generalised seizure.

Generalised seizures

- Non-convulsive
- Convulsive.

The most important part of the history is a clear account of the seizure, ideally from an eye witness. In someone with known epilepsy, poor adherence to medication is the most common reason for presenting with a seizure. Epilepsy may be precipitated by sleep deprivation, drugs/alcohol, TV screens, strobe lighting, or an emotional upset. A clear diagnosis of the type of epilepsy should be made based on the classification above. During the seizure a variety of signs may be observed:

- A typical simple partial seizure may cause jerking of a limb (motor cortex involvement) or numbness of an arm (sensory cortex involvement). Sometimes the seizure progresses from fingers, to hand, to arm, to face in a so-called Jacksonian march. The patient is conscious.
- A typical complex partial seizure may arise in the temporal lobe and be associated with visual, olfactory or gustatory hallucinations, impaired consciousness, behavioural disturbance, repetitive activities (automatisms) such as chewing, walking and lip-smacking.
- A typical non-convulsive generalised seizure or absence seizure is usually found in children. The child maintains posture, does not shake, but speech and movement are arrested as the child stares into space. Seizures are very brief but may recur frequently and be associated with poor school performance blamed on day-dreaming.
- A typical generalised convulsive seizure is associated with loss of consciousness and extension of the neck, back and limbs (tonic phase) for about a minute. The patient may cry out, bite his tongue or urinate and become cyanosed. This is followed by shaking of the limbs (clonic phase) which can last a few seconds or minutes. Following this the person is usually drowsy and confused before recovering.

Clinical management and plan

Figure 8.8 shows an approach to the use of medication. The golden rule is for monotherapy and to increase to the maximum possible dose before substituting or adding another drug. Avoid continual increases and decreases in dose. Generally, the best medication for a woman who wants to become pregnant is the one that best controls her seizures at the lowest possible dose, but specialist help should be sought. Choice of medication or dosage may need adjusting when combined with contraception or TB treatment due to the drug interactions.

When monotherapy fails to control seizures satisfactorily the following factors should be considered:
- Poor adherence
- Seizures not caused by epilepsy (20%)
- Psychological problem
- Underlying neurological problem
- Use of wrong medication.

The following factors may predict intractability:
- Onset of seizures at young age (< two years)

- Frequent generalised seizures
- Evidence of brain damage
- Severe EEG abnormality
- Low IQ
- Atypical absence seizures.

Figure 8.8 A stepwise approach in the management of generalised epilepsy

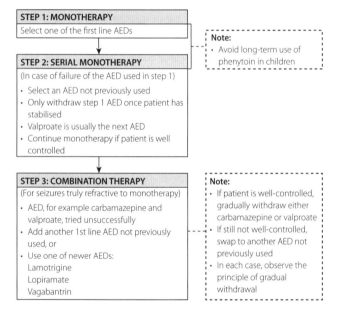

The diagnosis of epilepsy is associated with stigma and often strong cultural beliefs regarding causation or treatment. Try to understand the patient's perspective and to clarify misunderstandings. Discuss issues related to adherence and the risks or benefits of treatment.

Contextual management and plan

Involving the family in understanding the disease, so that they know what to do during a seizure and can support adherence to treatment, is essential. Frequently the person with epilepsy has problems at school, at work or with finding employment. Consider the implications for driving vehicles and for disability grants. Link the patient with any organisations that help with skills training or employment such as the South African Neuro-Epilepsy League (SANEL).

Alcohol use disorders

Alcohol use disorders can be classified as

- Dependency with loss of control, strong desire, tolerance and withdrawal symptoms
- Harmful alcohol use with significant effects on health (for example dyspepsia, injuries, sexual problems and hypertension), psychological wellbeing (for example depression), social wellbeing (for example relationships, marital problems, financial problems and legal problems) and occupational well being (for example absenteeism, warnings and dismissal)
- Heavy or binge drinking over the recommended limits of less than 14 units per week for women and 21 units per week for men. The rate of absorption is fastest and leads to more rapid inebriation in the following instances:
  - Drinking on an empty stomach
  - Drinks high in alcohol (20-30% such as sherry)
  - Aerated drinks (such as champagne)
  - Women or someone who is naïve regarding alcohol
  - Drinking faster than approximately one unit (10 g alcohol) per hour.

The consequences of alcohol use disorders are huge and include:

- Inter-personal violence: Intimate partner violence, homicide and assault are all related to high blood alcohol.
- Road traffic accidents: Traffic fatalities (in drivers and pedestrians) are associated with a blood alcohol concentration above 0.08 g per 100 ml in 40–45% of cases (Parry, 1999). The legal limit for driving in South Africa is under 0.05 g per 100ml (Parry, 1999). Most adults will be over the legal limit with two cans of 375 ml beer with five percent alcohol drunk in one hour (Paton, 2005).
- Medical complications: Foetal alcohol syndrome, hypertension, cirrhosis, cancers of the oropharynx, larynx, oesophagus and liver. The increased risk of unsafe sex, teenage pregnancy and HIV has not been quantified.

Individual treatment

Heavy drinking

Review the quantity and frequency of current drinking. For example if Peter drinks seven beers (375 ml) with five percent alcohol content and two bottles (750 ml) of red wine with 14% alcohol content per week, he consumes 341 g in one week ($7 \times 375 \times 0.05 = 131.25$ g plus $750 \times 2 \times 0.14 = 210$ g). At 10 g per unit he is over his safe limit of 21 units or 210 g.

A brief intervention such as FRAMES (Table 8.13) in a guiding style can help.

Table 8.13 FRAMES approach to a brief alcohol intervention (Bien, 1993)

Feedback	Feedback of personal risk or impairment	"Your liver is enlarged and not working properly and too much alcohol is the most likely cause for this."
Responsibility	Emphasis on personal control and responsibility for change	"I care about your wellbeing and therefore feel concerned about you, but it is really up to you to do something about this."
Advice	Clear advice to change	"I suggest that you stop drinking."
Menu	A menu of alternative change options	"I would like to help and support you as far as possible. If you believe that you can stop by yourself, you can try on your own. If you don't manage or if you want help, I could arrange for you to see someone to talk more about this."
Empathy	Therapeutic empathy as a counselling style	Attempt to understand the patient's ambivalence or readiness to change. Explore importance of change.
Self-efficacy	Enhancement of patient self-efficacy or optimism	Affirm patient's strengths and believes in possibility of change. Elicits possible changes.

Harmful drinking

The Alcohol Use Disorders Identification Test (AUDIT) helps identify people with harmful drinking (Mash, 2006). Assess the patient for any other psychological problems such as depression or anxiety disorders. Again a brief intervention and follow up is called for using a guiding style.

Dependency

The CAGE questions help identify people with alcohol dependency:
- Have you ever felt you should **cut down** on your drinking?
- Have people **annoyed** you by criticising your drinking?
- Have you ever felt bad or **guilty** about your drinking?
- Have you ever had an **eye opener** first thing in the morning to steady your nerves or get rid of a hangover?

A brief intervention may be needed to motivate the patient to commit to detoxification and rehabilitation. If alcohol intake has been under 15 units per day for men and 10 units for women the withdrawal process can be handled in ambulatory care with explanation and use of diazepam for symptom relief (Ritson, 2005). Others with a higher alcohol intake, other concomitant problems and a history of significant withdrawal symptoms will need in-patient detoxification.

The SA National Council on Alcoholism (SANCA) offers rehabilitation and counselling. Alcoholics anonymous (AA) does seem to have a role in improving abstinence at two year follow-up. Disulfiram is a well known deterrent substance that switches off alcohol metabolism leading to a build up of acetaldehyde and resultant toxic symptoms of flushing – you cannot drink while taking this and may be helpful in some patients (Enoch, 2002).

Depression

Only about 50% of depressed patients in primary care are recognised. Depressed patients often present with somatic symptoms, such as headache or back pain, or non-specific symptoms such as tiredness and sleep problems. Non-verbal cues in the consultation may be obvious such as a depressed affect, poor eye contact and slow speech. Contextual cues may include a recent loss such as unemployment, bereavement or loss of health (for example HIV or cancer). There may be a history of frequent attendance without a clear diagnosis. Depression is a clinical diagnosis and tests are done to exclude other causes of the symptoms.

It is important for clinicians to consider mental problems along-side physical problems when assessing patients and to be confident in screening for depression. Family physicians can use two screening questions (Mash, 2001):

- "Do you feel sad or like crying for no reason?"
- "As a person there are things that you enjoy doing -- do you find that you no longer enjoy these things?"

This is to detect the hallmark symptoms of low mood and loss of interest. If either symptom is detected, then the other symptoms should be looked for. A number of rating scales can be used to screen for depression.

In children and adolescents, depression may present through a change in behaviour such as refusal to go to school, withdrawal from the peer group or antisocial behaviour. In the elderly it may be confused with dementia or psychosis.

Clinical assessment and plan

A diagnosis of depression requires five (or more) of the following symptoms to be present on nearly every day during the same two-week period and to represent change from previous functioning. Both symptoms of depressed mood and loss of interest or pleasure must be present.

1. Depressed mood most of the day
2. Markedly diminished interest or pleasure in all or almost all activities
3. Significant weight loss when not dieting or weight gain (a change of five percent of body weight in a month) or a increase or decrease in appetite
4. Insomnia (early morning waking) or hypersomnia
5. Psychomotor agitation or retardation
6. Fatigue or loss of energy
7. Feelings of worthlessness or excessive or inappropriate guilt
8. Diminished ability to think or concentrate, or indecisiveness
9. Recurrent thoughts of death, recurrent suicidal ideation with or without a specific plan. Suicidal risk must be specifically assessed.

Classification of depression is as follows:
- *Postpartum:* Onset within four weeks of giving birth
- *Depressive disorders:* Major depression (single or recurrent episode), adjustment disorders with depressed mood, and dysthymia
- *Bipolar disorders:* Manic and depressive episodes.

Consider whether other medical conditions could be causing the symptoms, for example anaemia, malignancy, hypothyroidism, hyper-parathyroidism, Cushing's syndrome or post-infective states such as encephalitis.

Consider whether the symptoms could be a side effect of medication, for example reserpine, methyldopa, clonidine, corticosteroids, anti-Parkinson's drugs, cytotoxic agents, NSAIDs or oral contraceptives.

Consider any co-morbidity with anxiety, substance abuse or other mental problems.

Management usually involves a combination of pharmaco- with psycho-therapy. The physician should always identify and manage any suicide risk.

Medication

Titrate up to the recommended target dose, while monitoring for side-effects (see Table 8.14). There is usually little additional benefit from using higher than the minimal effective dose. Give an adequate trial of treatment before changing medication, for example 12 weeks at moderate to high dosage. The new drug should affect a different mono-amine neurotransmitter mechanism. If the response is greater than 30% rather augment treatment by adding another drug.

Table 8.14 Antidepressants, actions and side-effects

Class of medication	Action	Common side-effects
Tricyclic antidepressants (TCAs), for example amitriptyline and imipramine	Majority act primarily as serotonin-noradrenalin reuptake inhibitors (SN-RIs) by blocking the serotonin transporter (SERT) and the noradrenalin transporter (NET)	Dry mouth, weight gain, sedation, urinary retention, glaucoma, decreased libido, postural hypotension, dizziness
Selective serotonin reuptake inhibitors (SSRI), for example fluoxetine and paroxetine	Block serotonin reuptake at presynaptic junctions	Nausea, anxiety, agitation, headache, diarrhoea, insomnia, sexual dysfunction, possible increased suicidal risk in children and adolescents
Selective serotonin noradrenalin re-uptake inhibitors (SNRI), for example venlafaxine	Block serotonin and noradrenalin reuptake	Insomnia, tremors, tachycardia, sweating

Class of medication	Action	Common side-effects
Monoamine oxidase inhibitors (MAOIs), for example phenelzine and moclobemide	MAOIs inhibit monoamine oxidase leading to accumulation of amine neurotransmitters	Postural hypotension, drowsiness, insomnia, confusion, sexual dysfunction, weakness, fatigue Accumulation of metabolites may cause a severe hypertensive crisis. Can be precipitated by other medication (for example cough syrups and decongestants) or foods (for example cheese, pickled herring, broad beans and Marmite)
Lithium salts are used in bipolar disorders	Mood stabilisers	Headache, vomiting, mental confusion, stupor, seizure
Serotonin dopamine reuptake inhibitors (SDRIs), for example bupropion		Headaches, insomnia, nightmares, seizures Less sexual dysfunction than SSRIs

Electroconvulsive therapy (ECT)

ECT is safe, effective and acts rapidly and can be used with anti-depressants. It is usually given in six to eight treatments over three weeks. Indications for ECT include psychotic depression, failure to respond to anti-depressants, substantial suicide risk or severe psychomotor depression, refusal to eat or drink, self-neglect and/or depressive stupor.

Individual assessment and plan

Family physicians are able to learn simple psychotherapeutic strategies such as problem-solving, dealing with negative thinking and simple behavioural techniques. If available, more sophisticated psychotherapy may be offered by psychologists or psychiatrists.

Cognitive-behavioural therapy (CBT) is often a short-term 12-week commitment and specifically designed to deal with a patient in the here and now. Patients are empowered to monitor and modify their own thoughts and behaviours.

Analytical longer-term psychotherapy suggests that depression is triggered by traumatic events (minor or major) experienced in the patient's life. This approach is suitable for patients with a trauma history or personality disorder.

Contextual assessment and plan

Explore the patient's social context for triggers to the depression (for example bereavement, unemployment, conflict, abuse or intimate partner violence) that need attention or supportive relationships that can assist the patient. It may be important for the family to understand and be involved in caring for the patient.

Palliative care

Palliative care is an approach that improves the quality of life of patients and their families facing problems associated with life-threatening illness. This is done through the prevention and relief of suffering, the early identification and impeccable assessment and treatment of pain and other problems, including the physical, psychosocial and spiritual domain (Sepulveda, 2002). To emphasise some key points:

- Palliative care is not only for people in the terminal phase of their illness or only for people with cancer.
- The goal of palliative care is quality of life. Quality of life relates to an individual's subjective satisfaction with life. Quality of life assessment usually looks at four domains: physical, social, emotional (psychological) and spiritual (existential).
- The unit of care is the patient and family. Patient-centred care requires open and honest communication with the patient, respect, sharing of information in words the patient understands, mutual agreement of goals of care and treatment options. The family's views are important, but should not supersede the patient's wishes.
- Palliative care provides total care – physical, psychosocial, and spiritual. No one element of care is more important than another, although it is true that when a patient is in severe pain, it is difficult for them to focus on psychosocial issues until the pain is controlled.

The requirement for a multidisciplinary team is clear in order to be able to provide this total care. Many health care professionals equate palliative care with withdrawal of care. However, palliative care is active therapy that assesses and manages difficult symptoms, as well as psychosocial and spiritual issues. Appropriate assessment of patient problems enables the care team to develop an individualised care plan for each patient in consultation with the patient. Often at the end of life, patients experience symptoms that are more distressing and more challenging to manage than at other times of life. These symptoms need to be effectively managed to promote patient comfort and dignity.

In our context, with limited resources and late presentation, disease-oriented care (for example chemotherapy, radiotherapy or antiretrovirals) is often not available to many people at the time of diagnosis, so palliative care is increasingly important. With more health care professionals training in palliative care, this can be integrated earlier into the caring process, with better outcomes for patients, families and healthcare professionals.

The result of early intervention with active palliative care is better quality of life for patients and families, a peaceful and dignified death for the patient and better bereavement outcomes for the family. The professional satisfaction of effective compassionate care results in a rewarding experience for the health care worker, both personally and professionally, and a lower incidence of burn-out.

The dying patient

The terminal phase of a patient's illness refers to the last few hours or days of a patient's life, the stage when death is imminent. A patient may have had a recognised terminal illness for much longer but the terminal phase may still be an unpredicted event for both family and professionals. Care provided to the dying patient is important both to the patient to ensure physical comfort in the face of challenging symptoms and dignity in death, and to the family as the experience of caring for a family member who is dying has an impact on the bereavement process. The fact that patients are particularly vulnerable at this stage of their illness seems self-evident but it is often at this stage that care is withdrawn with the attitude of there is nothing more that can be done on the part of the doctor. In fact, the patient may need more accurate assessment and management of symptoms, and especially the assurance of ongoing care and non-abandonment.

The palliative care team has a role in supporting the patient and family through the terminal phase in whatever setting the patient chooses for receiving palliative care. A patient does not need to be admitted to hospital to die. In fact, the majority of people choose to die at home in familiar surroundings. When patients are in hospital or in a nursing home, it is important that family members are given the opportunity to be present during the dying process.

Explanation

- Fears – patients may be concerned about the dying process and there may be a particular symptom that worries them, for example pain or shortness of breath. It is important to elicit these concerns and to reassure the patient and family members about symptom control.

- Advance directives – the patient may discuss the fact that they do not want the dying process to be prolonged by medical interventions but that they would choose to receive medication to promote comfort.
- Resuscitation – the patient's views on resuscitation may be inferred from discussion about the advance directive but it may be necessary to inform both the patient and their family that resuscitation measures are not available in the home or hospice and to discuss that resuscitation would be inappropriate.
- Unfinished business – palliative care staff may identify that a patient is troubled and anxious/restless and a sensitive discussion may reveal the source of concern. Although some situations are not possible to resolve, discussion of the situation may assist the patient.

Symptom control in the terminal phase

- Rationalise regular medication: The burden of taking many tablets should be reduced and most regular medication discontinued, for example thyroxine, antihypertensives, vitamins.
- Route of administration: As the patient deteriorates it may be difficult to administer oral medication and it is important to use alternate routes such as subcutaneous or rectal. The use of a syringe driver facilitates delivery of medication essential for symptom control.
- Planning care: It is important to anticipate symptoms that may develop in the terminal phase so that medication to relieve these symptoms is available when required. Common symptoms in the terminal phase are:
  - Pain – regular analgesia is still needed but requirements for pain medication do not usually increase significantly. Morphine sulphate can be delivered by syringe driver at half to a third of the oral dose and can be combined in the syringe driver with other essential medication.
  - Nausea and vomiting – can be controlled by regular medication, such as cyclizine, haloperidol or metoclopramide. Haloperidol is commonly used as it also reduces anxiety and agitation.
  - Anxiety, restlessness, agitation – these symptoms can be very distressing to the family and carers and can be difficult to control. The escalation of opioid dosage is not appropriate. It is important to try and identify a cause of this distress which may be a simple reversible cause such as urinary retention, constipation or infection. Agitation and restlessness respond to benzodiazpines, such

as diazepam and midazolam, which are also useful for easing breathlessness and as an anticonvulsant. Haloperidol combines well with midazolam and morphine in the syringe driver to give good control of symptoms experienced in the terminal stage.

— Respiratory secretions – hyoscine butyl bromide is useful in reducing excess respiratory secretions.

— Dyspnoea – this is an extremely distressing symptom, reversible causes should be determined and treated. Congestive cardiac failure should be treated aggressively. Bronchospasm can be treated by nebulised bronchodilators. Low-dose morphine is useful in reducing the sensation of dyspnoea. Benzodiazepines may be required to relieve anxiety resulting from and exacerbating dyspnoea.

— Mouth care – patients may have dry mouth because of the illness or because of drug therapy. It is important to keep the mouth clean and moist and to treat infections such as oral candidiasis. Sodium bicarbonate solution or soda water are effective as mouth wash. Partially frozen drinks or chips of ice can be sucked to keep the mouth moist and petroleum jelly prevents sore, cracked lips.

— Pressure care – special mattresses and frequent turning and lifting of the patient are important and the family needs careful explanation of the importance of preventing pressure sores.

Psychosocial support

Psychosocial support facilitates the patient's and family's expression of emotional pain, fear, anger; assists in the containment of these emotions and allows end-of-life tasks to be completed. The family is facing uncertainty, emotional strain, and experiencing the distress of watching the deteriorating condition of the patient. They need reassurance that they are doing a good job of caring for their loved one, support in adjusting to the alteration of their role, for example husband to nurse. They are also experiencing the increased physical demands of nursing the patient, additional household tasks, interrupted sleep, and the emotional burden of care. Families need to be with dying patients, they may need to care for the patient themselves, they need information about the illness, impending death and what to expect. They need to express emotions and to receive comfort. We need to respond to the particular needs of the children of the terminally ill parent and the parents and siblings of a terminally ill child.

Spiritual care

The diagnosis of a terminal illness brings the individual and their carers face-to-face with questions regarding spirituality and the search for meaning in illness. As health care professionals we are also faced with the recognition of our patients' and our own mortality. To truly provide holistic care we need to acknowledge spiritual aspects of care and be open to engaging with our patients and their families in the discussion of their concerns. We may be fortunate in having colleagues who are trained in spiritual counseling, but many discussions that are initiated by patients are opportunistic. The responsibility we have to our patients, especially in the times of crisis that present as a result of a terminal diagnosis, includes being prepared to accompany them through their final journey and to face the difficult times with them. We need to recognise that whereas some patients will be well supported within their own religious framework, others may not have developed this support system. Ideally, the patient should receive spiritual care from a pastoral carer from their own faith.

Disability

Definitions

Disability is the presence of impairments, activity limitations, and participation restrictions. Impairment is a manifestation of pathology that leaves one with abnormalities of body structure (for example amputation) or function (for example hypothyroidism). Impairments can be temporary, permanent, progressive, regressive, static, intermittent, continuous, slight or severe. An activity limitation is when these impairments have an impact on the ability to carry out daily activities, such as washing, dressing, grooming, walking and speaking. Participation restrictions are when one is unable to participate in society and life situations.

Rehabilitation is achieved through modification of an impairment by medical or surgical means, compensation for loss of function with assistive devices and techniques, facilitation of social adjustment and acceptance, and modification of the environment.

Environmental factors make up the physical, social, and attitudinal environment in which people live and conduct their lives. These can facilitate function or be barriers, causing disability.

All these components interact, influencing a person's functioning, disability and health as summarised in Figure 8.9.

Figure 8.9 Interaction of the factors affecting disability

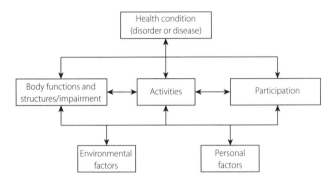

Role of the doctor in primary care

Every consultation provides an opportunity for the following:
- Confirmation of the diagnosis and prognosis
- Monitor the maintenance of previously achieved levels of functioning
- Assess abilities and reinforce positive life roles rather than a sick role
- Identify current problems (medical and functional)
- Identify potential complications (medical and functional)
- Treat appropriately at primary level
- Make appropriate referrals to medical, therapeutic and community resources
- Coordinate all interventions
- Organise follow up
- Advocate the needs of persons with disabilities, be it the supply of suitable continence devices and medications from medical aids and community health centres or return to work.

A systematic approach

A systematic approach using the following suggested framework facilitates comprehensive patient management. Complications often develop insidiously and the list below (Table 8.15) ensures that, potentially, nothing is missed.

Table 8.15 Comprehensive assessment of a patient with disability

Medical related aspects:

1. Optimal medical management
2. Nutritional requirements met
3. Skin and pressure care
4. Bladder and bowel
5. Pain and discomfort
6. Vision
7. Sexual dysfunction

Therapeutic related aspects:

1. Behavioural and psychosocial adaptation, cognition and perception
2. Community re-integration, work, leisure activities
3. Activities of daily living and mobility
4. Transport
5. Communication (including reading, writing, facial expression)
6. Feeding, swallowing and dentition

Other:

1. Finances
2. Education and training of patient and carer.

The following section is a brief overview of key issues in each of these problem areas to which the family physician should attend.

Optimal medical management

Ensure an accurate diagnosis to guide the prognosis and appropriate management. Medical problems generally fall into the following categories:

- Underlying cause and risk factors for the disability
- Complications of deconditioning and immobility (for example pressure ulcers, deep vein thrombosis, contractures, aspiration, reduced fitness, postural hypotension and osteoporosis)
- Secondary effects of the underlying pathology (for example seizures, spasticity, neuropsychiatric disturbances and incontinence)
- Secondary complications (for example urinary infection, bladder stones and depression).

All impairments across all systems must be optimally managed to afford the patient the best possible outcome.

Poly-pharmacy, drug interactions and the effect of prescription and recreational substances on functional ability must be considered.

Nutrition

Patients with pressure sores have an increased need for protein, calories, vitamins (especially vitamin C) and minerals (such as zinc). Immobile patients become constipated, often aggravated by poor fibre and fluid intake. Patients who have urinary accidents may limit their fluid intake. Sedentary patients have reduced energy needs, while patients who mobilise actively have increased energy demands.

Skin and pressure care

Patients, with or without sensory disturbances, who maintain the same position for prolonged periods of time, are at risk of developing pressure ulcers. Pressure mattresses and wheelchair cushions alone do not prevent pressure sores. The patient or carer must take responsibility for doing pressure relief every two to four hours, day and night. Precipitating and aggravating factors are:

- Wet skin
- Friction (spasms, pulling the patient across the sheet)
- Anaemia, debility (for example diabetes and HIV)
- Contractures
- Crumbs and creases in the bedding
- Substance abuse
- Pressure from orthoses, prostheses, assistive devices and clothing.

Once a pressure sore has developed, moist wound healing must be applied and the patient kept strictly off the affected area.

Bladder and bowel management

Exclude pre-morbid causes of incontinence. Ensure regular and adequate bladder emptying without reflux. In patients with spinal cord afflictions consider urological referral for complete bladder and sphincter function assessment. Patients with brain injury may be functionally incontinent due to cognitive impairment (do not recognise the need for the toilet), poor mobility (access to toilet, commode or urinal bottle), or inability to manipulate clothing in time. A regular voiding schedule is then indicated.

Facilitation of regular bowel empting is critical from the first day of injury to prevent complications of constipation and to promote social continence. Chronic constipation may lead to proximal liquefaction of stools with the patient presenting with diarrhoea.

Pain and discomfort

Spasticity and pain should be treated early and vigorously. Any change from previously controlled levels needs to be investigated. Spasticity is aggravated by infections, urinary stones, ingrown toenails, change in psychological status and pressure sores. Common causes of stump pain in amputees are infection, neuroma and ischaemia.

Vision

Diabetics should be aggressively monitored for cataracts and proliferative retinopathy. Brain-injured patients with hemianopia and hemi-neglect, should be approached from the hemiplegic side to provide maximal stimulation. Prism spectacles may improve hemianopia, but only perceptual retraining and not spectacles will help hemi-neglect. Visio-motor disorders can be treated with visual therapy which exercises the muscles involved in eye movements and accommodation. If diplopia is causing headaches and dizziness, alternative eye patching can be done on a daily basis.

Sexual dysfunction

The physical and relational aspects of sexual performance need to be assessed. Altered sensation may have an impact on the sexual experience. Impotence may be related to the lesion (for example spinal cord afflictions), medication or vascular disease.

The ability to maintain menstrual hygiene and the need for family planning must be assessed. Pregnancy may not be contraindicated, but spasticity and deformity may have an impact on child birth, and functional ability on child-rearing ability.

Behaviour and psychosocial adaptation, cognition and perception

The family needs to be counselled regarding probable behavioural patterns in persons with brain injury. For example, the loss of internal motivation may be seen as laziness, aggression as deliberate rather than loss of impulse control and poor memory may be seen as manipulative. Comatose patients often become restless and aggressive when their level of consciousness improves and they start interacting with their environment. The use of sedation needs to be used judiciously to avoid having an effect on cognition.

Depression may be pre-morbid, reactive or organic following brain injury. Patients with severe cognitive impairments are often not suitable for rehabilitation programmes if they cannot retain learned information. Families should be taught how to create a structured therapeutic home environment. This includes discouraging inappropriate behaviour such as manipulation and dependency.

Community reintegration, work, school and leisure

Patients should become integrated members of the family and community, fulfilling defined roles and participating in pre-morbid activities such as shopping, socialising and religious activities. An occupational therapist or clinical psychologist can assess children for either mainstream or special school placement. Patients interested in sport can be referred to the Sport for the Disabled organisation. Structured activity within the open, sheltered, or protected labour markets, a weekly activity group or within the domestic environment serves physical and emotional therapeutic goals.

If the person was employed at the time of onset of disability, this employment should be kept if at all possible and an occupational therapist consulted. Termination of work should be carefully considered taking into account the prognosis, natural history to date and the completion of all rehabilitative interventions. Families may insist on boarding for financial reasons. Alternatives (for example sick leave, temporary disability, unemployment insurance fund (UIF), insurance and state disability) should be considered.

Activities of daily living and mobility

A home visit will provide insight into the environmental challenges such as unpaved outdoor surfaces, outside toilets, lack of running water, narrow passages or inaccessible baths and toilets.

Enquiry into personal self-care includes eating (cutting food, bringing food to the mouth, chewing and swallowing), washing the upper and lower body with adequate quality, getting into and out of the bath, dressing the upper and lower body (including fasteners, underwear, putting on orthoses and prostheses), toileting (getting to the toilet, adjusting clothing timeously and safely, getting on and off the toilet, cleaning oneself), grooming (washing and combing hair, shaving, make-up) and sleep.

An occupational therapist can attend to problems with domestic tasks (for example sweeping, washing, hanging, ironing, making beds, preparing food, gardening) and childcare (such as holding a young baby, changing nappies and bathing an infant).

Loss of dominant hand function requires dominance retraining. If functional hand movement has not returned within three months after brain injury, it is unlikely to happen. Patients with increased tone must NOT squeeze a stress ball as this will aggravate flexor tone.

Mobility assessment can range from mobility in bed to playing sport, and transfers in and out of the wheelchair, to bed, toilet, chair, ground, and car. Bedridden patients are encouraged to sit up out of bed for limited periods. In neurologically impaired patients, walking is only advised when it is learnt in the correct neurodevelopmental sequence, to promote correct walking patterns. Enquire as to safety, distance, speed, need for assistive devices, ability to negotiate stairs, curbs, obstacles and uneven terrain.

If assistive devices or orthoses have been prescribed assess if the patient is correctly seated in their wheelchair, with the hips, knees, and ankles at 90 degrees with the pelvis positioned so that the spine follows its normal curvatures.

Transport

Can the patient access transport to attend the health facility and fulfil personal needs? Can they transfer in and out of the vehicle and stow assistive devices?

A patient requires competent physical and mental functioning (for example concentration, insight, judgement, reasoning, and the ability to cope in an emergency).

Do they have access to transport for the disabled if locally available? Do they have a disabled parking disc if they use private transport?

Communication

If the patient attempts to give the history then dysarthria, dysphasia, comprehension, and cognition problems can be detected. Patients are encouraged to talk, rather than the accompanying carer. If the history needs to be taken from the carer, maintain the patient as the primary focus of the interview. Establishing an accurate yes/no response, followed by naming of common objects, is the first therapeutic step in communicating with an aphasic patient.

A communication board is only effective for persons with adequate cognitive ability.

An ear specialist or audiologist's opinion may be required to ascertain if a hearing device will benefit the person.

Feeding, swallowing and dentition

With a facial palsy, dentures may no longer fit comfortably and may need to be altered or remade. Assess oral and dental hygiene. Oral thrush is often a reason to avoid feeding. Patients who drool are encouraged to suck back the saliva rather than dab the side of the mouth as this aggravates further drooling.

Does oral intake of solids and fluids match energy demands (increased or decreased)?

Can the person chew and swallow solids and liquids? Is there choking, regurgitation through the nose or aspiration? Has the person had repeated lower respiratory tract infections? In patients with unilateral brain lesions, choking is more likely due to poor positioning than neurogenic causes. Once positioning is corrected, patients who continue to choke should be evaluated by a speech therapist or ear, nose and throat specialist, with videoflouroscopy. A nasogastric tube does not eliminate aspiration of upper gastrointestinal secretions. A PEG feeding tube is an option for long-term assisted feeding.

Finances

Interventions need to be planned within the limitations of the patient's financial resources. An applicant will usually only qualify for a disability grant if they are unable to do any work. Some applicants are referred to a work assessment unit for further assessment of their disability. If a disability grant is not awarded, the patient can appeal within 90 days.

For many impoverished people a disability grant would provide a means of sustaining themselves and their families where there are no other means. The application carries high stakes for the patient and conflict may arise when the family physician and the patient disagree on the extent of the impairment and disability or on entitlement to government support.

Education and training of patient and carer

The doctor plays an important role in communicating the diagnosis, prognosis and management plan to all parties involved, including the patient, family, carers, health funders, employers. Consider the need for a family conference (see Chapter 4).

9   Community-orientated primary care

Steve Reid
Primary Health Care Directorate
University of Cape Town

Introduction

This chapter is about making a difference to the context within which our patients get ill and get better. In other words, it is about acting with and beyond the individual patient to bring about change in the wider factors that affect health. This involves family physicians in preventive and health promotion aspects of care outside a health facility. This is a situation in which doctors are often uncomfortable and involves using a detailed knowledge of illness and disease in individuals as a springboard for action at a community level, extending the scope of practice to community-wide health issues as part of a team.

Simply put, community-orientated primary care (COPC) is the *combination* of front-line clinical medicine with public health, the emphasis being on combination. It is defined as follows (Abramson, 1988):

> "A continuous process by which primary health care is provided to a defined community on the basis of its assessed health needs, by the planned integration of primary care practice and public health."

This idea was first championed at the University of Natal by two doctors, Sidney and Emily Kark, in the 1950s as the central strategy of the Institute of Family and Community Health, which arose out of their experiences at Pholela Health Centre in rural KwaZulu-Natal (Kark, 1942; Kark and Cassel, 1952). The objective of the centre was to "explore the practice of family and community health care in a number of neighbourhood health centres" (Kark, 1981; Tollman, 1991; Kark and Kark, 1999). The basic principles of COPC have been central to classic public health for decades, and were incorporated into the Alma Ata Charter on Primary Health Care in 1978 (WHO, 1978). The underlying assumption of this theory, which informed the current health policy of post-apartheid South Africa, is that health and illness have more to do with the social, economic, and political determinants of society than with the health care system itself.

More recent proponents of family medicine have held the same view. McWhinney (1981) states that the family physician seeks to understand the context of the illness, views her/his practice as a population at risk, is part of a community-wide network of supportive and health care agencies, and is a manager of resources. Each of these principles emphasises the family physician's responsibilities outside the consulting room (see the Introduction).

Common problems in practice can be dealt with efficiently at an individual level, for example HIV, tuberculosis, sexually transmitted infections, diseases related to smoking and alcohol abuse, trauma, malnutrition, obesity, atherosclerosis, and anxiety or depression. However, it is not enough to simply continue treating each individual patient as an individual, without looking at the issues underlying these illnesses at a wider level. In the management of trauma, for example, excellent standards of surgical practice will make no impact on the road traffic accident rate, and the mortality rate can even rise. A family physician can spend his/her whole life seeing those patients who attend the practice for care, without making any difference at all to the health of the community that the practice serves. In fact, it is possible that the health status of the community can deteriorate despite his/her best efforts, excellent clinical standards and practice, and careful attention to each patient. Excellence needs to be redefined in terms of contributing to the health of the whole community, not just those who are able to attend the clinic, health centre, hospital, or private practice. In the words of Bryant (1969):

> "The world is moving on, and in many countries, including my own, the medical profession and medical educators can no longer remain aloof to the unmet needs of vast numbers of people. The old arguments that we are preserving a standard of excellence are wearing thin, not because that standard is invalid but because there has been so little effort to extend the knowledge derived from that standard to the unserved. Another definition of excellence needs to be added, namely, that excellence in health care for a population is to be found in gaining maximum improvement in health and relief from suffering within available resources."

Population-based health planning requires the involvement of all health care professionals in order to cater for the priority needs of the defined population. The National Health Service in the United Kingdom is based on this system: each general practitioner in a district is responsible for the health of a certain number of people, whether they are well or ill, and care is taken to ensure that no one is left without access to health care.

In South Africa, the *district health system* gives us the framework within which it is now possible to plan health services more equitably, and to respond to community-wide issues affecting the health of the people in that community. It is now possible to define the geographical boundaries and demographic denominators of communities, and to plan to cater for the needs of all, not just those who present themselves for help. "Health for All" means exactly that, health, not treatment of illness, for all the people in a defined district or community, not just for those who can afford it. Once again, Bryant (1969) defines the Health for All approach:

> "Every apparent success must be measured against the needs of all. Every effort, every cluster of resources must be divided by the total number of people. The insistence of using this denominator – all the people – has profound social, political, ethical and educational implications."

The health care system is obligated to ensure equitable access to health care services for the poor and marginalised people of society. In South Africa, now more than ever before, there is a political imperative towards equity, and this provides the political will and support for COPC. At an international level, the 2008 World Health Report of the World Health Organisation (WHO, 2008) celebrated the 30th anniversary of the Declaration of Alma Ata with the title "Now More Than Ever", emphasising the relevance and need for the primary health care approach to address inequities in the field of health. Significantly, it includes a chapter entitled "Putting People First" indicating the importance of integrating personal care with community-wide activities to improve health at a collective level.

What is COPC?

In the same way that clinical medicine gives us the tools for treating the individual patient effectively, COPC gives health care professionals the tools for tackling health priorities in a district, in partnership with community representatives. The combination of these approaches, the individual and the collective, comprises effective COPC.

Table 9.1 demonstrates the differences in approach and application between primary care and community care. The link between these areas of activity is the family, which is the focus of the principles of family medicine. It is important to understand that COPC is neither primary care only nor community care only, but is concerned with the linkages and integration of these activities at a family level (Nutting, 1987; Rhyne *et al.*, 1998).

Table 9.1 COPC is a combination of primary care and community care

Domain	Primary care	Community care
Focus of care	Patients seen as individuals Focus on active users	Members of a population Active and inactive users
Assessment methods	Patient-orientated clinical skills	Epidemiological skills
Planning basis	Utilisation by active users	Health needs of community
Personnel	Family physicians, clinical nurse practitioners, and ancillary staff	Community groups, community health workers, family physicians and nurses
Interventions	Individualised patient education and treatment	Community outreach prevention programmes
Evaluation	Health of the individual patient	Health status of an identified population

COPC starts with the individual patient and works outwards, firstly to the patient's family context, and then to the broader community. In practice, this shift does not happen overnight but is often a gradual process over a number of years. For example, a family physician or group of family physicians who are interested in improving the care of diabetic patients might begin with those who are regular attenders, and then establish a diabetic clinic and a patient care group. This could be extended to infrequent attenders, and then to those in the area who need care but do not attend the local health care facility. Finally, a plan could be developed by an -appropriate team of people to focus on those at risk of diabetes in the whole community through primary preventive and promotive measures.

A step-wise approach is used in this chapter that is appropriate for active family physicians and for students as part of a learning exercise. The energy generated in family medicine through the family physician's interactions and commitment to the person who is the patient, is often the driving force for a wider involvement in community-based health projects.

There are numerous practical examples of this approach. For example, the acute shortage of health professionals in a rural area, which had a significant impact on the quality of medical care in that area, stimulated Dr Andrew Ross at Ingwavuma in rural KwaZulu-Natal to establish a community-based scholarship scheme to support local students through university. The lack of potable water lead Dr Victor Fredlund to play a leading role in the building of a pipeline and water reticulation plant for his community at Mseleni.

A step-wise approach

A framework for a step-wise approach to COPC is given in Table 9.2 and described in detail below.

Table 9.2 A step-wise approach to COPC

Step 1 **Practice profile**	Work out the (ten) commonest clinical problems presenting to a practice, clinic, ward, or hospital
Step 2 **Individual assessment**	Find a patient (or patients) with that problem, and understand the individual(s) in detail
Step 3 **Home visit**	Visit that patient's home, then describe the family and the context in which the illness developed
Step 4 **Community assessment**	Define/describe the community, e.g. denominator data, resources, structures, and functioning
Step 5 **Priorities**	Identify and prioritise health problems in the community
Step 6 **Team formation**	Convene a team appropriate to the priority issue in consultation with the district management team or interest groups
Step 7 **Plan of action**	Plan and implement activities that address the most important problems
Step 8 **Evaluation**	Evaluate what has happened in terms of the experiences of individual patients

For students, this step-wise approach assumes that a group of medical or nursing students has between four and eight weeks in total, either continuously or in stages, to become involved in a COPC learning programme. It may be called a community-based learning experience or a rural block, and it may not contain all the steps listed here. However, there are elements that are common to such programmes, and this framework suggests a logical progression of experience and learning. The steps can be undertaken sequentially by successive groups of students, each group building on the achievements of the previous group. The disadvantage of this approach is lack of continuity as each group does not experience the process from beginning to end and it is therefore less meaningful. It is better for one group to see the process right through, even though the time available may not be continuous.

After a number of years in practice, family physicians in both the private sector and the public sector tend to become involved in community projects intuitively. When they undertake postgraduate study, they often are surprised to find that what they have been doing all along has an academic basis, and they acquire new skills to augment their extensive experience. The first step may be stimulated by a routine home visit, or by a particularly powerful experience with one patient, or even by a personal experience of illness. The practical experience of the three-stage assessment can be complemented by a conceptual understanding through the discovery of the principles of family medicine. As family physicians come to appreciate the importance of the context of each patient on their health, they are more likely to try to influence some aspect of the context.

Step 1 Practice profile

Based in a health facility, be it a clinic, private practice, community health centre, or a hospital ward, the busy family physician will intuitively identify the commonest clinical problems. Ask a few family physicians what the ten commonest problems are that they see, and they will be able to list them easily. However, they need to be quantified, and can be ranked in order of frequency of presentation by gathering data from the daily attendance register over a month. The diagnostic categories for each entry need to be standardised and agreed upon by each family physician in a district in order for this data to be meaningful. The International Classification of Primary Care (ICPC) or the International Classification of Diseases (ICD-10) are two of the commonest tools used for this purpose.

The commonest problems presenting to clinics or private family practices will be different from those seen at health centres or hospitals as patients select their level of care according to their own perceptions. Unless there is a strict gate-keeping system, which ensures that patients are seen in hospitals only if they have first been seen and referred by a primary care provider, the hospital outpatients data will include a large number of problems that could be addressed at a primary care facility such as a clinic.

Every patient presenting to a health facility needs to be regarded as a representative of a group of people in that same community at risk of the same illness. This means that a profile of the commonest presenting problems will indicate the most pressing health needs of a district. However, it is not as simple as that, since frequently occurring illnesses such as the common cold are relatively unimportant, whereas other illnesses are relatively rare but are life-threatening. In this latter group, hospitals attract the sickest and the most seriously ill patients, but again this profile is limited to small numbers.

How do we decide on priorities? Is the deciding factor the problems affecting the largest number of people, or the most frequent cause of serious morbidity or death? Discuss this question.

What are the ten commonest problems presenting to private practices, the local government or provincial clinics, and community health centres in your district? Admissions to hospital will give an idea of the most serious morbidity, and death certificate registers held by the magistrate's office will give mortality data. The ten commonest reasons for admission to hospital and the ten commonest causes of death should therefore be relatively easy to establish in your district. (This exercise works well for students working in groups, with each gathering data from a different source.)

Step 2 Individual assessment

In the course of routine primary clinical care, typically seeing between 20 and 60 patients a day, the experienced nurse or family physician will have established relationships with a certain proportion of patients over the course of time. In government clinics, there is relatively little continuity of care with specific patients by specific family physicians, whereas general practitioners in private practice see a high proportion of known patients. In patient-centred medicine, relationships are important (see Chapter 2).

This intimate knowledge of patients over a period is often taken for granted by experienced family physicians. For the student, however, it requires a conscious and explicit effort to explore and understand the patient's experience of the illness, without the benefit of a previous relationship.

The purpose of this step of the COPC cycle is to understand the individual's experience of his/her illness qualitatively, in all its individuality. Each person responds to illness or adversity in a different way, often subconsciously, through a complex interaction of previous experiences, fears, expectations, and beliefs.

We have legitimate access to patients when they attend a health facility for care. They often give health professionals permission to do extraordinary things, such as agreeing to remove their clothes in front of strangers. Students are usually given similar access, provided they explicitly ask for the patient's permission, and thus they can learn an enormous amount by gaining the patient's trust at an early stage. It is crucial from an ethical point of view to ensure that you get the patient's full co-operation and consent before asking probing questions.

How can you, as an outsider, really understand someone else's experience of their illness? Should you start with your own experiences of illness in the past? What questions should you ask? Discuss these questions.

Q Identify a patient with one of the ten commonest problems. Patients with chronic problems are often suitable as they appreciate the extra attention and are willing to allow students to learn from them. Carry out a clinical and individual assessment. The clinical assessment is exactly what students have been taught so well at medical school, namely to make a clinical diagnosis. However, this is not enough in family medicine. We need to understand the individual better, and find out what she/he understands and feels about the illness. It is the aim of this exercise to try to understand the patient's experience of her/his illness.

Remember that family physicians recognise disease, whereas patients experience illness. Chapters 2 and 3 will help you with this exercise. (If students are working in groups, each group can find a patient with a different problem.)

Step 3 Home visit

Home visits were traditionally an important aspect of the work of family physicians in many countries, but the frequency of home visits has declined over the years. The reasons for this are numerous, including rising costs, and the improvement in communications and emergency services. Nevertheless, the home visit is a crucial link between clinical practice and comprehensive care, and it creates a physical and psychological bridge between facility-based and community-based interventions. So much insight can be gained from a single home visit that not only is the time spent justified, but the effect on other patients is often significant. McWhinney (1989) states that "the family physician sees patients at the office, at their homes, and in the hospital", since she/he is committed to the person who is the patient.

A home visit can be compared to the time and expense of a common elective surgical operation, with similarly dramatic results. It can be either diagnostic or therapeutic, and is often a combination of both. While the ostensible reason for a home visit may be that the patient cannot travel, or the medical problem is an emergency, the experienced family physician may often take the opportunity to understand a patient's context better, or demonstrate her/his commitment to the patient by making a home visit. As a learning exercise, students would undertake a home visit primarily as a "diagnostic" exercise, in the hope that they can learn more about the context of the illness, but they may be called upon to give advice. Whether it is requested by the patient or suggested by the family physician, entering a patient's home and family is an intimate experience, and must be approached with due respect and consideration.

Frequently in the rural situation in South Africa, there are cross-cultural issues to deal with. Even in ethnically homogeneous communities, every interaction between a family physician and a patient is to a certain extent a cross-cultural event. Family physicians have their own language and body of knowledge, while patients use their own language and norms to understand their illnesses. However, it is important to respect the norms of the patient's culture; for example, greeting, sitting, and eliciting information all require prior knowledge of these norms in order to avoid unintentional offence. Whereas experienced family physicians acquire these understandings over years, students may need to be introduced to cross-cultural issues explicitly.

Q How should you approach a patient's family in their home? Discuss this question. Role-playing different situations (for example, suspicion from the family) is a useful exercise.

Q Make plans to visit the home of the patient identified in the previous step, or another patient with a similar problem. (Students should work in pairs or groups.) It is important to obtain the patient's consent by explaining who you are, why you want to visit the home, and what you hope to learn. Most patients will be willing to allow a group of students to visit their home and family in return for a lift home from the health facility if they rely on public transport. Patients with chronic problems are often only too happy to have health workers visit their homes, as it is an opportunity to gain information and improve the situation for them.

What are the goals for the visit? Firstly, gather information on the index patient and their illness. What makes it worse? What makes it better? What started it? What could change? What is the effect of medication or other medical interventions on the illness? Look for help-seeking behaviour. What does this family do when someone is ill? Who gets involved in caring and who does not? How could this be different?

Secondly, look at the family. Gather information on the family structure, dynamics and relationships, values, daily activities, educational level, sources of income and stability, support systems (extended family, neighbours, and church or other groups), and other resources. For example, a traditional healer or a particular friend may be a significant person to the family. It is often useful to draw a genogram or ecomap (see Chapter 4) while you are at the home in order to help elicit further information about the family. Make an assessment of the family that draws all the important findings together.

Thirdly, look at the home. Look at the physical infrastructure, hygiene and sanitation, water sources, distance to schools and shops, means of transport, communications, environment, security, and stability of tenure.

Finally, make a difference to the patient, to the family, or to any other factor that influences the illness. For example, if you find other family members coughing at the home of a tuberculosis patient, you need to make plans to get the whole family screened. Or, if you find carpeted floors or pets in the home of a chronic asthmatic, you could suggest that specific information and action are needed for that family.

Step 4   Community assessment

The community in COPC is the equivalent of the patient in individual care. Knowing the characteristics of the community both qualitatively and quantitatively is an essential component of COPC practice. Just as we take a history and examine individual patients, so we must enquire about and examine the community that we serve, if we are to make any meaningful interventions beyond the individual level. This is basically a situational analysis of the community or district.

What is a community? How could it be defined or described? It could be:

• A group of people residing in a geographically defined area

- Members of a certain ethnic, language, age, or other demographically defined group who share certain characteristics
- The patients who attend a particular clinic or private practice, or members of a health maintenance organisation or medical scheme
- A group of people brought together by a school, church, workplace, shared interest, or necessity, who have the opportunity to interact with one another.

The district health system operates on the basis of distinct geographical districts, and all health workers within that area share the responsibility for the health of its residents. In South Africa, this gives us the opportunity to plan the utilisation of resources more equitably and rationally than ever before. Defining the parameters of a community in terms of its length and breadth, its boundaries and limits, is an essential first step in COPC, as it sets the denominators on which later assessments will depend. The whole population of a geographically defined district is the focus of the health care services, rather than select individuals within that district, such as those who can afford to attend a health facility. In managed care, or a health maintenance organisation, the community is defined as those members who subscribe to the scheme, either through their employer or individually. This effectively excludes the majority of unemployed people and those who cannot afford a monthly health insurance premium, an exclusion that the district health system seeks to avoid.

This stage of the COPC process is based on the collation and analysis of existing data. Sources of information include the health services themselves, census data, and the local magistrate or council offices. It can be carried out over a defined period by a small group of people, depending on the size of the area (district, sub-district, or smaller).

Use the patient's home as a starting point and explore the neighbourhood from there. Draw a map of the area, and describe the various components qualitatively and, where possible, quantitatively. Find the basic "denominator" (demographic) and health data at the district health office or the magistrate's office.

Q First, look at the *physical environment*. Describe the location, size, topography, climate, business areas, natural resources, communications and transport systems, housing, sanitation, water supply, shopping and educational facilities, and so on. Then, look at the *socio-demographic characteristics*. Here you will look at age and gender, population size, average income, educational level, literacy rate, ethnic characteristics, family structures, history, political structures, leadership, crime, employment, religious affiliations, recreation facilities, welfare, and so on. Third, describe the *health status*. Include the general mortality rate and its main causes: the infant, under-five, and maternal mortality rates; the HIV prevalence; the tuberculosis incidence and cure rate; the birth rate; the teenage pregnancy rate; the abortion rates; any substance abuse; the effects of violence; the number of road traffic accidents; the prevalence of chronic diseases and disability; immunisation coverage, and so on. Lastly, look at *health services*. This will include personal and non-personal health services, hospitals, clinics, community health centres, general and specialist practices, welfare services, environmental health services, and health programmes.

Step 5 Priorities

Once you have described the characteristics of the community, including its health status, the next step is to identify and prioritise the main health problems. This step is the equivalent of making a diagnosis on a patient, and can be called a "community diagnosis". Since communities are complex systems, and face many different health problems simultaneously, they are forced to compete for limited resources. Decisions regarding what, where, when, and how personnel and other resources should be deployed in a given community will depend on what are identified as the most important health needs.

The identification of health needs begins by listing all the health problems identified in the situational analysis and ranking the ten most compelling problems through an open discussion between the members of the district or sub-district primary care team. 'Brainstorming' in -response to the question "What are the most important health issues in this community?" will generate a long list, which can be subsequently whittled down by the application of criteria.

While health professionals can identify the major causes of morbidity and mortality by the analysis of health status data, these decisions cannot be made without the users of the health system, that is, the community itself. In the words of Sidney Kark (1981), the pioneer of COPC in the 1950s, we need to *"explore what the community feels, thinks and does about its health needs, since interventions need to be directed towards those aspects about which people can do much themselves"*. Thus, community involvement in this stage of identification and prioritisation is considered essential. Community representatives from formal representative structures such as local, district, or tribal councils should be invited to participate, as should key figures in the community, such as religious leaders or school principals.

However, if true community participation is aimed for, the best method is a participatory learning-in-action approach. In this method, ordinary community members are invited to a central venue, and a process of dialogue is started that aims at gaining insight into their felt needs. By drawing a "time-line" of the history of the development of health services in that area over the previous few decades as members relate it, a sense of continuity and ownership of the health services can be created. Mapping the community resources for health on the ground of a sports field is a good way to gain a spatial overview of the gaps and needs geographically. Experienced health practitioners who have lived in the community themselves, or who through home visits have become sensitive to the needs of the community, will hear and support emerging needs as they are expressed. Once these needs have been listed in a qualitative manner, they can be compared and combined with the quantitative health status information to present a comprehensive picture. For example, many communities will be reluctant to identify HIV and AIDS as a major issue, but the mortality figures from the hospitals can be presented objectively, and priorities can be agreed upon based on the whole picture.

Alternatively, a formal survey of community opinions can determine felt community health needs, but this keeps the initiative in the hands of the health professionals and does not engender community ownership and participation. Without community involvement, any subsequent intervention is unlikely to succeed.

The process of prioritisation of the identified health issues amounts to a "community diagnosis", equivalent to the 'problem list' of the individual patient (Williams *et al.*, 1995). To determine priorities, the parameters that need to be considered are:

- The magnitude of the problem, as measured by the prevalence or incidence
- The severity of each problem, as measured by the case fatality rate
- The level of concern of the community
- The feasibility of intervention
- The efficacy of intervention.

The application of these criteria to the list of health issues will help to identify priorities and the highest priority issue can be selected for initial attention in the next step.

Q With the guidance of the district health manager for the given community, list and prioritise the health issues based on the information gathered in the previous step. Each major issue needs to be weighted according to the criteria given above, and reasons should be given for its weighting. The highest-priority issue can then be selected for the next step.

Step 6 Team formation

It is likely that the selected issue is important enough so that there is already a group of people working on it either in an official capacity or as volunteers. It is therefore essential to connect with those in the government departments, the district management team, non-governmental organizations, private practices and organisations, or interest groups in the area that are concerned with the issue under consideration. In many areas of South Africa, it is important not to exclude traditional healers from the team. If a team does not already exist, this needs to be formed around the identified issue.

In a large regional hospital in South Africa some years ago, doctors in the paediatric ward became alarmed by the increasing number of measles cases and deaths in their wards. Clearly, vaccinations were not being given as they should at the clinics and health centres in the community, but this was not the job of the hospital doctors. Confronted with an epidemic, however, they convened a team of people who were involved in immunisations. These included the clinic nurses and their supervisors, the pharmacist, the community health services manager, the transport manager, and the trainer of the community health workers in the area. Together as a team, they devised a plan that was put into action, and the documented incidence of measles was shown to have started its decline from that point onwards. As hospital doctors in isolation of the team they were powerless to effect change, and the rest of the team did not appreciate the seriousness of the epidemic until the team was formed and information was shared.

Team formation requires initiative, leadership, commitment, and vision. If COPC is to be effective, the formation of a strong team composed of the right people for the task is the most crucial issue. Many community projects have failed because the most appropriate people have been overlooked during the formation of the team. Key community members with a stake in the issue may be crucial, as may be the inclusion of a technical expert where possible. You can improve the whole focus of the team by including a disabled person in a team working on disability or a person living with HIV in a team working on the issue of HIV and AIDS. Building a common vision for addressing the health issue forms the first part of the next step.

Q Draw up a list of the most appropriate people to form an action team around the identified priority issue. If there is already a committee or organisation dedicated to the issue, ask the convenor in what ways you might be able to contribute to their efforts. Otherwise, call a meeting and invite all those on the list. Ask them to identify others who might contribute to the process. Elect a leader and secretary, and establish a communication system.

Step 7　Plan of action

Once a team has been formed, it may be necessary to gather further detailed information on the specific health problem in order to record a baseline. For example, a project in the area of maternal health care may require the infant mortality rate to be accurately validated before beginning an intervention. Specific information on the reasons for a high infant mortality rate would need to be investigated. Focused surveys of a specific target population may be necessary.

Start the planning cycle by answering the following questions:

- What do we ultimately want to achieve – what is our vision?
- What are the broad aims or goals of the project?
- What are the objectives or components of these goals?

These questions will determine the project's activities, which need deadlines and people to carry them out. Finally, a budget needs to be allocated to each goal. The planning grid in Table 9.3 may be helpful for formulating a plan of action.

Table 9.3 A framework for planning objectives, goals, and activities

	Objec-tives	Activi-ties	When	Who	Indica-tors	Assump-tions	Budget
Goal A	1. 2. 3.						
Goal B	1. 2. 3.						
Goal C	1. 2. 3.						

Q Complete Table 9.3 for your selected priority issue, and check out the feasibility of its implementation with local health managers. Present it to the appropriate group or committee that can make use of your proposals.

Step 8 Evaluation

The initial detailed assessment of the problem gives a baseline for evaluation, and the inclusion of indicators in the planning process will ensure that evaluation is an integral part of the COPC project.

Similar to a quality improvement cycle (see Chapter 10), the process of COPC needs to be a cyclical one. The evaluation of a team's efforts after six months or a year should lead to further efforts to correct deficiencies in the plan, or to replan altogether in order to sustain improvements. A new team may need to be formed, new members may need to be co-opted, and a fresh mission statement may need to be drawn up.

A question that is often asked is "how far should we go?". In other words, what is the role of the clinical practitioner in addressing the social, economic and political determinants of health? Gruen (2004) provides a helpful model, defining the professional responsibility of the clinician as extending beyond the personal care of the individual patient to addressing issues of access to care, as well as those factors in the community that have a direct influence on health. The clinician need not be the leader of the team, but should at least contribute a clinical perspective to active efforts by a team to address the "upstream" factors that result in the most pressing health problems.

It is essential, however, that family physicians remain committed to people and not to abstract plans. This is their unique advantage – that they remain in direct contact with the users of the health system, and are able to receive direct feedback of the effect of any community-wide interventions on the people at whom they are directed. The strength of COPC is in the linkages between primary care practice and community-wide efforts to change the context in which it operates.

Conclusion

COPC offers an approach to involvement in the context of the families and communities of our patients, with a view to making a difference beyond the individual level of care. Through a gradual accumulation of successive experiences in families and the community over a number of years, family physicians often become involved in COPC-like activities without realising it. Students, however, with a limited time for this kind of activity, can get an initial understanding of the process through following a stepwise approach over a number of weeks.

The challenges of HIV, particularly, will test our skills and our resources to the limit in the following decades. It is abundantly clear that attention to the individual patient only, even with antiretroviral drugs, will not stem the tide of new infections. All health professionals need to support families and communities to explore jointly ways of preventing further infections, and of tending to those already infected. This is likely to be the nation's greatest single challenge in the area of health, and COPC provides some of the tools to address the needs.

The appealing aspect of COPC is the linkage of the personal with the collective, from individual patient, through family, to community. Students and practitioners are motivated by their commitment to the person who is the patient, and this commitment can be carried through to a wider involvement in district-wide initiatives to improve health. Enjoy the journey!

Recommended reading

Epstein L, Eshed H. (1988). *Community-oriented primary health care: the responsibility of the team for the health of the total population.* South African Medical Journal. 73: 220-223.

Gruen RL, Pearson SD, Brennan TA. (2004). *Physician-Citizens – Public Roles and Professional Obligations.* Journal of the American Medical Association. 291: 94–98

Kark, SL (1981) *The Practice of Community-Oriented Primary Health Care.* New York: Appleton-Century-Crofts.

Kark, S and Kark, E (1999) *Promoting Community Health: From Pholela to Jerusalem.* Johannesburg: Witwatersrand University Press.

Neuwelt P, *et al.* (2009). *Putting population health Into practice through primary health care.* New Zealand Medical Journal. 2009, 122: 98-104

Nutting P. (ed) (1987). *Community Oriented Primary Care: from principle to practice.* Washington DC: US Dept of Health and Human Services Public Health Service, Health Resources and Services Administration, Office of Primary Care Studies.

Rhyne, R, Bogue, R, Kukulka, G and Fulmer, H (EDS) (1998) *Community-Oriented Primary Care: Health Care for the 21st Century.* Washington DC: American Public Health Association.

Starfield B. (1998) *Primary Care: Balancing health needs, services and technology.* New York: Oxford University Press.

World Health Organization (2008). *World Health Report 2008: Now More than Ever.* WHO, Geneva.

10 Organisational and management principles

Nzapfurundi Chabikuli
Family Health International, Nigeria
and
Hon Lecturer, Department of Family Medicine
University of Pretoria
Sam Fehrsen
Former Head of Department of Family Medicine
MEDUNSA
Hon Lecturer, Department of Family Medicine,
University of Pretoria
Jannie Hugo
Head of Department of Family Medicine
University of Pretoria

Introduction

Most doctors entering the private or public sector do not have the skills needed for managing a practice. As undergraduates, students are totally occupied by clinical medicine and most find it difficult to be interested in the details of management systems sustaining clinical practice. As students may not have an opportunity to apply these skills, if taught at undergraduate level, they are likely to forget what they learn. Many *management courses* are available to people in the public and private sectors. Students are advised to attend such courses nearer the time when they will use these skills of managing people, health care, and financial systems.

The purpose of management in family medicine is to organise the work of the practice or health district so that the vision, principles, and core values of family medicine can be realised in a cost-effective and sustainable manner. These values and principles need to be applied within the possibilities created by South Africa's policies and values for health system transformation. These values and principles are not necessarily different from those in family medicine.

This chapter offers an introduction to the key principles in health systems management. The purpose is to provide enough information to help *identify* in what kind of health system a particular public or private practice is operating – that is, to understand what you are seeing. This will hopefully raise key issues for *debate* among students and future family physicians about the development of our health system in South Africa. This will no doubt emphasise that the world is struggling with runaway costs in health care and cost efficiency, and that we are all compelled to *work creatively* for a better system. One of our main aims is to *point to sources of help* to use when you are ready to assume management responsibilities.

Management opportunities

All doctors in South Africa undergo community service in rural and district level hospitals around the country. It has been suggested in a recent review of the community service programme that support from senior staff is limited in these settings. Perhaps for this reason, community service doctors do more than their scope of skills would allow. It is therefore an ideal moment to start learning about management while working in the health system and to develop further. The first lesson a community service doctor learns relates to the management of scarce resources in the health system in general. Young doctors are confronted almost immediately with the lack of adequate staff, equipment, support services, and even amenities. This problem is not confined to South Africa.

After community service, some doctors will opt to become registrars in family medicine. While training to become family physicians, registrars will learn about management during their academic programme and have the opportunity to participate in the management of health centres and district hospitals.

Family physicians in the public sector have management responsibilities as part of their job description and these usually focus on the co-ordination of clinical care, team leadership and clinical governance. Family physicians may also participate in the facility, sub-district and district management teams where decisions about issues such as service delivery, human resources, drug supply and health information systems are taken.

Family physicians in the private sector are usually involved in all aspects of practice management.

Health care system reforms

Health care delivery systems are changing worldwide as a result of a concern about runaway costs in the provision of health care and the need to expand access to health care. Both market-driven and socialist systems are experiencing rapid change influenced by increasing globalisation and the need to address the challenge of cost efficiency. From experiences of other countries and the published literature, there is no clear blueprint on how to transform and manage the health system efficiently; furthermore, there is no quick answer for developing countries.

South Africa has the additional concern of reducing inequity for the benefit of previously disadvantaged communities. Our current national policies emphasise equity whereby continuity of care should be equally available to all. However, resource constraints such as the lack of facilities in some areas, poor staff-to-patient ratios, and rapid turnover of staff make this personal continuity difficult to provide in an equitable manner.

In South Africa, the government is a key actor in the health care system, a role that stems from the government's regulatory, financing, and service provision functions. South Africa is in the process of restructuring its health service. Three key reforms are worth noting:

1. The establishment of a National Health Insurance (NHI)
2. *The strengthening of the District Health System,* which has been chosen as a managerial strategy to implement primary health care services in a manner that benefits most citizens
3. The increasingly regulated operation of private practices to fit into the vision of a unitary health system.

A previous restructuring of the public service administration and financing has established managerial efficiency measures in the public sector (for example performance management systems). Opponents of the transformation of the health sector argue that it has cost implications the economy cannot bear. Health care services are funded from taxes, by contributions from the household, as well as from employers. An effort is being made however to achieve greater integration and rationalisation of both the public and private systems of care in a manner that minimises costs.

Engaging with policy debates

The *transformation process* gives us an opportunity to find new ways to implement the broad aims of national policies within the district health system and in our practices. The NHI, for example, is one such reform inviting informed debate among students, practising family physicians, the public, and politicians. The debate is often influenced by vested interests and perceptions sometimes built on misconceptions. For instance, private health care funders and specialists in South African medical schools are experiencing major upheavals and change in the transformation process. In pursuance of equity, national funding policies are shifting to disadvantaged populations and to primary health care – a previously neglected area.

In an attempt to maintain the status quo, influential private health care funders and specialists groups fight these changes on the basis of dropping quality and standards. By doing so, they imply that the policies for transformation will inevitably make matters worse and that future patients will have less quality of care, for example access to specialists and the latest technology. However, if we can deliver more and better quality primary health care, the work of specialists and sub-specialists would be more focused and insurance claims reduced. Specialists' days would not be cluttered with inappropriate referrals and providing primary care at a tertiary institution. They would have more time and could serve the interests of their patients better.

Misconceptions may determine what kinds of reforms are possible when stakeholders make their inputs into new laws and regulations. The perceptions of health professionals also influence the ways in which they put the laws and regulations into practice in their particular environment. If our perceptions are based on the best available information, we can creatively work to influence our future. At the time of writing, issues around the NHI are being hotly debated. We can influence our circumstances as health professionals and as patients in the foreseeable future. Enlightened self-interest dictates that we all read and debate as best we can at this time. For this reason, this chapter emphasises understanding, evaluation, and discussion.

The *principles and core values* that should guide our policies and management aim at organising the practice or health district for equity of care and access in an affordable and sustainable way. We should manage to make it possible for the family medicine clinical process to be practised in the public and private sector, and to create a system for primary health care that is fit for patients, while maintaining job fulfillment and fair remuneration for health professionals. We need to protect those managerial processes that make for a relationship of trust between the patient and the health professional within which healing and care take place.

A note on terminology

The term *provider* will be used in the rest of this chapter, as it applies equally to students, nurses, other primary care clinicians, and doctors.

The term *practice* refers to primary care (or family medicine) services and applies to public health centres and private practice. We have chosen this term to emphasise the similarity of values and purpose in family medicine although the context in the private and public sectors may be very different.

Ten questions

These ten questions will help you understand the health facilities where you are doing your clinical family medicine training. You can then constructively take part in the debate that will shape your own future working environment. The questions explore if both the patient and health care provider are being dealt with fairly.

1 *Would I gladly be a patient in this place?*
   Consider why you would or would not be happy to be a patient in this facility, be it a clinic, health centre or hospital.

2 *Is an ongoing relationship of trust between the patient and provider possible here?*

3 *Who intrudes into the relationship between the provider and the patient?*
   To answer this question, you need to note all the people or third parties that stand between the provider and the patient and so influence the doctor–patient relationship. Are any of them exploiting the patient?

4 *Will I get job satisfaction and fair remuneration if I work here?*
   Here you may consider such things as clinical and administrative freedom or scope for participation and creativity within the practice. Will I be exploited here and by whom? Is the system promoting and sustaining the best for the patient, the community, and the provider, given the circumstances?

5 *What are the core values and vision of this practice?*
   These may be written and available for all to see, or may be implied in what you hear the people saying and what you see them doing. Check your impressions with the providers and the patients, or people in the local community.

6 *Who are all the people involved in this practice?*
   To find the role-players or stakeholders, you can think of those who control what happens, who make the decisions, who use the services, and who influence what happens in the practice. How is the community served and/or involved? Is this involvement meaningful, in the spirit of community-oriented primary care?

7 *If you work here, to whom are you accountable and how?*
In facing this question, you are likely to discover which people are truly participating in and influencing the process of service delivery. In one community hospital, for instance, records were not available on ward rounds, as the ward nurses were accountable to the matron for keeping patient records correctly. The matron thus kept the records in her office and marked them like examination scripts. Accountability to the patients and colleagues who also used the records to provide comprehensive and humane care was thus secondary to the requirements of completeness and tidiness of the records.

8 *How does the money move in this system? Who controls the budget?*
If you trace the money in the health system from its source to the end of its journey and note all those who live off it in its long trail, you will discover many issues for debate. This is true of both the private and the public sectors.

9 *Is this practice cost-effective and sustainable within the context of South Africa?*
Every practice has a policy to do certain things as a matter of routine, for example, recording the weight and height of all new patients at their first visit. Any practice routine should be evaluated to see if it is affordable over time in terms of the funds available, if it is effective, and if it is offered on an equitable basis. In such an evaluation, for example, you could ask what the implications would be of doing a cervical smear on all women in the practice every three years. In terms of equity, would this be possible for all women in your practice or health district?

10 *Is there a functional quality improvement (QI) system in this practice?*
Quality improvement is described later on in this chapter.

The complexity of systems in health care

Health care systems are complex and not easily transformed. Patients, the end users, have less control over what happens than in most other social systems. The information at patients' disposal, which is needed to make choices, is limited. For example, patients buying bread or meat in a store may exert more control over what they eat than over what medications they take when they go to the doctor. In the store, their knowledge of what they want and what they can afford enables them to make decisions. In the medical system, patients are often denied the opportunity of making informed decisions and just accept what health workers decide for them. Even if they are given the opportunity to participate, they may still rely on the attitude that the doctor knows best.

The organisation of health care can thus not be left only to market forces, bureaucrats, politicians, or health professionals. Systems need to be organised in order to encourage the participation of potential patients and community groups. We need to safeguard the interests of patients and their providers, who are often the weakest members in the health care system.

In this section, we will look at some of the elements of the South African system and their interrelationships to get a better understanding of the system as a whole. (Some of the key terms used in this section are described in a box at the end of the chapter.) The section is organised along the framework of the WHO's six building blocks of a health system (see Box 1).

Box 1: WHO's health systems building blocks:

1. Leadership and governance involves ensuring strategic policy frameworks exist and are combined with effective oversight, coalition-building, the provision of appropriate regulations and incentives, attention to system-design, and accountability.

2. A good health financing system that raises adequate funds for health, in ways that ensures people can use needed services and are protected from financial catastrophe or impoverishment associated with having to pay for them.

3. A well-performing health workforce, one that works in ways that are responsive, fair and efficient to achieve the best health outcome possible, given available resources and circumstances.

4. A well-functioning health information system, one that ensures the production, analysis, dissemination and use of reliable and timely information on health determinants, health systems performance and health status.

5. Good health services which deliver effective, safe, quality personal and non-personal health interventions to those who need them, when and where needed, with minimum waste of resources.

6. Equitable access to essential medical products, vaccines and technologies of assured quality, safety, efficacy and cost effectiveness, and their scientifically sound and cost effective use.

1. Leadership and governance

1.1 Laws and regulations

Society has given to government, at all levels, from local to national, the task of creating systems through which we will get the care we want. We safeguard our future as patients and providers by remaining vigilant and active in the debate. The purpose of laws and regulations in the health sector of relevance to this chapter, are primarily to:

- Make the services available to all
- Strive for equity
- Manage the risk to individuals
- Protect quality.

These laws and regulations (see Figure 10.1) have an impact on all the role-players. It is not only the National Health Act that affects operations in the health sector – so too do others, such as the Labour Relations Act and the Companies Act. All the parties involved may influence the laws, as they are made or adapted in light of experience, through their feedback and submissions.

Q What are the main laws and regulations that affect patients and providers in your practice?

How will the NHI affect your practice?

1.2 Control and accountability

One of the difficulties in the South African health system is that there are many who control health care without accountability to the patient and the public (see Figure 10.2). The Patients' Rights Charter and Complaints Procedure (see pages 359 to 360) was drawn up and propagated to increase public awareness of their rights and the role they have in improving the quality of care. The Charter consists of twelve rights, ten responsibilities, and a complaints procedure. It is good to see that many of these items support the core values of family medicine, especially the right to an ongoing relationship with a particular provider.

Q To which persons and organisations/institutions are providers in your setting accountable? How is accountability made practical? Will the Charter ultimately make matters better or worse for patients and their care?

Figure 10.1 Legislation and regulations that affect health care

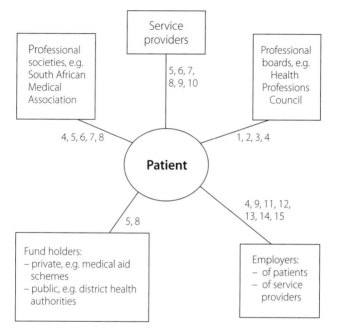

Key

1 Health Professions Act 56 of 1974
2 Nursing Act 50 of 1987 amended 1997
3 Pharmacy Act 53 of 1975 amended 2000
4 Constitution of the Republic of South Africa Act 108 of 1996
5 Medical Schemes Act 62 of 2002
6 Companies Act 61 of 1973
7 Medical, Dental and Supplementary Health Service Professions Act 56 of 1974 (containing the Rules of the Medical and Dental Council)
8 National Health Act 61 of 2003
9 Labour Relations Act 66 of 1995
10 Income Tax Act 34 of 1953
11 Basic Conditions of Employment Act 11 of 2002
12 Occupational Health and Safety Act 85 of 1993
13 Compensation for Occupational Injuries and Diseases Act 130 of 1993
14 Occupational Disease in Mines and Works Act 60 of 2002
15 Mine Health and Safety Act 29 of 1996

Figure 10.2 Control and accountability

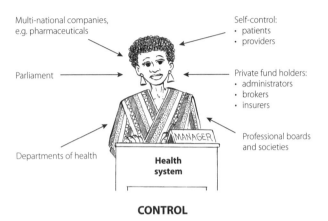

Multi-national companies,
e.g. pharmaceuticals

Self-control:
• patients
• providers

Parliament

Private fund holders:
• administrators
• brokers
• insurers

Departments of health

Professional boards
and societies

MANAGER

**Health
system**

CONTROL

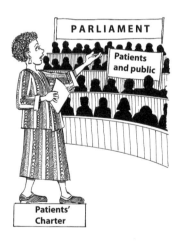

PARLIAMENT

Patients
and public

Patients'
Charter

ACCOUNTABILITY

2. Health financing system

2.1 Means of payment

Most patients receive care without paying the service provider directly. Payment is effected through a third party. In 2008 about 7,1 million people contributed towards a medical aid society and got their care within the private sector. The uninsured either pay cash for their services in the private sector or make use of the services offered by the public sector. In the public sector, services are free for all children, pregnant women, and people with infectious diseases such as HIV and pulmonary tuberculosis, as well as for the indigent. For the rest, there is a charge that is related to the person's means. Many move between the public and private sectors, depending on their needs at the time. The public health service is financed from taxes. All people contribute to a portion of this through value added tax (VAT). Others also contribute through income tax and other forms of taxation. The government is exploring the possibility of financing an NHI that will provide cover to all people, by pooling resources from employers, employees, and those who are self-employed, whilst government will provide for the indigent. These health funds will be administered by a single agency, contracting public and private health care providers. From the beginning of the discussions, treasury and professional groups have raised concerns that the NHI is costly and lacks flexibility. In response, the government has proposed a two-phased approach: start with a social health insurance (benefits to contributors only), and later an NHI (benefits to both contributors and non-contributors).

Since January 2000, all medical aid schemes have to cover people for a minimum benefit package of specified conditions, and for their diagnosis and treatment. This does not yet include primary care (see the Medical Schemes Act 62 of 2002 and the Regulations).

Providers are paid in three main ways (see Figure 10.3):

Figure 10.3 Methods of payment for health services

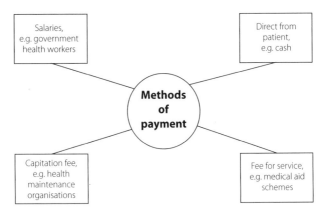

- Salary: Those working for the state are paid by means of a salary.
- Fee-for-service: The majority of those in the private sector are paid on a fee-for-service basis directly in cash or have their services reimbursed via a third party, such as a medical aid society.
- Capitation: In managed care organisationss, providers are paid an amount per person registered with them and then deliver a defined package of care. These organisations are usually for people in the lower income brackets who cannot afford the premiums of the fee-for-service system, which gives them access to any service or provider.

Q Examine and evaluate the route taken by money in your practice. Are the service providers realistically aware of costs? Are the patients aware of costs? How are services paid for in your practice? How are service providers paid in your practice? Are there better ways of arranging payments?

2.2 Risk sharing and risk taking

The concept of risk is core to the design and reform of health system financing mechanisms such as the NHI described in the previous section. This concept acknowledges that the young and people fortunate enough to have a hardy constitution seldom need health care outside of health promotion and prevention services, such as vaccinations. The elderly and those with less robust constitutions are often ill and in need of medical care. Those who need the most help can seldom afford the cost of care on their own. This is also true for many individuals who do not have sufficient money available at the time of a serious illness, although they have not needed help for many years. For these reasons, risk sharing mechanisms have been developed.

Risk sharing is a bottom-up process whereby a group, or the whole population, through a process of solidarity, pool resources and risk so that the group carries the cost of caring for all when illness strikes. In this way, the contribution made during the healthy periods in one's life helps to carry the cost of the sickness for oneself as well as for others in the community (cross-subsidisation). The NHI envisages making membership and contributions compulsory from all who are able to make payment, the government contributing on behalf of the indigents.

Risk taking is a top-down process in which shared contributions are redistributed and in which various people take risks (see Figure 10.4). For example provincial government and their departments of health take a risk that the funds allocated to health and budgeted for specific services will be sufficient for the year. If they are not assisted with more funds after overspending, they normally transfer their problem to their patients by stopping or reducing services. Many facilities have experienced shortages of supplies and medications at the end of the financial year when the funds dry up. One year the entire Free State ran out of funding for antiretrovirals when funds were exhausted. Poor planning, poor management, poor use of resources by health workers and misuse of health services by patients can all contribute to an adverse risk profile.

In the private sector medical aid societies and insurers manage the funds and bear the risk of going bankrupt when expenditure on health services exceed contributions. This money comes from their members' contributions. If they go bankrupt, the members lose their health cover. It should be noted that medical aid administrators, brokers and consultants make a living out of providing expertise to the medical aid societies and as they live off commission do not take any direct risks themselves.

To decrease the possibility of people being left without care there are many laws and regulations that aim to prevent this situation (see Figure 10.1). Increasingly, managed care organisations (MCOs) are being established in South Africa to manage the risk in health care.

Figure 10.4 Risk sharing and risk taking

Risk sharing
Where is the money coming from?
Bottom-up solidarity

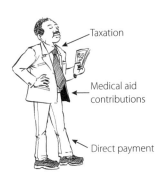

Taxation

Medical aid contributions

Direct payment

Patient
In need of health care
Taking and sharing risk

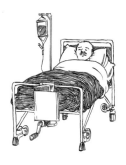

Risk taking
Who takes the risk of distributing the money?
Top-down distribution

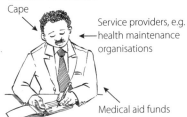

Department of Health, e.g. Provincial Administration of the Western Cape

Service providers, e.g. health maintenance organisations

Medical aid funds

The government has introduced a *Risk Equalisation Fund* (REF) that has two key elements. For example, one medical aid society could have young healthy members with low risk and another many pensioners with a large burden of chronic illness and high risk. To level the playing field and encourage medical aid societies to compete on quality and competitive prices rather than on looking for low-risk members, the REF first converts the whole population of people on medical aid into one risk pool by collecting money from low-risk pools and giving money to high-risk groups from the REF. The next phase for institutions is to ensure that low-income earners pay less and high-income earners pay more for basic services as determined by the Basic Benefit Package so that all employed people will ultimately be able to take up medical aid insurance.

Q Who is sharing the risk in your practice? Who is the solidarity group?

Who is taking the risk in your system?

2.3 Managing money

Financial management means knowing the resources at your disposal to generate income, and how return on these resources can be improved either by increasing income or cutting back on costs. In the process of making such decisions, a manager must think about possibilities of bringing in new activities (for example new clinical procedures in the practice) or enhancing the performance of staff to increase productivity or outsourcing certain non-profitable services. Financial management therefore requires not only information about costs and prices, but also information related to staff performance, quality and productivity.

Information produced by your accountant can be used to fulfill three basic roles:

1   *Financial accounting.* This means recording all monetary transactions and the subsequent production of summary financial statements reflecting the performance and financial standing of the organisation, for example income and expenditure accounts, balance sheets, and cash flow statements.

2   *Budgets and management reporting.* This provides information to managers that enables planning, monitoring and control. This entire process introduces accountability in the practice by agreeing with clinicians on targets to be achieved. These targets are set after costing services and allowing for the different types of patients seen.

3   *Cash flow management.* This is about ensuring the practice has

sufficient cash to meet all its current obligations. Should there be any cash surplus, it should be invested wisely. In case of cash short-fall, the information will determine the amount of loan the practice should raise to remain viable.

Detailed financial management courses are offered in many private institutions and students are encouraged to enroll in such training when they enter management positions.

Q Do you have an idea of the costs of your decisions and actions?

Do the patients understand the cost implications of their help-seeking behaviour?

3. A well-performing health workforce

3.1 Types of service providers

Family physicians have many options to consider when planning a career. For example, they can choose to work in the public or private sector. As the government is encouraging integration between the public and private sectors, it is expected that family physicians will increas-ingly work in both sectors. In the private sector, there are many options, from solo to group practice. Doctor networks (independent practitioner organisations and companies) are increasingly playing a role in securing the future of family practice by contractual relationships between prac-tices. These relationships vary from informal societies to formal business structures. Individual group practices may be in the form of associations, partnerships or incorporated companies.

The literature is increasingly promoting the multi-professional health team. Even in solo practices consisting of a family physician and a nurse practitioner, there is a rudimentary form of a multi-professional team. In the district health system and larger group practices, however, it is possible for multi-professional teams to share responsibility in primary care. Here not only doctors and nurses work together but there is potential for physiotherapists, occupational therapists, social workers, pharmacists, and other mid-level health workers to become part of the team (see Figure 10.5).

Figure 10.5 Service providers and the multi-professional care team

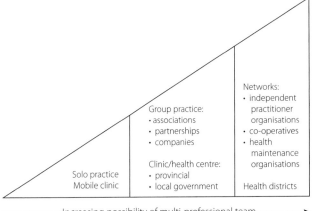

Networks:
- independent practitioner organisations
- co-operatives
- health maintenance organisations

Health districts

Group practice:
- associations
- partnerships
- companies

Clinic/health centre:
- provincial
- local government

Solo practice
Mobile clinic

———— Increasing possibility of multi-professional team ————→

Q How would you describe or categorise your practice? Who are the service providers in your team? What are their professions?

3.2 Practice trends

The main thrust of the restructuring of our public health service has been the establishment and strengthening of the primary level of health care within a *district health system* that will ensure basic care for all. This primary care service is linked to other levels of care in regional (secondary) and central (tertiary) hospitals through a referral system. Everything from home-based care up to the level of the district hospital is included in the primary health care concept. Each district therefore has a network of community-based organisations, day clinics, 24-hour health centres, and district hospitals. The numbers of these institutions has increased in the past ten years to expand coverage, particularly of previously disadvantaged communities.

Health districts are managed by a district health manager who may be appointed from any of the health professions. The district health manager is assisted by a team of senior professionals in the district from the various health professions. There are also various forums or community committees that meet with the district management team to give community input and assist with population-based planning, and the development and running of the service. It is essential for accountability that such bodies are not just consultative, but that they are taken seriously. Such committees are found at clinic or neighbourhood level, as well as at the level of the district as a whole.

Legislation makes integrated development plans mandatory for all districts. This means that the health sector, together with other government departments (such as education, justice, and agriculture), are required to formulate development plans with the community for each district.

The government has encouraged experimentation with various models for delivering health care through the district. Several universities and the Health Systems Trust have undertaken research in this regard. You are therefore likely to meet people during your clinical block who are looking for ways to make the work they do in their health district more cost-effective. Find out what they are doing and get involved if you can. Help build the future.

In the *private sector*, there is little shift from the old established solo practice to a larger partner practice structure. Major changes in the future will be around the location of practices due to the Certificate of Need. The effect of the Single Exit Price for medicines and the increased regulation of dispensing doctors will still show its effect, especially in areas where patients have previously obtained an affordable service by means of an inclusive package deal for a consultation and medicine.

In the *private sector*, the trend towards managed care and capitation-based payment systems is increasing, and third parties or outsiders are increasingly trying to decrease or control costs. For example, entrepreneurs form companies that control chronic medication, referrals to specialists, and hospital admissions to reduce costs for a particular medical aid fund. This can result in outsiders controlling the doctor–patient relationship, or in third parties managing and determining what may or may not be done by patients and providers. A third party (or outsider) can thus be seen as a person who intervenes between the patient (the first party) and the provider (the second party) and thus may interfere with the doctor–patient relationship to the benefit or disadvantage of the patient and the provider. This is also currently happening in the development of the district health system and the Essential Drug List. For example:

For 10 years a patient has received neostigmine to control his myasthenia gravis (a debilitating chronic illness) locally in the district. He now has to travel at great cost to the nearest state neurologist. His local family physician has been and still is quite capable of caring for him but third parties have decided this may not happen. To have the rule adapted for this patient and family physician takes much effort, many meetings, and much frustration for both the family physician and the patient. Third parties can make it difficult to practise cost-effectively and maintain local access for specific individuals and groups who have special needs.

Q   What are the new ideas and models being tried out in your health district, if any? What is the vision of this model/research?

How are the providers in your practice responding to the developments around the management of care by third parties?

If you are in some kind of group practice, what are the benefits?

3.3 Managing people

In the South African *public sector* there are white papers on the transformation of public service, human resources, and service delivery in order to put people first – the so called Batho Pele principles (http://www.dpsa.gov.za/batho-pele/Principles.asp).

In Meadows' view (1997), every district or practice management team should periodically review their vision. This should constantly direct what happens. A vision is something that changes more readily than core values and should always be looked at for its congruence with these values. Today, it is essential that the end user, the patient, be heard in this process of guiding what happens. As far as possible, management teams should have patient representatives, especially at the neighbourhood level. In other words, we need *participatory management* that includes the patient and is led by people who understand their own core values. People should be guided by a common vision. The developing of shared values and a shared vision are perhaps the most helpful things we can do to improve people's performance. This can be done for smaller functional units, as well as for an organisation as a whole.

Some authors draw a distinction between leaders and managers. They describe leaders as innovators, and managers as those who maintain systems once they are developed. In the management of people or personnel, many systems need to be maintained. Advertising for vacancies, the selection of personnel and negotiating their contracts and service conditions such as remuneration, leave, and other benefits, compiling job descriptions, formulating and supervising disciplinary and grievance procedures, and dealing with dismissal and retirement are all management activities.

In most situations today, there is an annual process of bargaining to negotiate new benefits for the year ahead. Those involved in this process need to develop skills in conflict management. There are companies that provide consultants who assist with negotiations and conflict resolution. Both the public and private sectors use their expertise.

Many complex systems attempt to improve job satisfaction and performance over and above the systems required by the labour relations laws. Such systems are generically known as *staff performance systems*. Some first world countries have intricate and expensive systems for monitoring staff performance together with a system of rewards and disincentives to increase performance. Martinez and Martineau (1998) concluded that these systems have not clearly shown that they actually enhance performance. To export such systems to developing countries is likely to make matters worse by diverting resources from needy people to a system that is more likely to discourage workers who already feel overburdened.

Apart from working with a shared vision, another way of improving matters is to ask each person to consider what they could do to contribute to a better working relationship between themselves and those they report to directly, and with those that report to them directly. Doing such an exercise on an annual basis is more likely to lift morale and prompt people to take personal responsibility, as opposed to a complex system requiring time, money and other resources to sustain it.

Staff performance systems can be seen as punitive and unfair. Whatever system is instituted in a particular working environment will do better if it generates some direction, hope, and personal development for the workers involved.

Q Describe some events you would call participatory in your practice.

Make some evaluation of the level of participation in your practice.

Does your practice have a clear, shared aim or vision?

How would you describe the level of hope and optimism or the morale in your practice?

Are there arrangements for staff development on an ongoing basis?

4. Health information system (HIS)

Health information systems should provide useful information to guide planning, monitor performance, evaluate outcomes, stimulate critical reflection and learning within the organisation. The overall health information system needs to be managed. Any form of practice needs time to plan and maintain its systems. These systems need to become part of the culture of an institution, but not become so entrenched that change and growth are prevented. Most health professionals are getting used to the idea that in clinical matters the best available evidence guides us and here we rely as much as possible on systematic reviews. In all forms of practice there is information that is collected, retained, and analysed in order to maintain the system. The information systems that need to be functional are those related to:

- People (patients, providers, and other stakeholders)
- Finances (capital, income, and expenditure)
- Clinical information.

Such systems need to be able to describe the practice population. At the very least, data about age and gender needs to be available, as well as the morbidity pattern. At a more sophisticated level, information required includes patient behaviour within the system, the cost of services, a comparison of different clinics or practices, and possibly a study of individual providers in relation to patient outcomes (such as number of people with hypertension whose blood pressures are controlled). Information systems should serve the purpose and priorities of the practice or the district. Information that is not used should not be collected as this wastes time and demotivates providers (see the box on page 361).

Information systems are necessary to plan new services and to improve the quality of current practice. Clinical information linked to individual patients and episodes of illness, the management undertaken, and the cost of care are important if a service is to be improved, especially in terms of quality. When it is not possible to gather this information on a routine basis, it can be done by means of surveys for the particular problem at a much lower cost than a large ongoing clinical information capturing system.

In practice you may come across systems at three levels; nationally, provincially and at the district level. Some systems select specific practices or facilities to provide additional surveillance of specific diseases. Disease notification, such as for TB and other specified diseases, is mandatory by all health workers; for example the 2005 typhoid outbreak in Mpumalanga was first notified by a GP. Notification allows the health services to rapidly respond to and contain an outbreak of disease.

Q Describe the information systems in your practice. Do they work?

Do you have a clear and informed picture of your practice population? Is the disease profile of your practice on record?

Is any time spent on feedback of the information gathered? Who gets the feedback? What is the time loop from gathering of information to feedback?

5. Good health services: managing clinical practice and quality of care

As described by the World Organisation for Family Doctors, "quality means the best health outcomes that are possible, given available resources, and that are consistent with patient values and preferences" (Wonca, 1999).

To achieve the best health outcomes, we need to make quality assurance a routine part of daily practice by allocating time and resources to continuous quality improvement.

In most of South Africa's health districts, family physicians work in poorly resourced circumstances. Many quality improvement systems, such as standard setting, audit, peer review and quality assurance, can be seen as controlling and even punitive. Punitive measures are eventually necessary in every system where people persist in practising in a systematically unacceptable way. However, such measures should preferably be separated from the quality improvement system, which needs to be a positive experience.

To do this, national or regional guidelines need to be adapted by local people into protocols in order to make them applicable and give providers some control and ownership. Quality is also provided when you do the best in your own context, and not necessarily for all circumstances in the country or world.

5.1 The quality improvement cycle (QI)

The quality improvement (QI) cycle also needs to become an integral part of continued professional development. The cycle consists of four steps (see Figure 10.6).

Figure 10.6 The quality improvement (QI) cycle

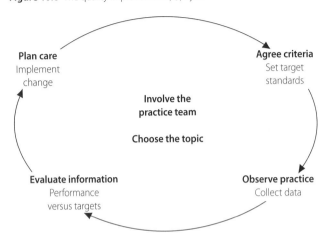

First, you need to agree on a topic to work with and you must form a team that will commit to the process of completing the cycle. Here we will use hypertension as an example.

Step 1: Agree on criteria

The team agrees on *criteria* to set for the chosen topic. Criteria may be chosen in respect of the structure, process, or outcome of care. Criteria may also be set for important principles and values of family medicine and primary care, such as continuity of care, accountability, accessibility, comprehensiveness, integration, and availability of care (Longo and Daugrid, 1994).

Structure refers to the staff and equipment that are in place – for example, are there a variety of cuff sizes to measure blood pressure in both children and the obese? *Process* refers to the activities that take place in the consultation or health facility, for example is the blood pressure taken at every visit? *Outcome of care* refers to the end-points of care, for example how many people's blood pressure is well controlled and how many suffer from complications such as heart failure or strokes?

Criteria are set with reference to the best available evidence and through discussion within the team. They should be important, measurable, and clearly related to the quality of care. It is important not to set too many criteria as this will make data collection a major task. For each criterion a *target standard* is created by setting a desired *performance level*. This level should be a realistic one in terms of the current quality of care and context, for example you might decide that in your situation it is realistic to aim for good control in 60% of your patients or (if you are already doing very well) in 80% of your patients.

Step 2: Observe practice

The next step is to observe your practice and collect data from direct observation of your actual performance. Common sources of data are the patients' records, routinely collected statistics, or encounter forms that are completed in the consultation. There are a large number of useful tools and methods for measuring and analysis described in the books by Grol and Lawrence (1995) and Alles *et al.* (1998).

Step 3: Evaluate information

Evaluate your actual performance by comparing it with your target standards, for example you may discover that only 50% of your hypertensive patients are controlled according to your criteria.

Step 4: Plan care and implement change

Reflect on and plan new ways to manage people with hypertension in your practice. This step should always end in an action plan that is put into practice, where working differently may improve care. You should also review and if necessary modify your target standards.

Finally, you need to repeat the QI cycle after an agreed period to see whether the practice has reached its target standards, for example improved from 50% towards the 80% target set by the team.

If a practice has made quality improvement an integral part of its work, there should be one or more quality cycles and teams working through these steps continuously. Quality improvement cycles may be set for "tracer" conditions in the following clinical areas (Longo and Daugrid, 1994), The quality of care for these "tracer" conditions is thought to be representative of the quality of care for similar conditions in that group:

- Acute self-limiting conditions, such as urinary tract infections and lower back pain
- Acute serious conditions, such as myocardial infarction and acute asthma
- Chronic conditions, such as hypertension and diabetes
- Prevention and health promotion, such as cervical smears and immunisations
- Pregnancy-related conditions, such as antenatal care.

The quality cycle needs to be practised. By doing so, both in under- and postgraduate education, we develop our quality-improvement skills until they become as natural as the skill of consulting with a patient. Quality work should ideally be integrated with continued professional development (see Chapter 13). Learning that is associated with problem-solving and changing and improving practice is cost-effective and results in deeper learning. In essence, quality improvement work is a reflective activity in which you become more conscious of your performance for the sake of your patients and yourself.

There are many commercial entities that offer to contribute to quality improvement and continued professional development. They have money available and skills that we may need. However, there is often a conflict of interest with them, especially if there is a product involved that you may not necessarily need in your context. One way to protect yourself is to see whether the activity is offered by or under the banner of the South African Academy of Family Physicians, the South African Medical Association, or a Department of Family Medicine. This also applies to guidelines and educational activities. Guidelines produced by other disciplines are not necessarily applicable or desirable in primary care. They need to be contextualised by those practising in primary care.

Q Does your practice spend time on quality improvement work?

Is there a punitive element in your quality improvement system? How can you lose your job in your practice because of your performance?

Is there a link between the quality improvement work and continued professional development in your practice?

What are the vested interests of those who provide the continued professional development for your practice?

5.2 Managing the support systems

Clinicians often make good clinical assessments and management plans, but the patient fails to get adequate care. Things may break down in one or more of the following support systems:
- The referral system
- The transport system
- The drug supply
- The stores

- The equipment
- The communication systems.

As a primary care clinician, you need to assist in making these systems work for your patients.

Career management

Many of you reading this book will be starting out on your career and making decisions about where to work within the health system. We will conclude this chapter with some advice on managing your own career.

Applying for a job

In the public sector, service conditions are more standard than in the private sector, and the job appointment process takes more time. In many parts of South Africa there is a growing number of family physician posts within the district health system and the number is expected to continue increasing in the immediate future. In a WHO/Wonca working paper (1994), a plea was made to deploy family physicians to their rightful place in primary care. Their view is that one of the factors in the failure of primary health care to deliver on its promise of "health for all by the year 2000" is the emphasis on nurses to the exclusion of the family physician in primary care. We need both in the team and others as well.

In the private sector, it is important to get advice before accepting a job or a contract, as these are not standardised. The South African Medical Association (SAMA) offers such a service for its members, and will review contracts. This service is worth making use of, especially for the novice. Consider the following when applying for a job:

- Can I make a contribution in this situation?
- Are there opportunities for me to learn and grow?

The district health system is not for the faint-hearted! Districts are still often poorly resourced and supported, but they are a challenge for those who wish to help build a health system that will deliver quality primary health care to all in South Africa.

Setting up in practice

Those who follow the recommended route to register as family physicians will have ample opportunity to prepare themselves appropriately if they are planning to enter or set up a practice. However, even qualified family physicians are well advised not to start a practice or join a group without getting sound financial and managerial advice and scrutinising contracts.

Patients' Rights Charter and Complaints Procedure

Standards

1. Each clinic displays the Patients' Rights Charter and a list of patients' responsibilities at the entrance in local languages.
2. The twelve patients' rights are observed and implemented.
3. The ten patients' responsibilities are displayed alongside the Patients' Rights Charter.
4. There is provision for the special needs of people such as a woman in labour, a blind person, or a person in pain.
5. Services are provided with courtesy, kindness, empathy, tolerance, and dignity.
6. Information about a patient is confidential and is disclosed only after informed and appropriate consent.
7. Informed consent for clinical procedures is based on a patient being fully informed of the state of the illness, the diagnostic procedures, the treatment and its side effects, the possible cost, and how his or her lifestyle might be affected. If a patient is unable to give informed consent, the family is consulted.

Patients' rights:

Every patient has the right to:

1. A healthy and safe environment.
2. Access to health care.
3. Confidentiality and privacy.
4. Informed consent.
5. Be referred for a second opinion.
6. Exercise choice in health care.
7. Continuity of care.
8. Participation in decision-making that affects her or his health.
9. Be treated by a named health care provider.
10. Refuse treatment.
11. Knowledge of their health insurance/medical aid scheme policies.
12. Complain about the health service they receive.

Patients' responsibilities:

Every patient has the responsibility to:

1 Maintain a healthy lifestyle.
2 Care for and protect the environment.
3 Respect the rights of other patients and the health staff.
4 Utilise the health system optimally without abuse.
5 Know the health services available locally and what they offer.
6 Provide health staff with accurate information for diagnosis, treatment, counselling and rehabilitation purposes.
7 Advise health staff about your wishes with regard to death.
8 Comply with the prescribed treatment and rehabilitation procedures.
9 Ask about management costs and arrange for payment.
10 Take care of the patient-carried health cards and records.

Complaints procedure

1 At the first point of contact with the health care provider, the user is informed verbally of the Rights Charter. The right to complain is emphasised and the complaints procedure is explained and handed over.
2 All clinics use a standard complaint form, which is filled in by the user who wishes to make a complaint.
3 The clinic has a formal, clear, structured complaint procedure and illiterate patients and those with disabilities are assisted in laying complaints.
4 All complaints or suggestions are forwarded to the appropriate authority if they cannot be dealt with in the clinic.
5 A register of all complaints and how they were addressed is maintained.
6 The name, address, and telephone number of the -person in charge of the clinic is displayed.

Health Information System Pilot Project

The following problems were found in the Health Information System Pilot Project on South African health information systems.

- Data is not routinely analysed by or reported back to those who collect it.
- Data flows to a variety of offices outside the district and is fragmented.
- A large amount of unnecessary data is collected and not analysed.
- Some important data is not collected.
- Data is inaccurate or missing.
- Data is difficult to interpret as useful information.

SOURCE: Mash and Mahomed (2000)

Definitions and terms

Medical aid schemes (or societies)

These are non-profit organisations formed under the Medical Schemes Act and regulated by the Registrar of Medical Schemes at the Department of National Health.

Medical scheme administrators

These are usually profit-making private companies that administer the benefits offered by medical aid schemes. They usually charge a fixed fee per member per month.

Brokers and consultants

These advise companies and trade unions on which medical aid schemes and administrators would be best for their purposes. Some brokers and consultants are independent and others are linked to specific groups as with insurance agents and brokers. They usually get a fee per member per month for recruiting and maintaining members with a particular medical aid scheme.

Managed care organisations (MCOs) and health maintenance organisations (HMOs)

These are new in South Africa. They are organised in many different ways and regulations are still being developed in the draft Medical Schemes Act. HMOs have been organised by insurers, administrators, and service providers or various combinations of these, for example groups of doctors have formed co-operatives. A co-operative may contract with a particular medical aid scheme to provide care to a group of patients for a fixed fee per month per person or beneficiary of the scheme. This is called a *capitation fee* and it is usually paid in advance. The risk is usually transferred from the medical scheme to the service provider, who now has to provide all the specified benefits the members enjoy under the particular scheme at no cost at the point of service. An unexpected series of high-cost health care needs (such as major operations and intensive care) may bankrupt this group of providers if they do not have sufficient funds to tide them over a period of exceptionally high expenditure.

Doctor networks

These are formed in various ways. An example is when doctors are contracted individually by a company or a medical aid scheme to be available to serve their members under specified conditions. Usually this means that patients are restricted to a particular doctor or group of doctors in such a network. Such networks of providers (for example doctors or physiotherapists) often organise themselves into independent practitioner associations or co-operatives.

Independent practitioner associations or organisations (IPAs or IPOs)

These have developed across South Africa in recent years in order to strengthen the bargaining and buying power of providers. Some also assist one another with peer review and continued professional development. Providers working in isolation cannot be as effective as a group when negotiating with government and medical aid administrators and schemes. These organisations may be voluntary informal associations. However, many have formed incorporated companies or formal co-operatives within the legal frameworks provided for companies and co-operatives. These groups are still to demonstrate their worth. In general, they are struggling to make decisions and act in a businesslike manner in the corporate world. With large numbers of members, it is difficult to make decisions and keep everyone participating.

Organisations and websites

So much is changing in the organisation of health care in South Africa and specifically in the district health system that the information in this book may soon be out of date. It is useful to be able to find the latest information on policies, laws, and regulations that shape our services on the various websites.

The National Department of Health – www.doh.gov.za.

The Essential Drugs List (EDL) – www.sadap.org.za/edl/. This site provides information on which drugs have been approved for use at the primary level and different levels of hospital care. The list is reviewed from time to time.

The South African Medicines Formulary (SAMF) – www.uct.ac.za/depts/pha/samf.htm. Here you will find information on medications available in the market place and an indication about their efficacy, uses, side-effects, and whether they are on the WHO essential drug list. No family physician in South Africa should be without this invaluable desktop aid.

The Health Systems Trust (HST) – www.hst.org.za. The HST has various newsletters and lists you can subscribe to that will keep you up to date with all developments in the establishment of the district health service. They can also help with providing articles and clinical information to remote practitioners via e-mail as an alternative to directly using the internet (for this service, contact them on www.healthlink.org.za).

The South African Medical Association (SAMA) – www.samedical.org. This site provides general information about the Association. The Foundation for Professional Development is the educational division of SAMA. Information about courses can be obtained from them at their e-mail address (foundation@samedical.org).

The South African Academy of Family Physicians (www.saafp.org) is the academic body for family physicians in South Africa and is affiliated to the world body for family doctors, Wonca.

MedLine – www.ncbi.nlm.nih.gov/entrez/query.fcgi. See Chapter 12 for a description of MedLine.

The site www.uib.no/isf/guide/guide.htm is a Norwegian site with a comprehensive list of other internet sites for primary health care.

11 The rural doctor

Ian Couper
Professor of Rural Health, Department of Family Medicine, University of the Witwatersrand

Introduction

Family physicians may choose to practise in many settings and contexts. However, in South Africa and around the world, the majority elect to work in cities or big towns, leaving a worldwide shortage of rural doctors. There are many obvious, practical reasons for this, which are related to career progression, family needs, education, socialisation, and so on. Yet, many doctors do not realise what rural practice has to offer, and do not try it. Those who do work there are often seen as the "mad, sad, and bad" of medicine, largely out of ignorance. In fact, there are many motives for rural practice, which include:

- A sense of vocation
- A sense of adventure
- A love of nature
- A need for experience
- A place to escape
- A place to focus on the family
- A way into the country
- A return home
- A worthwhile incentives package.

> "Nearly all countries – rich and poor – face a critical shortage of competent health workers in rural areas, where the need for basic care is usually greatest."
> *Dr Margaret Chan, Director-General, World Health Organisation*

Where is rural?

Firstly, we should try to define rural. It is important in terms of allocating resources, providing services, ensuring services are affordable, and protecting disadvantaged people from further disadvantage because of where they live (Smith, 2004). However, it is difficult to define and there is little consensus.

Rural areas have been defined in terms of population density, distance from a city, and available facilities or lack thereof (for example, using an "inhospitality index" (Deloitte and Touche, 1994)). Internationally, definitions have been based on population size, access to health care, occupation and other socio-economic variables and political proclamations (Muula, 2007). The most common definition uses a population cut off of 5 000 people, as in India, but often it is 2 500 persons or fewer, as in Mexico, or 10 000 or more, as in Nigeria. Other countries, including Brazil and China where rural villages are often very large, do not use population size but rather a range of characteristics related to facilities and legal or political status (IFAD, 2001). Statistics SA uses the concept of "non-urban" (StatsSA, 2003), namely outside of an urban area. The USA similarly defines rural areas as being outside urbanised areas, the latter being defined as built-up areas with populations of at least 50 000 people (Rosenblatt, 2001). Australia has developed a clear categorisation of rural areas that is based on population per square metre, and of remote areas that is based on distance from major centres (Australian Health Minister's Conference, 1994). Thus we can conclude that there is no agreed-upon international definition (Wilson *et al*, 2009).

Ultimately, the definition of rural is subjective. People who live in rural areas feel they are rural. They feel this because of the services not available to them (for example water, electricity and telephones) and the facilities not available to them (for example shops, banks, restaurants and cinemas). Rural communities feel strongly that they are different from urban areas and have special qualities not found in cities; city and government is often seen as distant and antagonistic (Wilkinson and Strasser, 2004).

Essentially, rural areas are underdeveloped areas. In the developing world, such as much of South Africa, these underdeveloped areas might be quite close to the city, as in informal peri-urban settlements. Whether or not they should be classified as rural is a moot point – they are still under-serviced from a medical point of view.

Rural people

Who then are these rural people? In South Africa, as is the case elsewhere, rural people are predominantly agricultural people, either commercial or small-scale farmers or, very often, subsistence farmers. Their livelihoods are frequently dependent on extractive industries, such as farming, fishing, forestry, and mining. Their livelihood is at risk from climate change, from droughts and floods, from illness and high mortality, and, in many countries, from war or civil disturbance (IFAD, 2001). The government is often a major source of support, either through direct employment or through social grants.

Rural people are often poorer than their urban counterparts due to insecure and low-paying occupations. For this reason, there is a high rate of temporary migration to other areas, especially cities, which is related to employment opportunities. Women, therefore, predominate in rural areas, as many men are away working. There is also a high proportion of children, both because of traditional practices that result in bigger families, and because children are often sent by working parents in the city to stay with their rural grandmothers, aunts, or other relatives.

Generally there are fewer resources available in rural areas, such as electricity, clean water or telephones. In these areas, people are likely to have less education, less money, less transport, less power even - than their urban counterparts. Yet, they are more likely to have their own piece of land, and more likely to have a home of their own, be it traditional or modern. They are more likely to be traditional and conservative, including their attitudes to health care, and have closer bonds to their cultural heritage. They are more isolated from technology and its advantages, yet are often better supported in crises by extended family and community networks.

They are also people in transition. With the influence of globalisation, the distinctions characterising rural people are less clear. They are suffering increasingly similar disease burdens to their urban counterparts, though they are more vulnerable to the problems associated with poverty and poor access to services. In South Africa, they thus also experience the quadruple burden of disease - communicable diseases (especially HIV/AIDS), chronic non-communicable diseases, maternal, neonatal and child deaths, and deaths from injury and violence (Coovadia et al., 2009).

The needs of rural people

Most rural communities are in dire need of clinics and hospitals. Over and above this, clean water, sanitation, jobs and education are often highest on their priority list (see Table 11.1).

Table 11.1 Priority issues raised by the community committees, Manguzi sub-district, 1996

Need	Number of times raised
Clean water	27
Clinics	15
Upgrading of roads	15
Creches	15
Radiophones to call the hospital	13
Toilets	13
Electricity	9

The basis for these needs is the fact that in the vast majority of developing and transitional countries, rural poverty remains at higher levels than in urban areas. Rural populations continue to experience higher levels of deprivation in terms of social indicators and access to basic services, despite general improvements over the last 30 years (Bird *et al.*, 2003). Almost everywhere, the incidence and severity of rural poverty exceeds urban poverty (IFAD, 2001)

In terms of health problems, rural people are more likely to need medical attention than urban people but often are less likely to seek it – their health seeking behaviour is strongly influenced by stoicism. They are more likely to consult traditional healers for health care and to treat themselves using folk remedies. They often only present for treatment when they are no longer able to carry on their daily tasks because of illness or disability (Smith, 2004).

Unsurprisingly, given the direct relationship between health status and socio-demographic factors, they have poorer health statistics. In South Africa, for example, infant and under-five mortality rates in rural areas are about 1.6 times that of urban areas. In 1998, the under-five mortality rate was 43 per 1 000 and the infant mortality rate (IMR) was 33 per 1000 in urban areas, while the under-five mortality was 71 per 1 000 and the IMR 53 per 1 000 in rural areas (Day and Gray, 2008).

Even in a developed country such as Australia, rural people, compared to urban, have up to 20% higher mortality rates from all causes, lower survival rates for cardiovascular disease and cancer, 50% higher mortality rates for men from occupational injury, more than double the deaths from road vehicle accidents and suicide, higher rates of morbidity and hospitalisation, and a higher incidence of domestic violence and sexual abuse (RDAA *et al.*, 2004).

Rural people generally suffer less violent trauma – accidents are related most often to agriculture and related occupations – but have greater exposure to toxic herbicides and pesticides. They are usually more often exposed to tropical diseases, especially malaria and parasitic infestations. They are often susceptible to natural and environmental disasters.

On the other hand, some rural areas are characterised by an influx of wealthy retirees, or of holidaymakers at particular times of the year, with their own needs and demands. Each rural community has its own particular set of health risks, with a health status directly tied to income, education, employment, race and ethnicity (Rosenblatt, 2001).

Rural practice trends

A commonly accepted definition of a rural doctor is one working as a generalist (whatever her or his background) whose scope of practice includes elements that in a city would be taken on by specialists. When compared to urban counterparts, rural practitioners usually carry a heavier workload and provide a wider range of services, are more likely to provide procedural services, and carry a higher level of clinical responsibility in relative professional isolation (Wilkinson and Strasser, 2004).

Why is there a fuss about rural practice? In South Africa, the majority of health professionals practise in cities, whilst almost half of South Africa's population lives in rural areas. The distribution of doctors across provinces shows a dramatic skewing towards the more urbanised areas (see Table 11.2). Rural areas have often been left, in medical terms at least, to the so-called madmen, misfits, and missionaries. In fact, rural hospitals have largely depended on foreign doctors; the majority of rural doctors, and certainly the senior doctors, are foreign graduates. The proportion of foreign-qualified doctors in the public health service is greatest in the most rural provinces – 20% in North West and Limpopo provinces compared to 5% in Gauteng and 2% in the Western Cape (Van Rensburg, 2004). In the allied medical and nursing professions, rural areas have generally been a second choice. Only local training of local people has been reversing this trend.

This is not a peculiarly South African phenomenon. Throughout many areas of rural Australia there is a shortage and maldistribution of health care providers, above-average population to health care provider ratios, high levels of health workforce turnover, and major problems of accessibility to services (Australian Health Minister's Conference, 1994). The 30% of Australians who live in the bush are served by 15% of the medical workforce (RDAA *et al.*, 2004). In the USA, 20% of the population lives in non-urbanised areas, but are cared for by 9.7% of the country's physicians; in primary care this equates to 49 physicians per 100 000 population in metropolitan counties, compared to 85 physicians per 100 000 population in non-urbanised counties (Larson and Hart, 2001). And this gap has been widening over time (Norris and Rosenblatt, 2003).

Globally, although the worlds population is split approximately 50/50 between rural and urban areas, only 24% of all medical practitioners work in rural areas and 38% of nurses (WHO, 2007). It is thus obvious that there is a great need for doctors and other health professionals in rural areas.

There is a range of factors affecting choices of practice location in rural and remote areas, commonly known as push and pull factors. Pull factors are those which attract health professionals to a new destination, such as improved employment opportunities and/or career prospects, higher income, better living conditions or a more stimulating environment. Push factors are those which make people decide to move, such as loss of employment opportunities, low wages, poor living conditions and lack of schooling for children (Lehmann *et al.*, 2008). Rural origin, personal values, relationship and role models must also be added in to this mix (Couper *et al.*, 2007).

Table 11.2 Distribution of population and health professionals in provinces

Province	% of total South African population (of 46.4 million), 2003[1]	% rural (= non-urban)[1]	All medical practitioners per 100 000 population, 1998[2]	% of total medical practitioners, 1998[1]	Public sector medical practitioners (excluding specialists) per 100 000 population, 2003[1]	Professional nurses in public sector per 100 000, 2005[1]
Eastern Cape	14.0	63.4	30.3	6.9	12.7	98.5
Free State	5.9	31.4	56.5	5.2	23.1	130.7
Gauteng	20.3	3.0	135.3	34.8	25.4	115.1
KwaZulu-Natal	21.0	56.9	54.4	16.0	21.3	107.3
Limpopo	11.7	89.0	14.8	2.6	14.3	119.3
Mpumalanga	7.0	60.9	33.6	3.3	17.9	93.7
North West	8.2	65.1	24.6	2.9	11.5	88.9
Northern Cape	1.8	29.9	43.0	1.3	28.4	127.1
Western Cape	10.2	11.1	152.9	21.2	31.9	113.9
Total	100.0	46.3	66.1	100.0	19.7	107.1

SOURCES: South African Health Review (2003/04), Van Rensburg (2004)

Rural practice

The main factors that distinguish the rural doctor are the context they practise in, the needs of the community, and the resources available.

Dr Robert Hall describes the uniqueness of rural and remote practice as follows (former senior lecturer, Monash University Centre for Rural Health, personal communication, 1998):

- The core concept of rural practice is the personal and professional relationship between the doctor and the patient in the context of their rural community.
- Rural practice involves the total bio-psycho-social management of individual, family, and community health problems, with implicit life-saving responsibility in emergencies as the bottom line.
- The rural and remote doctor needs to be appropriately trained to manage the majority of problems patients have, including chronic problems and performing diagnostic and therapeutic procedures, while involving other health professionals, as needed and where available, through referral and teamwork.
- In small rural communities, sensitivity to the local culture, patient confidentiality, and good communication skills are of paramount importance.
- Rural doctors need to be knowledgeable about the context of their patients. They also need to be an advocate for their community in acquiring resources so that comprehensive medical care can be provided for the area.

Broadly speaking, rural practice includes three main areas, each of which will be discussed below.

Family medicine (general practice)

Most rural doctors are generalists. The nature of rural practice means that sometimes even specialists find themselves too narrowly focused to continue exclusively in their specialty. Thus, most rural doctors, whatever their background, become generalists, who are able to deal with most of the wide range of problems that come their way, even if they concentrate on particular areas of medicine. In fact in South Africa, the Health Professions Council of South Africa (HPCSA) has stated, as part of its decision that family medicine should be registered as a specialty, that rural medicine should be seen as a specific discipline within the domain of family medicine (HPCSA, 2003).

In the USA and Australia, specialists are increasingly becoming involved in rural areas, particularly in disciplines such as internal medicine, paediatrics and obstetrics. Those specialists who do work in rural areas often take on the role of supporting, teaching, and training colleagues in a particular region or district.

HIV medicine and the care of patients with AIDS is now a very important aspect of the work of a rural doctor. Included in this is palliative care and the management of antiretroviral therapy, which is the responsibility of the family physician in the rural context.

The rural doctor may work in hospitals, in clinics, or in private practice (or a combination), with the numbers of private general practitioners in rural areas steadily increasing. The setting will obviously determine the exact nature of the practice. However, the rural doctor, unlike his or her urban counterpart, is expected to be able to deal with everything a patient brings to him or her.

Public health

Because the rural doctor usually lives within a defined geographical area, and the patients usually come from a particular district, location, or town, they are uniquely placed to play an extended role in working towards health, rather than simply treating disease. For example, if many patients have malaria, it would make sense for the rural doctor to become involved in water protection, bed net programmes, community education, and so on. Also, many rural communities do not have designated and employed officials tasked with looking after the health of communities, so it falls to the rural doctor to do this. Rural medicine is in fact only one part of rural health. Rural doctors need a broad vision of health care and their role in the health care system, as opposed to the conventional and narrow focus on clinical medicine. This is exactly what primary health care, as a broad philosophy, is all about. The principles of primary health care can be summarised as follows:

- Equity
- Availability
- Accessibility
- Affordability
- A focus on prevention and promotion
- Community participation
- Inter-sectoral collaboration
- Appropriate technology.

The basic understanding of a rural doctor is, or should be, that they are responsible for the health care of a group of people. Their practice management becomes more focused on this. So, while individual patient records are still important, systems that allow for good immunisation, for screening for disease, for ensuring access to health care, for appropriate referral, and so on, become more important. (All of this should be an integral part of family medicine in any situation, but it is brought into sharper focus in a rural context.)

Extended procedural skills

This applies more to the public service doctor than to the private doctor, but still includes both. Certain skills are basic to rural practice in most places, simply because patients cannot be passed over to specialists. Areas in which rural doctors usually develop procedural skills include the following:

- Obstetrics and gynaecology: labour ward procedures, Caesarean sections (virtually a requisite for rural practice in South Africa and many other parts of the world), tubal ligations, uterine evacuations, and so on
- Surgery: biopsies, removal of lumps and bumps, debridements, skin grafting, hydrocoelectomies and laparotomies
- Anaesthetics: spinal anaesthesia, ketamine anaesthesia, and often general anaesthesia
- Paediatrics: the resuscitation of neonates and intraosseus infusions
- Orthopaedics: the application of plaster casts and the closed reduction of fractures
- Psychiatry: the management of the acutely psychotic, aggressive patient, and so on.

Skills related to palliative and home-based care have become increasingly important in the context of the HIV/AIDS pandemic.

Many rural doctors acquire specific skills to enable them to offer additional services related to the needs of their particular context, such as cataract surgery or family therapy, and even hip replacements! (Fredlund, 2003). Often, the rural doctor also functions as the district forensic medical officer and thus requires skills in medico-legal work, for example forensic autopsies, the examination of survivors of assault and rape, disability grant reviews, and court appearances. Small towns often do not have pharmacies, so rural doctors are often self-dispensing, and hospital doctors often work without pharmacists. Thus skills in managing drug supplies and dispensing drugs are frequently needed (see Chapter 6).

Procedural skills of rural doctors may be used as an index of a wider picture. For example, surgery in rural hospitals is an important support to first level care and a helpful basic indicator (Jacques *et al.*, 1998).

The role of the rural doctor

Another feature of rural practice is teamwork. Because of the extended demands on the doctor, the shortage of other health professionals, and the desire to promote health and develop health services for a community, the rural doctor seeks out or takes the initiative in a team of health professionals. The rural health team is characterised by the willingness of its members to function in an undifferentiated way and to extend themselves beyond their traditional scope of practice to meet the needs of their patients.

Usually, the most basic rural team is formed by the doctor and the professional (or enrolled) nurse. The patient's first contact is often the primary care nurse. The doctor gives secondary care to patients referred to them by nurses, or acts in a supportive and training capacity to nurses. This only happens effectively if there is a sense of teamwork and a common understanding.

There are many other members of the team with various specialist areas, for example therapists, radiographers, dentists, pharmacists and community health workers. Where there are gaps, these need to be filled by doctors or other team members. Thus, many doctors in rural hospitals take on the job of extracting teeth, of ordering and issuing medicines, or of taking X-rays.

It often seems that everyone in a rural hospital functions at a level higher than their post: the doctor plays consultant to the professional nurse, who acts as a doctor, assisted by the enrolled nurse, who functions as a sister and is supported by a cleaner acting as a nurse. Because of this shifting of functions to lower levels of health worker, a process of delegation of duties is needed. This process has its own rules that determine its effectiveness.

The realities of rural practice

Dr Will Mapham, Madwaleni Hospital, Eastern Cape

I was called to casualty to see an elderly woman on the Saturday morning of the Easter weekend. She was lying on a bed with a scarf around her face and head. We removed this and found that her entire face had been chopped off. Her cheeks, nose and upper lip were hanging from a thin piece of skin connected to the right side of her mouth. She needed a plastic surgeon. The referral hospital was contacted and I spoke to the surgeon on call. His hospital was overwhelmed with emergency cases and he said that there would be no time for my patient. This left me with the problem – as rural doctors, we are often called upon to deal with health issues that are beyond our scope of practice. Being the only doctor in a large area places responsibility on your shoulders. It took three hours of cleaning, careful suturing, and local anaesthetic to repair the woman's face. I was the only doctor on call and had to act as anaesthetist and surgeon – multi-tasking is common for a rural doctor. Eventually the woman's face resembled normality. She spent a further week in hospital and I subsequently was able to discuss with a plastic surgeon what I had done. She is now able to breathe through her nose and, importantly, is able to smile.

Rural medicine can be professionally lonely, but also provides a challenge. You learn to become as self-sufficient as possible and the job becomes increasingly satisfying.

Rural medicine also involves working with families; this includes the hospital staff, the patients and the community. On another occasion, a 25-year-old woman was brought into the casualty, accompanied as is often the case by at least three or four family members. I recognised one of the family members, who was the hospital driver, before I saw the patient. The patient had been tied up by her hands and had been stabbed 26 times in her chest and back. She had bilateral pneumothoraces and a likely stab wound to the heart. We were lucky to have two doctors present, but despite our best efforts at resuscitation the patient did not survive.

Major trauma such as this is extremely uncommon in our area. This was the first case of what seemed like deliberate murder which we had dealt with in two years. The family was extremely distraught. The patient's brother, the hospital driver, was especially upset because he was the one who had initially found her. It had taken him some time to find a taxi willing to transport the patient to hospital. He blamed himself for her death and I asked him to come back for counselling.

Over the next few months the hospital driver slowly became less and less reliable. He turned to alcohol. However he was given no time off and each day he was forced to drive the three hour round trip to the referral hospital. The hospital only has one transport vehicle and it is always packed with patients. Luckily he was never involved in an accident.

We were eventually able to arrange for him to take some time off. He improved after the person who attacked his sister was seen in court.

As this story illustrates, the rural doctor may have to take on a lot of responsibility and is very important in the community. The doctor is often the proverbial big fish in a small pond. This can result in a sense of being valued and of making a difference, which is satisfying. Certainly, it is rewarding to come across patients in the street and see that they have improved, to be thanked by mothers because their children are now well, to see the recovered alcoholic hospital driver or the smiling scarred face of the assaulted woman. This familiarity also helps you in the consultation, as it gives you that extra insight and information.

The negative aspect is that the rural doctor struggles to step outside this role – that is to live a life outside of medicine. It can be a burden when people in the shop stop you to ask about health problems, or when you are watched very carefully when you go to the bottle store. Often your patients are your friends or colleagues, or relatives of colleagues. This can have negative effects. Burnout is an important risk for rural doctors, with the usual stress of medical practice being compounded by the fish bowl experience, limited social engagement, having to do more than you were trained to do, the lack of referral support and the pressure that comes from treating people you know, sometimes friends and colleagues. Rural doctors need to ensure they have support structures in place and to recognise that rural medicine is not for the faint-hearted!

Training for rural practice

Ideally, the process of preparation should start in medical school. Students should be exposed to rural practice throughout their training, thus learning to apply their knowledge to rural practice situations and challenging their teachers to be relevant to the rural reality.

Many students choose to do their electives in rural hospitals, where they report rich learning experiences, as the following quotes from student elective reports confirm:

> "My visit to [a rural hospital] really taught me more than factual knowledge. It exposed me to the lives of my future patients and the context in which they live."

> "I was exposed to such a wide range of medical and social knowledge and was able to put the theory I have learnt into practice."

> "Rural medicine is a discipline in its own right, requiring the doctors and staff involved to be highly flexible and

knowledgeable in every aspect of health care … I have gained far more from these two weeks than I could ever have expected. I learnt so much about medicine, I learnt so much about myself, but above all else I can say with unwavering confidence: this is what I am meant to do!"

"This elective has been a time which I can truly say was life changing. The impact that [M] Hospital had on me as a person and as a professional is astronomical and the work that is done for the community there is greatly honourable … My time at [M] has been one of great discovery not just of my own potential but also of the potential of others".

"An invaluable part of being in a rural hospital is being forced out of your comfort zone. Nothing is familiar or easy, however, there is a motivation to take risks … I am astounded at the magnitude of benefits I gained. I have developed a new sense of respect for human kind – for their struggle and their course whether doctor or patient. "

"The most important thing I have learnt is to love what I am doing. The hospital has about 250 beds, theatre is not properly functional, accommodation for the three doctors is not that good, the laboratory lacks some equipment, and pharmacy and radiology staff is short. Yet these doctors enjoy and love their work. They told me if I went into medical school for the love of money and not for the love of my job I will find it difficult to work in rural areas. They told me they never care how many people they are seeing each day. For them happiness is brought by putting a smile on their patients faces at the end of the day."

(Extracts from University of the Witwatersrand MBBCh 3 and 5 Student Elective Reports)

Internship is best served in regional hospitals where lots of hands-on experience leads to the acquisition of skills in a context where supervision and handing over of responsibility are balanced. Community service can be a time either to experience rural practice firsthand or to acquire more skills (for example in orthopaedics, surgery, and anaesthetics) that will be required for rural practice. Many skills can be learnt on the job, but this depends on the context and the amount of support available. Often there is not the volume of work in a particular field to enable a new doctor to gain sufficient experience of a particular procedure in a rural hospital. This is where regional hospitals can play a vital role.

As part of the development of full time registrar training for the specialty of family medicine, there are increasing numbers of rural training programmes, assisting graduates to acquire the necessary skills. There are also specific skills training courses and modules in rural health.

The process of preparation for rural practice is ideally integrated, and can be seen as a pipeline – sequential rural training experiences which include programmes to attract rural students to medicine and prepare them for medical school, programmes based in medical schools to select appropriate students and enhance health science curricula, programmes oriented to equip qualified doctors through postgraduate medical education, and programmes designed to place and retain doctors in rural practice, with support and training (Norris and Rosenblatt, 2003).

Increasing the rural doctor workforce

Many stakeholders involved in health care in South Africa have realised the need for targeted interventions to train, recruit and retain doctors for and in rural practice. Universities are increasingly placing emphasis on this aspect of training, as well as looking at the recruitment of students from rural areas.

A systematic review of 110 published scientific articles on recruitment and retention for rural and remote health care found that current evidence only supports the implementation of well-defined student selection and education policies. Coercive strategies address short-term recruitment needs, but there is little evidence to support their long-term positive impact, whereas incentive and support schemes may have some value.

In 2003 the Department of Health implemented rural and scarce skills allowances to try to attract doctors, and other key health professionals, to the public sector in general and to rural hospitals in particular (Reid, 2004). While the Occupation Specific Dispensation (OSD) has since replaced the scarce skills allowance, the rural allowance continues to provide an important incentive. The community service programme, whereby all health professionals are required to work in the public sector for one year, also seeks to increase the number and range of health care workers in rural areas. The extent to which these incentives and programmes are having an impact is difficult to say. However, what is certain is that a co-ordinated strategy is needed to address this problem, because the inequitable distribution of health care professionals is the result of multiple factors with complex interactions (Grobler *et al.*, 2009). The pipeline concept mentioned above is an important example of such a co-ordinated strategy.

Rural practice in the world

Over the last 15 years, a new international awakening has begun as rural doctors from all over the world have started to make stronger connections with each other and discover their common strengths and challenges. Despite major differences in resources and health needs between developed and developing countries, there are features of rural practice that are common to all. Because of this, there has been a series of conferences organised by the Working Party on Rural Practice of the World Organisation of Family Doctors (Wonca), starting with the First International Conference on Rural Medicine in Shanghai, China, in 1996 and the Second World Rural Health Congress hosted in Durban in 1997. These conferences have continued to take place approximately every two years and have been important in raising the profile of the rural health agenda.

The first two conferences developed a set of recommendations for rural practice, governments, medical bodies, and individuals. At the second conference, the Durban Declaration was adopted, which called on all nations to work towards the dream of health for all rural people and called for affirmative action on behalf of rural communities.

This was taken forward by a joint WHO and Wonca-sponsored consultation in 2002, called Health for All Rural People (HARP), which has produced an action plan for rural health (Wonca-HARP, 2003). This provides a set of key actions needed to improve rural health, grouped into five broad areas:

- Supporting capacity building within rural communities
- Supporting the development of linkages between patient care and public health through primary health care
- Improving health outcomes by improving quality and access of health services to people living in rural and remote areas of the world
- Fostering research to advance knowledge in the field of rural health
- Improving education and training for rural health practice.

In 2010, the WHO launched its "Guidelines on access to health workers in rural and remote areas though improved retention". These guidelines indicate the need for a co-ordinated package of strategies to address rural health worker shortages, including intervention in the areas of education, regulation, financial incentives and personal and professional support (WHO, 2010).

The US Institute of Medicine's Committee for the Future of Rural Health Care outlined eight principles as being critical for high-quality, appropriate health care for rural people in the USA. These are to focus attention on improving population health in addition to meeting personal health care needs; to provide a core set of health services within rural communities with links to services in other localities, based on the population health needs of the local community and guided by local rural community organisations and institutions; to develop teams of well-trained health care clinicians, managers and leaders working together, with health training institutions taking responsibility to select, educate and support health professionals for rural practice; to address the special circumstances of rural areas in health care financing; and to focus attention on rural communities in developing health information technology infrastructure (Institute of Medicine, 2005).

The potential for development in rural health care is enormous: the need is for more dedicated doctors and other health professionals to take on the challenge!

Recommended reading

Articles in the international journal, *Rural and Remote Health*, accessible free, after registration, at http://rrh.deakin.edu.au/

Articles in *Rural Health Matters* – the October 2002 issue of CME, vol. 20 and CME vol. 29, 2011.

JP Geyman, TE Norris, LG Hart (Eds). (2001). *Textbook of Rural Medicine.* New York: McGraw-Hill.

Websites

Some useful South African websites for further information:
The Rural Doctors Association of Southern Africa, www.rudasa.org.za
Africa Health Placements www.rhap.org.za
The Rural Health Advocacy Project www.ahp.org.za
The Wits Centre for Rural Health http://web.wits.ac.za/Academic/Health/Entities/RuralHealth/
The Ukwanda Centre for Rural health, University of Stellenbosch
http://sun025.sun.ac.za/portal/page/portal/Health_Sciences/English/Centres%20and%20Institutions/Ukwanda_Centre
The UKZN Centre for Rural Health http://crh.ukzn.ac.za
Health Systems Trust, www.hst.org.za

12 Family medicine ethics

Keymanthri Moodley
Bioethics Unit: Tygerberg Division
Faculty of Health Sciences
University of Stellenbosch

Introduction

According to Christie and Hoffmaster, "family medicine requires an ethical model with the richness and complexity of the clinical model it has introduced to medicine" (1986). This chapter looks at ethical models for family medicine and discusses the evolution of moral thinking during the pre-modern, modern, and post-modern eras. A brief overview is given of important theories, codes of conduct, and principles of ethics. The principles of family medicine are examined within the context of post-modernism and a parallel is drawn. Finally, a practically relevant framework is proposed to help resolve ethical dilemmas.

Ultimately, this chapter aims to develop an ethical model for family medicine in which ethics are combined to produce a practically relevant approach.

Clinical ethics?

In 1979 Siegler posed an interesting question: "If one practises good clinical medicine, does this not imply that one practises ethical medicine?" This might have been true when medicine was less complicated than it has become in the past three to four decades. However, the advent of new technologies, profit-driven medicine, managed care, and the information revolution has influenced medicine significantly to create options and choices that previously did not exist. The result is a need for special attention to the subject of ethics.

A definition of ethics

Ethics is a generic term for various ways of understanding and examining the moral life (Beauchamp and Childress, 2001). The World Medical Association (WMA) defines ethics as "the study of morality – careful and systematic reflection on and analysis of moral decisions and behaviour, whether past, present or future" (WMA, 2005). *Morality* refers to social conventions about right and wrong conduct that are so widely shared that they are accepted by the majority of people in a stable society. The purpose of *ethical theory* is to enhance clarity, systematic order, and the precision of argument in our thinking about morality.

Ethics is a matter of knowing what the best thing is to do in a particular situation; morality is about what is actually done in practice. In practical terms, when we are faced with two or more equally important but competing values, how do we make the right choice?

The role of the law

We might ask why the law is not sufficient. Should the law not guide us in our decision-making? Why do we still need ethical guidelines? The reality is that:

- The law is often *silent* on important issues such as physician-assisted suicide and HIV/AIDS.
- The law *changes* from time to time (such as the abortion laws in South Africa) and from place to place (for example, physician-assisted suicide is legal in Oregon in the United States but not in South Africa).
- The law might *condone unethical practice* (Kantor, 1989). The apartheid laws of our recent past bear testimony to this. The Choice on Termination of Pregnancy Act (1996) also contains issues that some members of the medical profession regard as being unethical.
- Various laws on similar issues may be inconsistent, for example, the age of consent for treatment in children differs significantly in the Children's Act, the Choice on Termination of Pregnancy Act, and sections of the National Health Act. Furthermore, some terms such as therapeutic research, non-therapeutic research and minimal risk are inadequately defined.

Hence, while the law is an important contributory factor in the solution of an ethical dilemma, it is clearly not enough in all situations of choice.

Intuition

Why is such a great deal of emphasis placed on ethics nowadays? Surely most family physicians have behaved and practised medicine ethically in the past? Yes, we have all made ethical decisions based on the Hippocratic Oath, but, more importantly, on *intuition*, which can be described as an immediate perception of the right way to act in a given situation. The problem with intuition is that it is subjective; it is neither systematic nor reflexive and can vary greatly from one individual to another (WMA, 2005).

Hence, we have lacked a systematic way in which to articulate our moral dilemmas, that is, a method or framework to guide us along the decision-making pathway. Ultimately, some of our actions have lacked justification, leaving us in lingering doubt about whether or not we have done the right thing in situations of moral conflict.

Consequently, much of the work thus far has been aimed at filling this void – at introducing a theoretical approach to aid clinical decision-making.

An approach to the evolution of moral thinking

Moral reasoning and thinking have evolved with the passage of time. A simple way in which to understand this progression of ethical theory over time is to consider three periods of ethical thinking:
- Pre-modern – before the seventeenth century
- Modern – from the seventeenth to the twentieth century
- Post-modern – from the late twentieth century onwards.

Pre-modern ethics

This represents the longest of the three periods and pre-dates the seventeenth century.

In ancient times, mythical thinking was a prominent feature. People used myths as a way of understanding or making sense of the world. As we understand it, a myth is usually a dramatic story. These stories were an integral part of a tradition or community and were transmitted orally from one generation to the next. The people in these stories were usually divine or supernatural forces and it was believed that they established the fixed order of the world. In order to please the gods and so protect themselves, people carried out rituals to maintain the status quo in keeping with the story of the myth. It was unheard of to question the content of these myths. They were accepted completely, without question or argument (Prof AA van Niekerk, Head, Department of Philosophy, University of Stellenbosch – personal communication).

During the pre-modern period, a sense of family and community was very important and tradition was valued. As such, a communitarian ethic was a prominent concept. The good of the community was valued above the needs of the individual. In fact, individuals allowed their lives to be directed by external forces such as the family, the community, or the supernatural forces of the myths.

Approximately 2 500 years ago, the Greek philosophers Socrates, Plato, and Aristotle engaged in independent theoretical attempts at understanding the world and this thinking was subjected to the demands of rationality. Theoretical insights had to be pursued in a rational way in order for them to be valid. Much of their time was spent in understanding the concept of happiness and what it meant to lead a good life. A dominant theory of this time was virtue ethics, which will be discussed later in this chapter.

In the years that followed, during the Middle Ages, Christianity became a dominant force and much ethical reasoning was influenced by the teachings of the Church.

Modern ethics

The modern period was heralded in by the Age of Enlightenment. The Scientific era extended more or less from the seventeenth century to the twentieth century, when Newton was the hero of the day, and when medicine took a sharp and irrevocable turn in the scientific direction. During the modern period, morality was not seen as a natural trait of human life but rather as something that needed to be designed and injected into human conduct (Bauman, 1993). Another significant outcome of this modern scientific era was the reductionist, biomedical model. Objectivity and pure rationality were valued above all else.

In keeping with this era, modern ethics were universal and objectively founded, and based on abstract theories, rules, codes of conduct and principles.

To begin with, we will discuss the various ethical theories. Although theories such as virtue ethics and casuistry were developed before the modern period, for the sake of simplicity and convenience, they will all be discussed as part of modern ethics.

Universal ethical theories

Much of the theoretical development started with broad-based universal ethical theories grounded in Western philosophy (Beauchamp and Childress, 2001). The following case study will be used to illustrate the important features of the major ethical theories, which are summarised in Table 12.1.

Table 12.1 The main features of traditional ethical theories

Theory	Basics	Main feature
Utilitarianism	Consequence	Greatest good/happiness for greatest number of people
Kantianism	Obligation-based theory	Intention, duty, or obligation to do the right thing
Liberal individualism	Rights-based theory	Positive and negative individual rights with obligations and responsibilities
Communitarianism	Community-based theory	Communal values, needs, and rights paramount
Ethics of care	Relationship-based accounts	Interpersonal relationships, care, and compassion emphasised
Casuistry	Case-based reasoning	Practical decisions based on real-life case studies
Character ethics	Virtue-based theory	Your personality and character (key traits and virtues) taken into account

Example

Mr Khomo has been your patient for two years. Originally from the Eastern Cape, he now lives in an informal settlement on the Cape Flats and works as a petrol attendant close to the day hospital. He is 34-years-old and is married. Previously, he has seen you for minor ailments such as coughs and colds. Today, he has come because his wife, who is 34 weeks pregnant, was referred by the antenatal clinic to the day hospital for treatment of syphilis. Her first appointment is in a week's time as she has already been given her first penicillin injection. The nurse at the antenatal clinic told her that she has a sexually transmitted disease and that her husband would need blood tests and possibly treatment.

Mr Khomo is concerned and confused as he feels very well and cannot understand how he could have a disease of this nature. However, he confesses that he has been having sex with other women during his wife's pregnancy. He is terrified that if his wife finds out, she will be very angry. He requests that you do not mention this to her during her visit the next week.

Under the circumstances, you decide to counsel Mr Khomo for HIV testing and he agrees to take a blood test for HIV in addition to syphilis.

Two days later, you receive his results. He has syphilis and is HIV positive. You call him at work and ask him to come in for a second HIV test. Mr Khomo is devastated to hear the results but is eager to have it repeated in case it was a mistake (false positive). The second confirmatory test is also positive. By this time, it is the day for Mrs Khomo's appointment and the couple is waiting to see you. You call Mr Khomo in first. He is very worried and is extremely upset to hear that his blood test is confirmed to be HIV positive. His biggest concern is that if his wife finds out, she will leave him and he will never see his only child as she has already threatened to go back to her family in the Eastern Cape if he is unfaithful. In spite of your pre-test counselling agreement regarding disclosure of his status to his wife, he begs you not to tell his wife.

Mrs Khomo comes in next. She is clinically well and has come for her second penicillin injection. You suggest that she should have an HIV test as she already has one sexually transmitted disease. She admits that she would like to be tested because she knows that her husband has been sleeping around. She knows that he must have given her syphilis as he refuses to use condoms. She tells you that her husband insists on having intercourse as he believes "the baby will not grow if she does not have intercourse while she is pregnant".

Mrs Khomo is HIV negative. It is now two weeks since Mr Khomo was told his result. He has not told his wife or his other sexual partners and is adamant that you do not tell her either, even though you have explained the risks to his wife and unborn child.

Q   How would you manage this situation?

Utilitarianism

This is a consequence-based theory. An action is described as right or wrong based on its outcome or consequences. This theory is based on the principle of utility where a good outcome is the one that produces the greatest good or happiness for the greatest number of people. People are viewed merely as a means to an end.

In the scenario described above, the ethical dilemma faced is one of maintaining the confidentiality of your patient, Mr Khomo, as opposed to breaking the confidentiality clause in order to protect third parties at risk, namely his wife and unborn child. Other third parties potentially at risk are his numerous sexual partners, but if you do not know who they are, the protection you can offer them is clearly limited.

The benefits of breaching confidentiality are as follows:

- It is more likely that Mrs Khomo will return for another test to make sure she is not in the window period (about twelve weeks) if she knows that her husband is HIV positive.
- If the baby is born before she has a second HIV test, she might opt to take a short course of antiretroviral treatment during labour.
- If her HIV status is not confirmed by the time she delivers, she might decide not to breastfeed, as this will further protect her baby. Alternatively she may decide to breastfeed and give the baby nevirapine until weaning occurs.
- If she is in the window period and later tests positive, it will give the medical staff directly involved in the delivery a chance to take full precautions to protect themselves, as it is well known that in South Africa, universal precautions are not always followed due to a lack of resources such as protective goggles and sometimes even gloves.

What are the disadvantages of breaching confidentiality?

- The doctor–patient relationship runs the risk of being eroded due to the resultant loss of trust.
- Mr Khomo might feel betrayed and might not return for any further treatment that he may need.
- The marital relationship runs the risk of disruption to the extent of separation or divorce.
- Mr Khomo could lose all his important support systems.
- He might never see his child again.

While this appears to be a difficult decision to make, a utilitarian approach would try to achieve the greatest good or happiness for the greatest number of people. On balance, therefore, a utilitarian approach would favour a breach of confidentiality.

Kantianism

This is an obligation-based theory where an action is supported not for its outcome, but for the underlying good intention, duty, or obligation to do the right thing. An action is regarded as right even if the outcome is unsuccessful, provided the intention at the outset was good. The theory was developed by Immanuel Kant, a well-known modern philosopher.

In the case study above, using a Kantian approach, you might feel a sense of obligation to your patient, Mr Khomo, irrespective of the consequences. You would therefore opt to preserve confidentiality. Alternatively, you might feel duty bound to do the right thing, that is, offer Mrs Khomo and her unborn child what protection you can from a life-threatening disease. You may also feel compelled to tell the truth. The decision then would be to breach confidentiality. However, even if this decision results in disruption of the family unit in the form of divorce, your action, using this Kantian theory as justification, cannot be regarded as bad because you acted out of a sense of duty and with good intentions.

Character ethics

This theory is virtue based. The focus is on the type of person that you are in terms of your character and personality rather than your actions. The good family physician must act ethically (based on principles and rules) but must also display certain key traits or virtues, such as compassion, trustworthiness, integrity, and discernment (Beauchamp and Childress, 2001). This is one of the oldest theories with its origins in the philosophy of Plato and Aristotle. In this case study, if the doctor valued the virtues of trustworthiness and compassion, they might opt not to breach the trust implicit in the doctor–patient relationship and hence decide not to disclose. If the doctor valued the virtues of honesty and integrity they might decide to breach confidentiality.

Liberal individualism

This is a rights-based theory, of Western origin, which is rapidly spreading throughout the world. We are all familiar with the human rights culture that has evolved globally. Both positive and negative rights are included. A positive right entitles a person to receive something, such as the right to health care, which the state has an obligation to provide. Conversely, a negative right allows a person to forego something, such as the right to refuse treatment for a terminal illness. In such a case, the family physician has an obligation to respect the right of refusal.

The link between rights and responsibilities is important. While one person might be entitled to enjoy a specific right, another person might be responsible for ensuring that the first person enjoys the particular right. At the same time, the person enjoying the privileges of a particular right also has responsibilities. For example, in the context of the doctor–patient relationship, the patient has certain rights, such as competent and confidential treatment from the family physician. On the other hand, the patient has responsibilities, such as to follow the family physician's advice in terms of taking the treatment prescribed correctly.

In considering the case of the Khomos, the rights of all parties would have to be considered. In addition, the meaning, scope, and weight of the various rights would be important. Mr Khomo has the rights of autonomy, privacy, and confidentiality regarding his diagnosis. He also has the right to adequate information, which he received during the pre-test counselling. His decision not to disclose his HIV status falls within his rights. However, in accepting this view, the rights of his wife and unborn child are being violated. While in general, liberal theory would protect the rights of the individual as far as is possible, in this particular case, the rights of the wife and child would carry significant weight also. Hence, even liberal individualism requires a delicate balancing of the various rights involved before a decision can be reached.

What about the rights of the family physician? Do you have a right of conscience and can this override the rights of patients?

Communitarianism

This is a community-based theory, which is on the other end of the spectrum compared with liberal individualism. This theory was mentioned in the discussion on pre-modern ethics. This is a relevant theory in the context of African tradition and culture where the needs of the community as a whole are placed above the needs of the individual.

The Nguni saying *umuntu ngumuntu ngabantu* (a person is a person through persons) describes how the individual is embedded within the community (Unpublished data. Augustine Shutte, Department of Philosophy, University of Cape Town). Unlike the Western concept of personhood that defines a person as rational, autonomous, individual and separate from others, the traditional African notion of personhood is relational, communitarian and extended. Reciprocity and inter-dependence are reflected in the African concept notion of *ubuntu* (I am what I am because of who we all are). The family or community are regarded as the moral agent as a result of the family being the most important aspect of identity. A horizontal and vertical dimension of being is described where a person is connected to the living, the ancestors, and those yet to be born. A deep respect for elders is cultivated and the authority of these elders is vested in a socio-moral responsibility to promote community and familial interests (Mkhize, 2004:46).

In the scenario described above, communitarians would not be interested in which rights are at stake, but rather would be concerned about how communal values and relationships would be affected. The family unit would be viewed as a small community in itself. Mr Khomo's request for non-disclosure would be seen as a lack of commitment to the welfare of his family. In keeping with this theory, HIV infection would pose a serious risk to the lives of the wife and child and, as such, infringements on the rights of Mr Khomo would be permissible.

Ethics of care

This has its origins in feminist theory where the relationship between people is emphasised. An attitude of care and compassion is stressed. The relevance of this type of theory to the doctor–patient relationship in family medicine is evident.

If we consider the Khomo family, an ethics of care would focus on relationships involving care, responsibility, trust, fidelity and sensitivity (Beauchamp and Childress, 2001). Mr Khomo has been unfaithful to his wife and now fears that his marital relationship will be jeopardised if he discloses his HIV status. He fails to display adequate care for and responsibility towards his unborn child who could be spared the risk of contracting a terminal illness if precautions are taken soon enough. The doctor–patient relationship is also crucial in this case. Breach of confidentiality might erode the relationship with Mr Khomo, while the relationship between the family physician and Mrs Khomo is likely to strengthen. Whatever your decision, both patients must be handled with the greatest care and sensitivity.

Casuistry

This refers to a case-based approach where real-life case studies are examined and generalisations are subsequently developed. Casuistry focuses on practical decision-making in particular cases.

In the case of the Khomos, you would examine features specific to their case rather than looking at universal principles and theories such as utilitarianism or rights. You would examine other cases in which a breach of confidentiality was necessary. The Tarasoff case comes to mind. Here, a university student told his psychologist, in the assumed confidence of their therapeutic relationship that he was in love with a young woman, Tatiana Tarasoff. He confessed that he intended to kill her due to unrequited love. The therapist decided to breach confidentiality and reported the threat to the campus police who did not succeed in preventing the perpetrator from actually murdering Miss Tarasoff. This has become a benchmark case in assessing the right and, sometimes, obligation to breach confidentiality in order to prevent harm to others. Personal privilege ends where public peril begins.

A more recent example is the case of Stephen Kelly in February 2001 (Chalmers J, 2002). Stephen Kelly was a 33-year-old intravenous drug user who became HIV positive while in prison. He received harm reduction counselling from a nurse while in prison. After his release from prison he became involved with Anne Craig. Stephen had a sexual relationship with her, but did not disclose his HIV status to her. Furthermore, he told her that using condoms was unnecessary. Anne subsequently tested HIV positive. The case was taken to the High Court in Glasgow in February 2001. Stephen Kelly was convicted of recklessly causing injury to another and was sentenced to five years imprisonment.

Three important questions arise from this case:

1. Did Stephen have a moral duty to inform Anne of his HIV status?
2. Did Stephen's health care provider have a duty to inform Anne of his HIV status?
3. Should this moral duty be reinforced by criminal law?

Professional codes of conduct or guidelines

Modernity also saw the development of various codes of conduct. The void left by the Church during the scientific, modern era had to be filled by rational rules; these had to be developed and taught so that they would be obeyed. Many medical oaths, declarations, and codes of conduct were developed towards the end of this period. In the 1940s, the WMA developed various declarations to inform and enforce ethical medical practice. Some of these declarations represent modifications of the Hippocratic Oath.

The *Declaration of Geneva* may be regarded as an updated version of the Hippocratic Oath and was originally formulated in 1948. As a family physician, it requires that you dedicate your life to the service of humanity; that you make "the health of your patient" your first consideration; that you respect the patient's secrets (even after the patient's death); that you prevent "considerations of religion, nationality, race, party politics, or social standing" from intervening between your duty and your patient, that you "maintain utmost respect for human life from its beginning", and that you not use your medical knowledge "contrary to the laws of humanity".

The WMA's *International Code of Medical Ethics* was adopted in 1949 and requires, among others, adherence to the Declaration of Geneva, the highest professional standards, clinical decisions uninfluenced by the profit motive, honesty with patients and colleagues, and exposure of incompetent and immoral colleagues.

In South Africa, the Health Professions Council (HPCSA) has various codes of conduct and the South African Medical Association (SAMA) has guidelines. With respect to disclosure of the HIV status of patients to partners HPCSA offers the following guidance:

> "Health Care Workers (HCWs) should encourage their patients to disclose their status to their sexual partners, so as to encourage them to undergo VCT and access treatment if necessary. If the patient refuses to consent, the HCW may, after carefully weighing up all the factors, use their discretion when deciding whether to divulge the information to the patient's sexual partner. Disclosure by the HCW without the patient's consent must still involve the patient and the patient must be counselled on the HCW's ethical obligation to disclose such information. After disclosure, the HCW must follow up with the patient and the patient's partner to see if disclosure has resulted in adverse consequences or violence for the patient, and, if so, intervene to assist the patient appropriately."

The guidelines of the South African Medical Association (SAMA) state:

> "These guidelines recommend that a patient's medical information should be kept confidential. However, if disclosure does occur, the following conditions must be met:
> * The sexual partner should be known and identified.
> * The sexual partner should be at real risk of being infected – the patient has refused to disclose or take precautions and the doctor must have substantial information of this. There should be no other way to protect the partner.
> * The patient must be warned of the intended disclosure and given a specified period of time to disclose.
> * After the above steps, the doctor may disclose.
> * If the patient firmly believes that their disclosure to a partner will place their life at risk, the doctor's duty is to protect the life of the patient and act in their best interests."

Using a modern approach to ethics, when faced with an ethical dilemma, you could use one of the theories described above to justify your final decision or you could apply rules from one of the codes of conduct. Alternatively, you could use a principle-based approach.

In spite of various rules and guidelines, unethical medical practice has occurred throughout the world in various different forms. Is this because such rules are simply ignored, or are these rules simply inadequate to inform ethical medical practice? Does the profession need more fundamental ethical principles to guide ethical behaviour?

The four principles of medical ethics

The problem with the theories and codes of conduct is that a wide gap developed between universal abstract theories and real-life ethical dilemmas in medicine. In an attempt to narrow this gap and to make ethical theories more applicable to clinical dilemmas, a principles-based approach was developed approximately 25 years ago in the United States (Winkler, 1993). These four principles are: autonomy, beneficence, non-maleficence, and justice.

Respect for autonomy

Autonomy literally means self-rule. It refers to the right of every individual to make their own decisions. In health care, this entails allowing the patient to make the final decision regarding their treatment, after having been given all the necessary and relevant information. The obligations created by respect for autonomy are described below.

Informed consent

Before subjecting a patient to any investigations or treatment, we need to obtain their agreement. It is important, firstly, that the patient is competent to consent and that the consent is voluntary. The patient must not be manipulated or coerced into consenting. Once this requirement is satisfied, it is essential that the patient is given all the relevant information related to the procedure or treatment in language that is easily understandable. Ensure that the information has been understood.

The risks and benefits of the intervention must be clearly stated and your recommendation is also important. This is especially relevant in our setting in South Africa where the concept of autonomy is not fully developed and where patients place high value on the advice of their family physician.

In cultures where Western individualism is not prominent, patients might want to discuss the issue with family members before making a decision. This must be allowed for and respected. Finally, the patient will make a decision, and either authorise the intervention or refuse to have the procedure/treatment.

Hence, it is clear that informed consent is not an event that is over in a few minutes. Truly *informed consent is a process* and may be unavoidably time-consuming. The pre-test counselling protocol used to obtain informed consent from patients prior to HIV testing is an excellent example of the process of informed consent (see Chapter 8). In practice, often, constraints limit the essential acquisition of fully informed consent. As levels of awareness and knowledge improve in South Africa, it will be possible to obtain informed consent more efficiently.

Table 12.2 The elements of informed consent

Threshold elements	Competence (to understand and decide)
	Voluntariness (in deciding)
Information elements	Disclosure (of information)
	Recommendation (of a plan)
	Understanding (of information)
Consent elements	Decision (against or in favour of a plan)
	Authorisation (of chosen plan)

SOURCE: Adapted from Beauchamp and Childress (1994:146)

Confidentiality

Medical confidentiality is another way of respecting the patient's autonomy. Family physicians explicitly or implicitly promise their patients that they will keep confidential the information confided in them. Without such promises of confidentiality, patients are unlikely to divulge highly private and sensitive information that is needed for their optimal care. In the context of the doctor–patient relationship, confidentiality should always be maintained, except if the patient consents to the disclosure or if you are forced to divulge information in a court of law or in situations where the life of a third party is at risk, as is illustrated in the Tarasoff case study.

Truth telling

Respect for the patient's autonomy requires us to not deceive them. This means telling them the truth about their illness unless they specifically indicate that they do not wish to know. This is especially important where terminal illness is concerned. Concealing the diagnosis from the patient is clearly unacceptable unless there are very good and exceptional reasons for doing so. Furthermore, Chapter 2 of the National Health Act, 2003 (Act 61 of 2003) specifies in section 6(a) that every health care provider must inform the patient of their health status except in circumstances where there is substantial evidence that the disclosure would be contrary to the best interests of the patient.

Communication

The patient-centred approach used in family medicine is in keeping with the principle of respect for autonomy. Listening to the patient enables the family physician to decide what information the patient needs, how this information should be transmitted to the patient, and what the patient's preferences are. Hence, it can be seen that good communication in the context of the doctor–patient relationship is an ethical requirement. See Chapters 2 and 3 for guidelines on communication.

Language barriers that are prevalent in many South African health facilities between patients and doctors have been shown to both prevent informed consent and break confidentiality either because the doctor cannot exchange information clearly or because other patients and community members are used as interpreters (Schlemmer, 2005).

Beneficence and non-maleficence

Beneficence refers to doing good while non-maleficence literally means do no harm. Whenever we try to help others, we inevitably risk harming them (Gillon, 1994). In medicine, it is essential to balance these principles to achieve the net benefit for the patient. In order to fulfil the requirements of these principles, we have certain obligations to our patients.

First, we need to be able to provide the benefits to our patients that we profess we are able to provide. This is why it is essential to have a rigorous and effective education and training before and during our professional lives (Gillon, 1994). We also need to be clear about risk and probability when we make our assessments of harm and benefit. For example, it is crucial that we know all the important side-effects of a particular drug before we decide to use it for its beneficial effect. We get such information from effective medical research, which is therefore also an important moral obligation. As is outlined in Chapter 13, the practice of evidence-based medicine and continuing medical education are obligations we have to our patients in order to offer them the best we are capable of at all times.

Finally, empowerment of the patient to take control of their health and health care is also seen as an obligation of beneficence.

Justice

This principle deals with the fair treatment of patients. Obligations of justice may be divided as follows:
- Respect for people's rights – rights-based justice
- Respect for morally acceptable laws – legal justice
- Fair distribution of limited resources – distributive justice.

While all categories are important, *distributive justice* is particularly relevant in South Africa where, especially in the public health sector, there are limited resources. At most state hospitals, the staff-to-patient ratio is extremely inadequate. Consequently, triage of patients is unavoidable so that only patients with the most urgent medical problems may be seen on a particular day. The number of patients admitted for care is determined by the number of patients it is humanly possible for the family physician to see. In the interests of justice, it is crucial that patients can compete on an equal basis for admission and that some patients are not favoured above others for reasons other than medical need. In tertiary care hospitals, resources such as dialysis machines and intensive-care beds are severely limited and it is essential that these resources are fairly allocated to patients.

Table 12.3 The four principles of medical ethics

Respect for autonomy	Informed consent, confidentiality, truth telling, and good communication
Beneficence	Doing good – ongoing education and training, empowerment
Non-maleficence	Do no harm – risk and probability
Justice	Fair treatment – rights-based, legal, and distributive justice

Criticism of the principles-based approach

This principle-based approach has played a valuable role in the evolution of biomedical ethics but has been criticised in various ways. Some people feel that the principles are too abstract; others find them difficult to interpret. Some critics say that the principles just are not enough in all situations of choice.

In assessing the four principles of ethics, we will often find ourselves in situations where two or more principles will conflict with each other (Winkler, 1993). In many clinical circumstances, the weight of respect for autonomy is minimal, and the weight of non-maleficence or beneficence is maximal. This is particularly relevant in the public sector where patients who are educationally disadvantaged and who have not been allowed to exercise their autonomy depend on beneficent treatment from their family physicians. The frequent saying "Doctor, you know best" is all too familiar in South African health care. Similarly, in the public health arena, the demands of justice can easily outweigh the demands of respect for autonomy. The triage system described earlier is testimony to this.

From our discussion of the theories and principles in ethics thus far, it might seem as if the application of these broad-based theories and principles to real life ethical dilemmas in family medicine can be confusing and difficult!

An ethics for family medicine

It is evident that we need to establish the nature of the ethical problems which we face in family medicine and decide how these theories and principles are applicable and relevant to our discipline.

According to Christie and Hoffmaster (1986), an applied ethics of family practice must be grounded in the underlying philosophy of the discipline. As such, the "nature of family medicine imposes constraints on an ethics in family medicine".

The philosophy of family medicine

Family medicine is based on specific principles as outlined earlier in the chapter (McWhinney, 1989). The approach to patient care is holistic and not merely disease-oriented. Subjectivity as opposed to pure objectivity is important, that is, the fears, feelings, and expectations of the patient are significant and are taken into account in the three-stage assessment of the individual. The patient is seen as a person rather than a disease and this person is seen in their context and not in isolation. This accounts for the contextual aspect of the three-stage assessment. Hence, the approach used is very specific and relevant to the needs and problems of the patient.

Is there another ethical model that is different from the universal theories and principles we have discussed so far? In order to develop such a model, we need to introduce the concept of post-modernism to our discussion.

Table 12.4 The differences between modernism and post-modernism

Modernism	Post-modernism
Reductionist biomedical model	Holistic bio-psychosocial model
Objectivity	Subjectivity
Concept of disease	Concept of the person
Individual in isolation	Context
Rules	Personal responsibility

Post-modernism

Family medicine is compatible with the definition of post-modernism, which is essentially a reaction against modernism. Post-modernism refers to a change in attitude and thinking that started in Europe in the late twentieth century (Bauman, 1992). This new thinking has influenced art, music, literature, architecture, and, yes, even medicine. In Table 12.4 the main differences between modernism and post-modernism are highlighted.

In post-modern thinking, the holistic bio-psychosocial model, based on systems theory, is strongly favoured. Subjectivity and the importance of the emotions are considered. The concept of the person replaces the concept of the disease. Furthermore, the person is seen not in isolation but in context. This post-modern approach parallels the principles of family medicine.

In keeping with this post-modern trend, the doctor–patient relationship has changed from one of monologue to one of dialogue, where the family physician no longer instructs the patient but rather is involved in negotiated management with the patient. The doctor–patient relationship of today has even been described as a "meeting between experts" (Barker, 1998) – the doctor as an expert on medical knowledge and skill;

the patient as an expert on their own experience of illness and context.

In addition, there is a move from universal theories to particular concrete cases and people start taking responsibility for personal choices instead of referring to the rules of institutions.

If family medicine is a post-modern discipline, then are post-modern ethics not best suited to this discipline?

Post-modern ethics

Post-modern ethics represent a new approach to ethics that is different from, but not exclusive of, the universal rules and theories typical of modern ethics. The main features of this approach are (Bauman, 1993):

- It is a move away from timeless abstract theories.
- It is sensitive to complexity.
- It focuses on the particular rather than the universal.
- It is concerned with reality rather than abstract theory.
- It engages in positive deconstruction of, for example, the doctor–patient relationship.
- It encourages scepticism.
- It has no single authority; authority is shared.
- It emphasises autonomy of the moral agent, that is, family physicians have the ability to decide for themselves where ethical issues are concerned and they have to take personal responsibility for the decision.

Post-modern ethics represent a practical approach:

- It is a move from *macro-ethical* issues to also incorporate *micro-ethical* issues (Sparks, 1998). Macro-ethical issues deal with traditional issues in medicine such as abortion and euthanasia. Micro-ethical issues refer to the ethical nature of the doctor–patient relationship, the consultation, and the nature of communication between the family physician and the patient. For example, it is unethical, in the process of the consultation, to delve unnecessarily into the private life of the patient.
- It is a move away from *abstract, single principled theories* such as utilitarianism or Kantianism to *pluralistic theories* such as virtue ethics, relationship-based ethics, communitarianism, and casuistry.
- The *four principles* – based on general ethical theory – are still important but are not relevant in isolation. Rather, attention is given to the scope of their application (Gillon, 1994), or they are used in combination with common morality theory (Beauchamp and Childress, 2001), relationship-based theory, and virtue ethics.

The five-step post-modern approach to resolving an ethical dilemma

Step 1: Identify the moral dilemma

As a starting point, it is essential to *identify the conflicting values*. For example, in the case study discussed earlier, the dilemma is one of maintaining confidentiality as opposed to obligations to third parties. Examples of other dilemmas that you may face include the following:

- A critically ill patient, who is a Jehovah's Witness, refuses a blood transfusion after a motor vehicle accident. Do you respect patient autonomy and omit the transfusion or do you adopt a paternalistic approach and administer the blood despite the patient's objection?
- A 40-year-old woman with three children requests termination of her fourth pregnancy. Do the rights of the foetus, the rights of the father or the rights of the patient take precedence?

Step 2: Establish all the necessary information

It is important to establish all the necessary information related to the case. We use the case study of Mr Khomo to illustrate this step.

- What are the *medical facts* surrounding HIV/AIDS? They are the life-threatening nature of the disease, its mode of transmission, the probability of such transmission occurring, the methods available to reduce transmission, treatment options, and so on.
- What *laws* or *Health Profession Council rules* will influence your decision? These would be the laws on confidentiality. The National Health Act supports confidentiality except in the following circumstances:
  - the patient consents to the disclosure in writing
  - a court order or any law requires disclosure
  - non-disclosure of the information represents a serious threat to public health.
- What is the *ethical standpoint*? How do the four principles interact? Here we consider autonomy versus non-maleficence/beneficence. We ask if a universal ethical theory such as utilitarianism can influence a decision or, in family medicine, is the ethics of care or relationship-based ethics approach more appropriate? The Declaration of Geneva has strict rules for confidentiality. Are these applicable to the case?
- What does the *patient* prefer? How does culture contribute to or influence the patient's preferences? In this case, Mr Khomo would prefer that his HIV status be kept confidential.
- What does your *personal value system* dictate? Usually, this will influence the final decision significantly. In South Africa, how are these value systems influenced by medical education, parental influence, political beliefs, and personal experiences?

- What are the *socio-political norms* of the day? Are they acceptable? How will they influence medical decision-making?

Step 3: Analyse the information

Considering all the information, you will go through a balancing process in which the various components are assigned different weights. In addition, you may use different approaches to the core problem and examine different outcomes.

Step 4: Formulate solutions, make recommendations, and then act

In this step you consider possible solutions, make recommendations, and then act on the decision.

Step 5: Implement policy

In medical institutions, such as a hospital, *policy* may have to be implemented, created, or amended. This will be based on how the case was handled in the end. In a private medical practice, guidelines may have to be drawn up so that the management of a similar problem in the future is much clearer because of a precedence being set.

Table 12.5 A post-modern approach to ethical decision-making

Step 1	Identify the moral dilemma – what are the conflicting values?
Step 2	Establish all the necessary information – medical, legal, ethical, socio-political norms; patient preferences; family physician's personal value system
Step 3	Analyse the information obtained
Step 4	Formulate possible solutions and make recommendations or take action
Step 5	In institutional settings, implement the necessary policies

SOURCE: Adapted from the curriculum in medical ethics, courtesy of Dr Eugene Bereza, family physician/clinical ethicist, Department of Family Medicine, McGill University, Canada

Using a post-modern approach

This framework is not intended to be a rigid approach to solving ethical dilemmas. In broad terms, it provides a guideline that does not necessarily have to be used in the above order. Using the framework as a guide, consider the following case study and then discuss the questions that follow.

Dr Goodfellow has a busy practice in a peri-urban area. There are a number of factories near the surgery and many of the employees are patients of the practice. Mrs Thomas is 28-years-old and has two children aged three and five years. Her mother lives 250 km away and takes care of the children. Her husband works in Johannesburg and she plans to join him there soon. Mrs Thomas has just received a message that her mother has taken ill. She has decided to come to see Dr Goodfellow to ask for a medical certificate for the next five days so that she can go to see her mother. She would also like Dr Goodfellow to give her some medication to take to her mother who has had a fever, diarrhoea and vomiting for the past two days. Her mother was last seen by Dr Goodfellow a year ago.

(Case study courtesy of Dr U Govind – University of KwaZulu-Natal)

Q   If you were Dr Goodfellow, what would you do?

What is the ethical dilemma facing you?

Do you require more information? If so, what else would you like to know? Consider medical, legal, ethical, institutional norms, patient preferences, and your personal value system.

Once you have collected all the relevant information, how would you analyse it?

Are you able to formulate a plan of action or make recommendations?

If you can use this guideline to decide how to respond to the above ethical problem, or to any other ethical problem, then it represents a practically relevant approach to ethical dilemmas for you. The advantages of using this approach to medical ethics are (Robertson, 1996):
- A heightened awareness of the ethical nature of our work
- A more democratic approach to addressing practical moral dilemmas
- Ultimately, better clinical decision-making.

In simple terms, post-modern ethics represents a practical but complex approach to solving ethical dilemmas. It is complex in that all the factors that interact and influence each other must be considered. Hence, it is clear that post-modern ethics provide an ethical model with the richness and complexity of the clinical model proposed by family medicine.

Health and human rights

Because of the atrocities committed during the Second World War, the United Nations proclaimed the *Universal Declaration of Human Rights* (1948). The declaration forms a foundation for the discussion on human rights. The right to health is a positive right that requires action on the part of the state. Rights may also be seen as being categorised in a three-tier hierarchy:

- Civil and political rights
- Social, economic, and cultural rights (for example, a standard of living adequate for health and well-being)
- Collective and international rights (for example, global disarmament).

Human rights are an integral part of any curriculum in medical ethics, especially in South Africa. This is because human rights violations have occurred at all levels in the medical profession in South Africa both during and after the apartheid era. These violations have affected medical students, health professionals, and, most importantly, black patients, and have taken place in hospitals, in private practices, in police custody, and in prisons. Within the profession, there is still much resentment and anger relating to past discrimination.

The Truth and Reconciliation Commission (1998) made history by holding health sector hearings that examined the role of the health sector in human rights abuses. They concluded that "the health sector, through apathy, acceptance of the status quo and acts of omission ... [a]llowed the creation of an environment in which the health of millions of South Africans was neglected, even at times actively compromised, and in which violations of moral and ethical codes of practice were frequent, facilitating violations of human rights".

Despite these findings, there were many health professionals who did not ignore human rights abuses, who worked in poor and under-served communities, and who actively campaigned for an end to discrimination.

Some institutions, such as the Faculty of Medicine at the University of the Witwatersrand, have examined their own history of human rights violations (Wits Internal Reconciliation Report http://www.wits.ac.za/alumni/irc rep.htm). A report has revealed that black medical students endured a host of discriminatory acts from the 1950s onwards and these included the following:

- They were not allowed to have contact with white patients.
- They had to enter and leave the Johannesburg General Hospital by back entrances.
- They were not allowed to attend post-mortem examinations on white

bodies. They had to wait outside the morgue until the body had been removed and they were then allowed to view the organs.
- They had separate facilities, including separate crockery and utensils.
- In 1987, they were allowed entrance to all sections of white hospitals, except the maternity and gynaecology wards.

Even today, in post-apartheid South Africa, there are some private medical practices in rural settings with separate entrances and separate waiting rooms for medical aid as opposed to patients paying by cash, which effectively separates white from black.

The need to cultivate a culture of health and human rights in South Africa, both within the profession and in the context of the doctor–patient relationship, is long overdue. Fortunately, medical undergraduate training has progressed significantly and the 1990s ushered in a new era of equality and dignity in medical education and medical practice in South Africa.

In order to prevent future human rights violations in South African health care, the Truth and Reconciliation Commission has made the following recommendations:
- More black graduates should be included in under- and postgraduate studies.
- Human rights issues and ethics should be taught as part of medical training.
- Health care workers should be made aware of ethical principles.
- Statutory health councils should proactively promote human rights and investigate unethical conduct.
- Fair and consistent disciplinary processes should be implemented.
- Autonomous and independent councils should ensure that policies and legislation do not violate the rights of patients.
- Professionals who oppose and expose human rights violations should be supported.

Today, as we traverse a new path into the twenty-first century in South Africa, it is indeed with a deep sense of relief and hope that we leave the many human rights abuses of the past behind us.

Solving ethical dilemmas is never easy. Doing the right thing is a matter of conscience and sometimes requires great moral courage. Ultimately, we are guided by fundamental principles common to all of humanity and by our personal value systems.

Recommended reading

Gillon, R. (1995) Medical Ethics: Four Principles plus Attention to Scope. *British Medical Journal*, 309:184–188.

Christie, RJ and Hoffmaster, CB. (1986). *Ethical Issues in Family Medicine*. New York: Oxford University Press.

Moodley K. (2011). Medical Ethics, Law and Human Rights: A South African Perspective. Pretoria: Van Schaik

Chalmers, J. (2002) The criminalisation of HIV transmission, *Sexually Transmitted Infections*, 78:448–451.

13 Continuing professional development

Michael Pather
Division of Family Medicine and Primary Care
Department of Interdisciplinary Health Sciences
University of Stellenbosch

Introduction

Family physicians need to do a lot more than merely update their knowledge, yet they are drowning in information. The current knowledge explosion and rapid advances in diagnostics and therapeutics are cause for concern. There is no logical means to choose what to read unless you use a systematic way of reading.

Family medicine is not confined to knowledge of a particular group of diseases and requires a breadth of knowledge and skills that is particularly challenging. The reflective family medicine practitioner will always encounter patients with stimulating questions, or who push the boundaries of current practice. In addition, there are always new approaches to care, new roles for the family physician (as business manager, negotiator, planner, and information broker) and new skills to learn (such as the use of information technology).

Doctors are trained and qualify only once. In South Africa at present, doctors can then make life and death decisions, and there is no formal reassessment of their continued competence. However, the Health Professions Council has made it a requirement for medical professionals to attend accredited *continuing professional development* (CPD) activities. Critics of CPD activities say that they often perpetuate medical school and favour knowledge acquisition. CPD should therefore take into account factors such as the topic, method of instruction, duration, convenience, relevance, and applicability.

The following trends may develop in the future:
- Patients will be increasingly well informed.
- Patients with disease will be members of support groups that provide high-quality information.
- Patients will increasingly want involvement in shared decision making.

- The disease spectrum will change.
- There will be a need to teach patients and family physicians how to cope with uncertainty.
- Diagnostic activities will become more sophisticated and equipment will become more portable.
- Family physicians will be held more and more accountable to their patients and their profession and will need to undergo further forms of re-certification and re-accreditation.

The implications for primary health care are profound. Family physicians can no longer assume that their position and livelihood are automatically assured. If they can demonstrate quality, imagination, teamwork, and development, they will not only survive, but they will also continue to grow and play a central role in health care.

In this chapter you will learn about a set of useful reader's guides that will help you to critically appraise the published evidence. In addition, you will be shown how to convert uncertainty around a patient into an answerable question, how to find the best evidence to answer that question, how to convert its critical appraisal into clinical action, and how to evaluate this process. This is essentially what the process of evidence-based health care entails.

The reflective practitioner

In South Africa, all doctors are now required to obtain CPD points in order to re-register with the Health Professions Council. Much of the CPD on offer, however, is of limited quality or unlikely to change clinical practice (Cantillon and Jones, 1999). For example, publishing new evidence in a scientific journal and giving a lecture, the two most common forms of CPD, are probably the least effective. Multifaceted approaches that use interactive workshops, accessible reminders or prompts for decision-making, and educational outreach visits may be more effective at bridging the gap between new evidence and clinical practice. Other forms of CPD that may be useful include quality improvement cycles, local adaptation of national guidelines, and patient-mediated interventions (Bero, 1998).

Acquiring CPD points does not necessarily lead to change in practice or improvements in quality of care. What is of central importance is for family physicians to develop a critical or reflective stance towards their practice – to become aware of the questions, uncertainties, and errors of everyday practice that require further learning or reflection. In some situations, the more formal quality improvement cycle may be used by family physicians to reflect on their own quality and actual performance (see Chapter 10). Various tools that may assist this self-directed learning and reflective stance are outlined in this chapter.

Critical reading in family medicine

Most doctors, especially in family medicine, receive a stream of journals, both solicited and unsolicited, in their mail. The huge information explosion requires the average family physician to read at least 19 articles per day in order to keep up to date with new developments in family medicine. Family physicians seldom have time to read, and it is therefore important for them to develop and maintain a systematic approach to reading and critically appraising clinical literature.

The following approach, called READER (see Table 13.1), can help you to make these choices (Macauley, 1994). This is a basic framework which can be used to initiate the critical reading process. It is not in itself an adequate critical appraisal tool. User-friendly critical appraisal tools for research articles on diagnosis, treatment, prognosis, harm and guidelines are presented later in this chapter.

When you receive a journal, scan the titles of the articles and apply the following criteria before you decide what to read in depth.

- Relevance: Does the article deal with family medicine? Is it written from a family medicine perspective?
- Education: Is the article likely to challenge my current practice and beliefs or to suggest alternatives? Is it likely to reiterate what I already know or believe? Challenging articles are more likely to help family physicians keep up to date and change behaviour.
- Applicability: Is the article applicable to my situation? For example, could the research have been done in my practice? Could I apply the results in my practice with its particular facilities, situation, and location? If the issue is applicable, then it may change behaviour.
- Discrimination: Is the article of high quality? Are the results valid? Was there rigorous peer review before publication?
- Evaluation: Evaluate your responses to the above questions. Should this paper be considered seriously?
- Reaction: If the article has passed the above criteria, you should read it in depth. Consider how you can use the information. Should it be implemented in your practice immediately? Should it be shared with your colleagues? Should a copy of the article be stored or filed for future reference? Should the citation be kept for future reference in a library?

Table 13.1 READER – an acronym to aid critical reading by family physicians

Relevance	Is it about family medicine?
Education	Does it challenge my knowledge?
Applicability	Does it apply to my situation?
Discrimination	What is the scientific quality of the article?
Evaluation	What is my evaluation, based on the above criteria?
Reaction	How can I use this information?

Evidence-based health care (EBHC)

In the past, the public had an implicit trust in the medical profession. This may no longer be the case as this implicit trust is gradually eroded. The public is becoming more and more informed and is increasingly more proficient in searching for information on the Internet. They may demand more explicit accountability and may insist that family physicians base their decision-making on sound, valid, contemporaneous, relevant, and accessible external clinical evidence.

The purpose of this chapter is to introduce the reader to EBHC and especially the skill of critical appraisal of published evidence for its closeness to the truth, practical relevance, usefulness, and applicability. By engaging with evidence in this way, you will be able to make sound, evidence-based decisions within your practice.

The literature has described EBHC as a paradigm shift, clinical epidemiology revisited, a neologism for informed clinical decision-making, and a panacea. It is a paradigm shift in that it will probably encourage a move away from an authoritarian (opinion-based) way of practising, to an authoritative (evidence-based) approach (Guyatt *et al.*, 1992). Although it has been described as a panacea, it is certainly not the wonder solution of all that ails medicine.

Definition

EBHC has been defined as the conscientious, explicit, and judicious use of current best evidence in making decisions with individual patients. It combines and integrates the external clinical evidence (in the form of scientific research) with the family physician's clinical experience, expertise, wisdom, judgment, and proficiency (Sackett *et al.*, 1998). EBHC therefore reduces the knowledge gap between clinical research and practice.

EBHC is all about quality – in finding the studies that address a particular question, in only selecting studies of acceptable quality, in distilling the information into knowledge, and in making the knowledge understandable. Another quality step is when the knowledge is combined with a family physician's education and experience and their knowledge of a patient and the values of people and society, in order to make sound decisions.

EBHC is a method of problem-solving that:
- Recognises that no individual person can know all that is needed to practise effectively across the spectrum of care
- Acknowledges that not all therapies or health care decisions that are used have been validated (Wallace, 1997).

The definition of key terms in EBHC are given in the box at the end of this chapter.

The rationale for EBHC

Family physicians act as witnesses to their patients' suffering, interpreters of their stories, and guardians against the over-medicalisation of their problems. They often have to carry out these tasks when the evidence for diagnosis and rational treatment is unavailable, absent, invalid, unreliable, or irrelevant.

Decisions about groups of patients or populations are usually made by combining three factors: values, resources, and evidence. At present, many health care decisions are based principally on values and resources, that is, opinion-based decision-making, and little attention has been given to evidence derived from scientific research. This, however, is changing as pressure on resources increases. Increasingly, decisions will have to be made explicitly and publicly, and those who make decisions will have to produce and describe the evidence on which each decision is based. It is hoped that this will encourage a transition from opinion-based decision-making to evidence-based decision-making (Muir Gray, 2000).

One of the ways we can deal with uncertainty in family medicine and be better family physicians is to become more quantitative in our clinical thinking (that is, quantify or explicitly state our diagnostic uncertainty) and to use a common language of critical appraisal. Sir William Osler stated that good clinical medicine will always blend the art of uncertainty with the science of probability. It is clear that the critiquing of clinical research therefore demands the application of both art and science. The art has been described as making sound and reasonable decisions in uncertain circumstances with imperfect or incomplete information. This is achieved by using and involving your judgement, wisdom, personal experience, and expertise that you have obtained over the years as well as intuition, common sense, and humanity (Charlton, 1995). EBHC de-emphasises intuition and unsystematic clinical experience, and stresses good quality, valid, and relevant research.

The five steps of EBHC

The EBHC process has five steps:
1 Convert needs for clinical information into focused answerable questions.
2 Track down the best evidence with which to answer the questions.
3 Critically appraise the evidence for its validity, importance, and usefulness.
4 Apply the result of the critical appraisal in your practice.
5 Audit your performance.

The whole process therefore starts and ends with a patient (Sackett *et al.*, 2000).

Step 1: Formulate a focused, answerable question from the patient's problem

This is the most fundamental step of the whole process. The clinical problem should determine the type of question you ask and the type of research evidence you seek. To qualify as a focused and answerable question, it must contain the following four components:
- A patient or problem: How could I best describe a group of patients such as this patient?
- An intervention (or exposure): Which main course of action am I considering?
- A comparison (where relevant): What are the alternative courses of action?
- An outcome: What can I hope to accomplish?

After identifying a knowledge gap or area of uncertainty, formulate a question to include the above-mentioned components. The following three case studies will demonstrate this step in the EBHC process.

Mr SH, a 40-year-old patient with chronic dyspepsia who has no other sinister features that suggest malignancy, prefers to have non-invasive investigations to establish the diagnosis. His chronic dyspepsia has responded well to H$_2$ antagonists in the past. You think that his condition may be associated with *H. pylori*, but he refuses to have invasive procedures done to confirm the diagnosis.

A focused question would be: 'In a 40-year-old patient with chronic dyspepsia (*patient*), what are the sensitivity, specificity and predictive values of a non-invasive test (*intervention*) compared to that of a gold standard endoscopic biopsy (*comparison*) in terms of diagnosing *H. pylori* (*outcome*)?'

This is a *question of diagnosis* (see Table 13.2). Other questions may deal with cultural and quality-of-life issues, but the whole process is initiated by questions arising from the consultation.

Mrs S, a 33-year-old woman with migraine headaches, requests a prescription for sumatriptan after reading a magazine article about this medication.

A focused question here would be: 'In a 33-year-old woman with frequent migraine attacks (*patient*), would sumatriptan (*intervention, exposure*) reduce the severity of her headaches (*outcome*)?'

This is a *question of therapy* (see Table 13.2).

Mrs B's one-year-old son had a febrile convulsion. She would like to know what his risks of developing epilepsy are.

A focused question here would be: 'Does the febrile convulsion (*exposure*) that this one-year-old infant (*patient*) had increase the likelihood that he will develop epilepsy (*outcome*)?'

This is a *question of prognosis* (see Table 13.2).

Well-built quantitative clinical questions usually contain four elements (as described above) and can arise from any of the eight possibilities listed in Table 13.2. These questions assist you in identifying the evidence needed to provide the patient with a clear answer. However, patients may also have other questions that are less readily answerable using the process of EBHC. These may be questions about the context itself, for example about why and how. These questions may need to take into account qualitative as well as quantitative evidence, that is, descriptions as well as numbers. Philosophical, existential, or reflective questions often arise during the consultation and are best dealt with by the family physician using the judgement, experience, and proficiency gained over the years.

Table 13.2 The foundation of clinical questions

1 Clinical findings	How to gather and interpret findings properly from the history and physical examination
2 Aetiology	How to identify causes for disease (including its iatrogenic forms)
3 Differential diagnoses	When considering the possible causes of a patient's clinical problem, how to rank them by likelihood, seriousness, and treatability
4 Diagnostic tests	How to select and interpret diagnostic tests, in order to confirm or exclude a diagnosis, based on considering their precision, accuracy, acceptability, expense, safety, and so on
5 Prognosis	How to estimate the patient's likely clinical course over time and anticipate likely complications of the disease
6 Therapy	How to select treatments to offer patients that do more good than harm and that are worth the effort and cost of using them
7 Prevention	How to reduce the chance of disease by identifying and modifying risk factors and how to diagnose disease early by screening
8 Self-improvement	How to keep up to date, improve your clinical skills, and run a better, more efficient clinical practice

SOURCE: Adapted from Sackett *et al.* (1997)

Step 2: Search for evidence

MEDLINE and EMBASE are the two main databases on the Internet that remain excellent general resources. These are general databases covering all of biomedical research and many other areas. The Cochrane Library is also a useful resource.

MEDLINE is compiled by the National Library of Medicine in the United States. It contains references from more than 4 000 journals published internationally. A number of companies supply access to MEDLINE, the most common being Ovid and Silver Platter. MEDLINE has a number of limitations (including a sensitivity of 50% and English language emphasis), and you need to use other sources in order to get a comprehensive list of relevant literature. The more experience you have of searching MEDLINE, the more skillful you will become at it and your searches will be more complete and precise. Remember that MEDLINE indexers use American spellings and phrases so for some questions you would need to list both English and American terms or spellings.

You can use the following criteria to search the MEDLINE database:

- A keyword or phrase from your focused question (for example, *H. pylori*)
- The MeSH term (medical subject heading), which are the terms used to index the articles
- The title (the search will look for words in the title of the paper)
- The author (the last name and initial)
- The name of the journal (for example, *South African Medical Journal*)
- The type of publication (for example, randomised controlled trial, meta-analysis, and so on).

When you are searching for evidence you should first look for a systematic review or meta-analysis. Systematic reviews of randomised controlled trials (RCT) represent the highest form of evidence available. Therefore, you should first search for a systematic review and then proceed down the hierarchy for the next best evidence available (see Figure 13.1).

Who can help you with your search if you get stuck? Try a librarian, an expert who practises EBHC, or a search engine on the World Wide Web (http://igm.n/m.nih.gov/index-html). Good user-friendly tutorials, which are regularly updated, are available on Pub Med to assist in improving your searching skills.

Step 3: Critical appraisal

Critical appraisal involves the assessment of the scientific quality of a research article, including its design, methodology, and analysis. This part of the process draws on biostatistical and epidemiological concepts. For research to be considered useful (see Table 13.3), it not only has to be valid (internally and externally) but also of relevance (to primary care and your patient) and reasonably accessible.

In assessing internal validity, you have to look at the possible influence of bias, chance, and confounding factors as rival explanations in explaining the association between an exposure and an outcome (for example, sumatriptan and reduced migraine frequency). Validity should not be seen as a dichotomy (that is, valid or not valid) but rather a spectrum with these judgements at either end. As with any other skill in clinical practice, the skill of critical appraisal improves with practice.

Formal critical appraisal training is becoming increasingly available and joining a problem-based journal club may provide you with an opportunity to practise.

The absence of excellent evidence does not make evidence-based decision-making impossible. What is required in such a situation is the best possible evidence available and not the best evidence possible, using the classification shown in Figure 13.1. A number of guides are available to assist you in critically appraising a research article (see Tables 13.4, 13.5, and 13.6).

Figure 13.1 The traditional hierachy of evidence

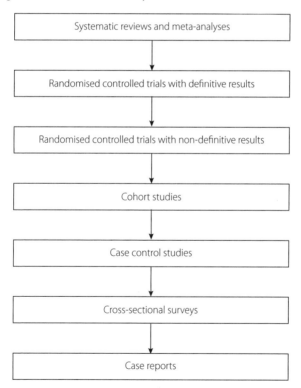

It may be unwise to assume that what is statistically significant to the researcher and clinically significant to the family physician will also be personally significant to the patient. These issues of statistical significance, clinical significance, and personal significance are illustrated in Tables 13.4 to 13.8.

The Graphic Appraisal Tool for Epidemiological studies (GATE) frame is another useful way to assist you in conceptualising an epidemiological study and provides a visual framework which illustrates the generic design of all epidemiological studies. This is a useful way to assist with the understanding of the different primary and integrated epidemiological studies and to improve the critical appraisal of such studies. (Jackson *et al.*, 2006)

Table 13.3 Assessing the usefulness of a study

Usefulness	Explanation
Accessibility	Can I easily obtain or retrieve the study?
Internal validity	Is it close to the truth? Is it accurate? Can I believe it? Consider whether the results are influenced by bias, chance, or confounding factors.
External validity	Can the results be generalised to my practice population?
Applicability	Are the results applicable to and acceptable to my specific patient?

SOURCE: Adapted from Evans (1997)

Table 13.4 A guide for assessing an article on therapy

Are the results of the study valid? (Statistical significance)

Primary guides

Was the assignment of patients to treatments randomised?

Were all the patients who entered the trial properly accounted for and attributed at its conclusion?

Was follow-up complete?

Were patients analysed in the groups to which they were randomised?

Was an intention-to-treat analysis done?

Secondary guides

Were patients, health workers, and study personnel blind to treatment?

Were the groups similar at the start of the trial?

Aside from the experimental intervention, were the groups treated equally?

What were the results? (Clinical significance)

How large was the treatment effect?

How precise was the estimate of the treatment effect?

Will the results help me in caring for my patients? (Personal significance)

Can the results be applied to my patient?

Were all clinically important outcomes considered?

Are the likely treatment benefits worth the potential harm and cost?

Table 13.5 A guide for assessing an article on diagnostics

Are the results of the study valid? (Statistical significance)

Primary guides

Was there an independent, blind comparison with a reference standard?

Did the patient sample include an appropriate spectrum of patients to whom the diagnostic test will be applied in clinical practice?

Secondary guides

Did the results of the test being evaluated influence the decision to perform the reference standard?

Were the methods for performing the test described in sufficient detail to permit replication?

What were the results? (Clinical significance)

Are the likelihood ratios for the test results presented or is data necessary for their calculation provided? (See Chapter 5.)

Will the results help me in caring for my patients? (Personal significance)

Will the reproducibility of the test result and its interpretation be satisfactory in my setting?

Are the results applicable to my patient?

Will the results change my management?

Will patients be better off as a result of the test?

Table 13.6 A guide for assessing an article on harm/aetiology

---

Are the results of this harm study valid? (Statistical significance)

1 Were there clearly defined groups of patients, similar in all-important ways other than exposure to the treatment or other cause?

2 Were treatment exposures and clinical outcomes measured the same ways in both groups (was the assessment of outcomes either objective (for example death) or blinded to exposure)?

3 Was the follow-up of study patients complete and long enough?

4 Do the results satisfy some criteria for causation?
   - Is it clear that the exposure preceded the onset of the outcome?
   - Is there a dose-response gradient?
   - Is there positive evidence from a dechallenge-rechallenge study?
   - Is the association consistent from study to study?
   - Does the association make biological sense?

Are the valid results from this harm study important? (Clinical significance)

		Adverse outcome		Totals
		Present (Case)	Absent (Control)	
Exposed to the treatment	Yes	a	b	
	No	c	d	
Totals		a + c	b + d	a + b + c + d

In a randomised trial or cohort study:

Relative risk = RR = [a/(a+b)]/[c/(c+d)]

In a case-control study: Relative odds = RO = ad/bc

Should these results change the treatment of an individual patient? (Personal significance)

1 Can the study results be extrapolated to this patient?

2 What are this patient's risks of the adverse outcome?

3 What are this patient's preferences, concerns and expectations from this treatment?

4 What alternative treatments are available?

Table 13.7 A guide for assessing a review article

Are the results of the study valid? (Statistical significance)

Primary guides

Did the overview address a focused clinical question?

Were the criteria used to select articles for inclusion appropriate?

Secondary guides

Is it unlikely that important, relevant studies were missed?

Was the validity of the included studies appraised?

Were assessments of studies reproducible? (that is, did the reviewers use explicit, consistent, transparent and standardised methodology in reviewing the article?)

Were the results similar from study to study (homogeneity)?

What are the results? (Clinical significance)

What are the overall results of the review?

How precise were the results?

Will the results help me in caring for my patients? (Personal significance)

Can the results be applied to my patient care?

Were all clinically important outcomes considered?

Are the benefits worth the harm and costs?

Table 13.8 A guide for assessing an EBM guideline

Are the recommendations in this guideline valid? (Statistical significance)

1 Were all important decision options and outcomes clearly specified?
2 Was the evidence relevant to each decision option identified, validated and combined in a sensible and explicit way?
3 Are the relative preferences that key stakeholders attach to the outcomes of decisions (including benefits, risks and costs) identified and explicitly considered?
4 Is the guideline resistant to clinically sensible variations in practice?

Is this valid guideline or strategy potentially useful? (Clinical significance)

1 Does this guideline offer an opportunity for significant improvement in the quality of health care practice?
2 Is there a large variation in current practice?
3 Does the guideline contain new evidence (or old evidence not yet acted upon) that could have an important impact on management?
4 Would the guideline affect the management of so many people, or concern individuals at such high risk, or involve such high costs that even small changes in practice could have major impacts on health outcomes or resources (including opportunity costs)?

Should this guideline or strategy be applied in your practice? (Personal significance)

1 What barriers exist to its implementation? Can they be overcome?
2 Can you enlist the collaboration of key colleagues?
3 Can you meet the educational, administrative and economic conditions that are likely to determine the success or failure of implementing the strategy?
   a Credible synthesis of the evidence by a respected body
   b Respected, influential local exemplars already implementing the strategy
   c Consistent information from all relevant sources
   d Opportunity for individual discussions about the strategy with an authority
   e User-friendly format for guidelines
   f Implementable within target group of clinicians (without the need for extensive outside collaboration)
   g Freedom from conflict with economic incentives, administrative incentives, patient expectations and community expectations.

The killer Bs

1 Is the Burden of illness (frequency in our community, or our patient's pre-test probability or expected event rate [PEER]) too low to warrant implementation?
2 Are the Beliefs of individual patients or communities about the value of the interventions or their consequences incompatible with the guideline?
3 Would the opportunity cost of implementing this guideline constitute a bad Bargain in the use of our energy or our community's resources?
4 Are the Barriers (geographic, organisational, traditional, authoritarian, legal, or behavioural) so high that it is not worth trying to overcome them?

Step 4: Apply the result of this appraisal in your practice

The fourth step in the process of using an evidence-based approach in the practice of health care is to decide how to apply the information obtained to the particular circumstances of your patient. It is not only a question of whether your patient would have fitted the inclusion or exclusion criteria of the trial; but also whether the beneficial effects of the intervention outweigh the harms and the costs. In addition it is important to decide how to take into account the patient's stated and perceived needs, the resources available, and the priorities that may be placed by the patient on different treatment options. This process requires a partnership between the doctor and the patient. If at the end of the process the decision is made not to apply the available evidence, that decision should be a shared and conscious one.

There are three ways in which results of trials can be presented: by relative risk reduction (RRR), absolute risk reduction (ARR), and numbers needed to treat (NNT). These measures of association are used to express the relative benefits of one intervention compared to another. Absolute risk reduction (ARR) is used to calculate the numbers needed to treat (NNT). You should try to calculate all three measures in order to get a true reflection of the strength of the association between the intervention and outcome. This would only apply if the outcomes are categorical and one is interested in determining whether an association (typically between a risk factor and a disease) is statistically significant and strong. If the outcomes concerned are not categorical but continuous (for example, measured on a continuous scale) one would look at correlation or regression techniques as an indication of the strength and significance of the associations between an exposure and an outcome.

In addition to critical appraisal of the evidence, the family physician should reflect on the context of the individual clinical encounter. The danger of EBHC is that the context often gets ignored or under-emphasised. The context may include the realities of the health system (that is, what drugs are available) as well as the individual patient. Reflection is therefore a way of putting back the context, allowing a more holistic approach, and attempting to anchor research in reality. For example, if you are appraising the evidence from a controlled trial, you should also take into account the unique situation of your patient.

Therefore, even if critical appraisal reveals useful evidence, its applicability is not a forgone conclusion as patients have different preferences and priorities which should be respected. Eliciting and respecting patients' preferences are especially important when there is reasonable doubt about the best course of action. Even good evidence can lead to bad practice if it is applied in an unthinking or unfeeling way (Naylor,

1995; Kassirer, 1994). Applying the results of the appraisal by involving the patient in a shared decision-making process is an important and underutilised step in the consultation process (Elwyn and Edwards, 1999).

Critical appraisal of the published research, critical reflection on context, and the way you practise will allow you to make the best use of EBHC, and stimulate continuing professional development.

Evidence-based decision-making

In clinical practice a junior doctor faced with a clinical dilemma would turn to a more senior doctor for the definitive answer to the problem. This answer to the problem, usually based on the many years of anecdotal experience of the senior doctor, would be taken at face value by the junior doctor, acted upon and not ever be tested empirically. This way of practice is gradually changing. Junior doctors now need to become proficient at searching for information themselves, assessing it for its validity and importance and applying it to the patient or practice setting, thus making evidence-based decisions.

At the end of any consultation the clinician usually has to make decisions regarding further management, ideally in consultation with the patient. Such a decision will need to incorporate important elements of evidence, resource availability and cost effectiveness of diagnostic tests or treatment offered, the patient preference, and considerations of the context in which the practitioner practices. Resources are dependent on whether one practices in a developed or developing country; private sector or public sector, or a tertiary hospital or primary care community health centre. Attempts should always be made to integrate these elements, as emphasising one over the other will detract from the overall quality of the decision-making process.

The element of evidence refers to whether there is sound, valid, and current research evidence available to support what is being offered to the patient in the form of a diagnostic test, therapeutic intervention, or advice on prognosis. The best research evidence can be quantitative or qualitative and will depend on the question asked. Quantitative evidence includes relevant patient-centred clinical research into the accuracy of diagnostic tests, the power of prognostic markers, the efficacy and safety of treatment regimens, and the effectiveness of clinical interventions. Qualitative evidence on the other hand, best describes the meaning of illness or patient experiences, understanding, attitudes, and beliefs. So evidence-based decision-making involves the application of the best evidence to practise, be it a randomised controlled trial (RCT) to evaluate a question on treatment interventions, a cohort study to evaluate a question on prognosis, a case control study to examine a question of causation (when an RCT or a cohort study is not feasible) or a qualitative study to learn about the meaning of illness. Such evidence is not just for clinicians, but is relevant to all members of the primary care team.

The element of resources looks at whether the patient or the practice can afford the diagnostic or therapeutic intervention being offered to the patient, as cost is always an important consideration. The potential cost of the medication or intervention offered to the patient, as well as the diagnostic test involved, should always be considered.

Patient preference deals with the unique ideas, expectations and concerns which the patient brings to the consultation and which need to be factored into the decision-making process if they are to serve the patient. In addition, it also refers to the underlying assumptions and beliefs that are involved when clinicians, along with patients, weigh what they will gain or lose when making a management decision.

To explain the application of evidence-based decision-making further, one could use the following examples of a patient seen in primary care.

Scenario

Mr Smith (42) presents to you with classical clinical features of acute maxillary sinusitis – nasal obstruction, purulent discharge and pain and tenderness over his maxillary sinuses. X-rays of his sinuses reveal mucosal thickening consistent with maxillary sinusitis. This is his first episode, which you ascribe to a recent viral upper respiratory tract infection.

In applying the elements of evidence-based decision-making one will have to consider the important points shown in Table 13.9.

The health care practitioner has a duty of beneficence towards patients, which involves making sure patients understand information and assisting them in making appropriate health choices based on sound research evidence. Evidence therefore is but one component of the decision-making process and is necessary, but not sufficient for delivering high-quality patient care.

By availing ourselves of the most reliable and up-to-date research information, we can free up our intellectual capacity to utilise our communication, examination and other diagnostic skills. We can also discuss clinical management problems with greater confidence, and make the most effective referral and commissioning choices. This approach is not restricted to decision-making in practice, but can also be used to inform health policy-making, decisions in public health and decisions facing hospital managers.

Table 13.9 Example of evidence-based decision-making in patient with maxillary sinusitis

---

1 Evidence

What is the diagnostic accuracy and predictive value of clinical signs, nasopharyngeal swabs and X-rays?

What are the efficacy, effectiveness and safety of the following advice and medication?

- Nasal douches and steam inhalation
- Decongestants
- Analgesia
- Antibiotics (for example amoxicillin seven to ten days) if symptoms persist.

Evidence is needed ideally from relevant, high-quality systematic reviews; EBM guidelines or randomised controlled trials

---

2 Resources – cost effectiveness

What are the costs of medication or other treatments?

Do the potential benefits of the treatment outweigh the harms and cost?

---

3 Patient preferences

What are the possible side-effects of the medication?

What is important to the patient?

What other options is the patient interested in?

Step 5: The audit of clinical performance

To what extent is the care of your patient evidence-based? This is a difficult question to answer and the methodology used to answer such a question should be both quantitative and qualitative. Remember that not all that is of value is measurable and not all that is measurable is of value (Greenhalgh, 1996; Kinmonth, 1995; Green and Britten, 1998). Auditing clinical performance with formal quality assurance is an important way of ensuring that evidence is implemented and that quality and high standards of care are continued.

The advantages of EBHC

- It allows for greater efficiency and quality of decisions.
- It reduces the gap between research and clinical practice.
- It improves family physicians' understanding of research and its methods.
- It improves computer literacy and data-searching skills.
- It attempts to diminish uncertainty.

- It provides a common language for critical appraisal.
- It promotes self-directed learning.
- It promotes effective and efficient family physicians.
- It is presented in synopsis form as protocols and guidelines.

Limitations and competing demands

The lack of time availability in primary care and the restricted resource allocations are important reasons for the slow uptake of the principles and philosophy of evidence-based practice. In addition, a vast array of unsolicited guidelines purporting to be based on evidence is becoming available. There is also a wealth of topics and problem areas where evidence is missing, inconclusive or based on less robust research methodologies.

Some opponents of evidence-based practice are sceptical about viewing the randomised controlled trial as the gold standard of clinical research evidence. It is more important though that the type of research question is matched with the most appropriate research methodology to answer that question. Green and Britten (1998) have presented a sound argument for the importance of qualitative research evidence within primary care that looks at patient experiences, service development, and other management and quality topics.

However robust the research, clinicians face the dilemma of applying group evidence on effectiveness to individual patients. Uncertainty is inherent in medical evidence when it is applied to individual patients. One of the ways we can deal with the uncertainty in family medicine is incorporating evidence-based practice.

EBHC in family medicine

There are obvious difficulties involved in integrating EBHC into family medicine. The family physician may lack the necessary skill and time to access and interpret the available evidence. In addition, few studies relate to primary care, negative findings are less likely to be published, and MEDLINE searches may only retrieve 50 to 80% of the relevant literature.

Family medicine is characterised by particular emphasis on the doctor–patient relationship and on biomedical, personal, and contextual perspectives in diagnosis (Jacobson *et al.*, 1997). EBHC predominantly addresses the biomedical perspective of diagnosis and principally from a doctor-centred paradigm. Family physicians need evidence that is derived from a patient-centred paradigm and that recognises the personal and contextual elements to decision-making in practice.

Research evidence dealing with quality of life measures, meaning, and a deeper understanding of patients' and doctors' attitudes is less readily available.

Emphasis on the biomedical perspective and the randomised controlled trial, which is often seen as the gold standard of EBHC, fails to do justice to the realities of family medicine, which is influenced by the subjective, anecdotal, patients' stories of illness and personal experience (Jacobson *et al.*, 1997). Personal experience and qualitative research are often characterised as being a poor basis for making a scientific decision (Greenhalgh, 1996). However, they are often more persuasive than scientific publications in changing clinical practice.

Evidence–based medicine initially aligned itself with the sort of research evidence that could be expressed as mathematical estimates of risk and benefit in the population sampled. There is however the need to expand our understanding of the patients' illness experience, the appropriateness and relevance of health services, and the barriers to change in patients and professionals.

Qualitative research in particular can investigate family physicians' and patients' attitudes, beliefs, and preferences and the whole question of how evidence is turned into practice. It also improves judgement, enriches imagination, enhances perspectives, sensitises family physicians to the illness experience of patients, and therefore broadens the scope of EBHC (Greenhalgh, 1996; Kinmonth, 1995; Green and Britten, 1998; Macnaughton, 1995; Rosenberg and Donald, 1995). In the absence of useful evidence, the family physician might be forced to make use of evidence that is only doubtfully relevant and generated perhaps in a different grouping of patients in another country, at another time, or using a similar but not identical treatment. This is called *evidence-biased* medicine (Grimley, 1995).

The time may come when health authorities require a minimum acceptable level of evidence-based decisions by family physicians and hospital doctors, and when failure to adhere to highly authoritative evidence-based systematic reviews or clinical guidelines will be deemed negligent. Family physicians have a responsibility to accommodate EBHC as a desirable feature of good practice. Patients have a right to receive medical opinions based, when possible, on the best available evidence. The message, however, is clear that reading, interpreting, and acting on published literature should become a routine part of clinical practice.

Recommended reading

Elwood, Mark (1998) *Critical Appraisal of Epidemiological Studies and Clinical Trials.* Second edition. Oxford: Oxford University Press.

Gabbay, Mark (1999) *The Evidence-based Primary Care Handbook.* The Royal Society of Medicine Press Limited.

Jones, Roger and Kinmonth, Anne-Louise (1995) *Critical Reading for Primary Care.* New York: Oxford University Press.

Muir Gray, JA (1997) *Evidence-based Healthcare. How to make Health Policy and Management Decisions.* New York: Churchill Livingstone.

Sackett, David L (2000) *Evidence-based Medicine. How to Practice and Teach EBM.* Second edition. Edinburgh: Churchill Livingstone.

Jackson R, Ameratunga S, Broad J, Connor J et al (2006). The GATE frame: Critical Appraisal with pictures. *ACP Journal Club* 144(2): A8–11

EBHC terms and definitions

Absolute risk reduction (ARR) The difference in risk of a particular event between two groups (the control group event rate minus the experimental group event rate).

Accuracy Without systematic error (bias); on average the results approximate those of the phenomenon under study.

Bias Systematic error that can occur in all study designs in the form of selection bias, information bias, or confounding bias. Bias reduces the validity of results.

Blinding Patients and researchers are unaware of the treatment given until the study has finished.

Categorical outcome An outcome whose values are categories (for example dead or alive; male or female).

Confidence interval (95%) One can be 95% confident that the true population value for the variable being estimated lies within this interval. The interval is defined numerically by the highest and lowest values at each end of the interval.

Confounding Error that occurs when groups being compared in a study are different with regard to risk or prognostic factors other than the factor (treatment or exposure) under investigation.

Continuous scale A scale used to measure a numerical characteristic with values that occur on a continuum (for example age).

Correlation A measure of the linear relationship between two numerical measurements made on the same set of subjects. It ranges –1 to +1, with zero indicating no relationship.

Critical appraisal The assessment of the scientific quality of a paper, including the design, methodology, and analysis.

Critical reflection The use of a family physician's knowledge, experience and judgement to relate research findings to practice.

Effectiveness The extent to which a treatment produces a beneficial effect when implemented under the usual conditions of clinical care.

Efficacy The extent to which a treatment produces a beneficial effect when assessed under ideal conditions such as a research trial.

Evidence-based decision-making Application of clinical research evidence, consideration of cost effectiveness and resource constraints, as well as incorporating the values and preferences of patients in deciding on patient management.

Gold standard The criterion used to unequivocally define the presence and absence of a condition or disease under study.

Hypothesis An assertive statement that an association or relationship difference exists between variables in the larger population from which the study samples are obtained.

Incidence The rate at which an event occurs in a defined population over time. The number of new cases divided by the total population at risk.

Intention to treat analysis Analysing patients in the groups to which they were randomised at the beginning of the study, even if they drop out of the study or withdraw. Failure to do so results in the loss of the randomisation effect and bias occurs.

Likelihood Likelihood is an expression of the certainty or uncertainty that an outcome will occur and is expressed as a probability or odds.

Loss to follow-up Patients often withdraw, crossover, move, die, or disappear during a trial. This should be minimal and preferably not be related to either form of treatment.

Meta-analysis A mathematical synthesis of the results of two or more primary studies that address the same hypothesis in the same way.

Number needed to treat (NNT) A measure of the impact of a treatment or intervention. It states how many patients need to be treated with the treatment in question in order to prevent an event that would otherwise occur. It is calculated as the reciprocal of ARR.

Odds ratio The probability that an event occurs divided by the probability that the event does not occur (the probability of an event divided by its complement) for example the odds that a person has Blood type O are: $0.42/(1-0.42) = 0.72:1$ but "to 1" generally is not stated explicitly.

Placebo An inert substance given to a study subject who has been assigned to the control group to make them think they are getting the treatment under study.

Practice guideline A set of recommendations for using or not using available interventions in clinical or public health.

Precision Without random error or variability from measurement to measurement of the same phenomenon (synonym: reproducible, reliable, repeatable).

Prevalence The proportion of people in a defined group who have a disease, condition, or injury. The numbers affected by a condition divided by the population at risk.

Publication bias The tendency not to publish small studies, studies with conflicting results or negative studies, which do not demonstrate a statistically significant difference between groups.

P value The probability of obtaining data at least as extreme as the data obtained in the investigation's sample set if the null hypothesis (of no difference, no relationship) was true.

Qualitative methods Methods that are committed to understanding and interpreting the experiences of individuals.

Randomisation The process of allocating treatments (patients) to the alternative treatments in a clinical trial. The purpose of randomisation is to produce comparable treatment groups with respect to important prognostic factors.

Randomised controlled trial A clinical trial where at least two treatment groups are compared. One of them serves as the control group and treatment allocation is carried out using a randomised unbiased method. (This is often referred to as the gold standard of EBHC.)

Regression The process of predicting an outcome (dependent variable) from a predictor (independent) variable.

Relative risk reduction (RRR) The proportion of the initial or baseline risk that was eliminated by a given treatment or intervention.

Systematic review An overview of primary studies that contains an explicit statement of objectives, materials, and methods and has been conducted according to explicit and reproducible methodology.

Validity An expression of how well a study actually measures the effect it is designed to measure. The degree to which the results of a study are likely to be true, believable and free of bias. When a study has deficiencies in its validity (and most do have some), this statement implies nothing about the sincerity or honesty of the researchers. Rather, it refers to the methodological flaws (often subtle) which may bias the results and outcomes of the study.

14 Integrative medicine

Maria Christodoulou
Division of Family Medicine and Primary Care
University of Stellenbosch

Introduction

Integrative medicine is a healing-orientated medicine that takes into account the whole person (body, mind and spirit), including all aspects of lifestyle. It emphasises the therapeutic relationship and makes use of all appropriate therapies and disciplines, in an evidence-based approach.

Integrative medicine is an emerging and evolving discipline. It extends beyond conventional paradigms to embrace the diversity of health systems, traditions and professions that exist in the world in a broader, more inclusive approach to health care. This approach is closely aligned with the core principles and values of family medicine whilst simultaneously challenging the family physician to expand their horizons beyond the confines of conventional medical knowledge.

In essence, integrative medicine seeks to combine the very best of conventional, complementary, alternative and traditional medicine. In doing so a new model of health care is emerging that not only incorporates existing practices, but transcends each of these to define an entirely new system of healing.

The terms complementary and alternative are used interchangeably with traditional medicine in some countries, but are generally considered to refer to *a broad set of health care practices that are not part of a country's traditional or indigenous practices, or not integrated into its dominant health care system.* In the South African context, the terms traditional medicine (TM) or traditional African medicine (TAM) will be used to refer to medicine practiced by traditional healers as defined by the Traditional Healers Act, and should be viewed as distinct from complementary and alternative medicine and the specific professions registered by the Allied Health Professions Council, for example chiropractic, homeopathy, traditional Chinese medicine and Ayurvedic medicine.

Important terminology

Some of the terms that will be used in this chapter are explained below.

Allopathic or conventional medicine: Western, orthodox or conventional medicine as practised by the scientifically trained medical doctor in hospitals and clinics throughout the world.

Alternative medicine: treatment, therapy or modality not recognised by allopathic medicine and which patients might use *instead of* conventional medicine.

Complementary medicine: any treatment, therapy or modality which may be used *in conjunction with* conventional medicine, for example a herbal medicine (made from herbs) to treat symptoms of nausea whilst a patient is having chemotherapy.

Cultural bias: take cultural context into account when defining something as complementary or alternative, for example to the doctor of Chinese medicine, Chinese medicine may be the convention, and anything else, including Western allopathic medicine, could be considered alternative or complementary.

Integrative health care: a healing-orientated paradigm that may be employed by a wide range of healing professions, including the allied health professions, for example chiropractic, homeopathy, nursing, physiotherapy, occupational therapy and dietetics.

Integrative medicine: used more narrowly than the terms integrative health or integrative health care and refers specifically to the education and practice of medical doctors within this paradigm.

Traditional medicine: "sum total of the knowledge, skills and practices *based on the theories, beliefs and experiences indigenous to different cultures*, whether explicable or not, used in the maintenance of health, as well as in the prevention, diagnosis, improvement or treatment of physical and mental illnesses" (WHO, 2000). Traditional medicine includes "health practices, approaches, knowledge, and beliefs incorporating plant-, animal- and mineral-based medicines, spiritual therapies, manual techniques and exercises, applied singularly or in combination, to treat, diagnose and prevent illnesses or maintain well-being, that rely on practical experience and observation handed down from generation to generation, whether verbally or in writing" (WHO, 1998).

CAM: Complementary and alternative medicine

TM: Traditional medicine

TAM: Traditional African medicine

TCAM: Traditional, complementary and alternative medicine

Integrative medicine in context

Across the globe there is evidence of a growing demand for complementary and alternative medical approaches. Deteriorating patient-provider relationships, the escalating costs of allopathic medicine, overutilisation of pharmaceuticals and technology, and the pandemic of chronic disease for which medicine has yet to find adequate solutions, are all contributing factors in this trend. Greater awareness of the risks and side-effects associated with medical interventions and pharmaceutical drugs is also causing patients to seek out approaches which they consider safer, less invasive, more natural and more cost-effective. Most importantly, research shows that "people find complementary approaches to be more aligned with their own values, beliefs, and philosophical orientations toward health and life" (Rakel and Weil, 2007).

In Africa, as in many other countries, traditional health practitioners have sustained the health of millions of people for many centuries, and patients continue to seek out their services despite the reservations of the scientific community. In South Africa it is estimated that 72% of the Black African population use traditional medicine, accounting for about 26.6 million people from a diverse range of age groups, education levels, religions and occupations (Mander *et al.*, 2007). WHO statistics confirm similar figures in other African and Asian countries, with approximately 80% of people depending on traditional medicine for primary care (90% in Ethiopia, 80% in Benin, 70% in India and Rwanda, 60% in Uganda and Tanzania) (WHO, 2002).

In China, traditional medicine accounts for 40% of health care delivery (WHO, 2002) and in Malaysia, an estimated US$500 million is spent annually on traditional, complementary and alternative medicine, compared to $300 million on allopathic medicine (WHO, 2002). Statistics show that South African consumers spent approximately R3 billion on traditional medicines and R4 billion on complementary and alternative medicines in 2006 alone (Visagie and Sapa, 2009).

Accessibility and affordability contribute significantly to this trend in developing countries. In South Africa there are an estimated 190 000 traditional health practitioners compared to approximately 34 000 medical doctors (Gqaleni, Moodley *et al.*, 2007). In Tanzania, Uganda and Zambia, the ratio of 1:200 - 1:400 traditional medicine practitioners to patients contrasts starkly with the ratio of 1:20 000 for allopathic practitioners. In addition, the distribution of allopathic services is often concentrated in urban areas, making it even less accessible (WHO, 2002). For many people in rural areas traditional medicine is often the only source of health care, or the only affordable source of health care.

Herbal medicines are usually cheaper than pharmaceutical drugs and may also be payable in kind and/or according to the wealth of the client (WHO, 2002).

In developed countries, higher income and higher education are guiding factors for patients who prefer complementary and alternative medicine. At the same time, for ethnic minorities who are often socially and economically disadvantaged in these societies, traditional medicine is often a primary health care choice rather than a complementary one (Bodeker *et al.*, 2010).

The need to recognise the role of traditional healers and traditional medicines in patient care has been acknowledged in both national and international policy. The WHO defined and recently reviewed a comprehensive "WHO Traditional Medicines Strategy" as part of the "Decade of Traditional African Medicine 2001-2010" (WHO Factsheet no. 134). This strategy includes a comprehensive set of aims for the health care sector:

> WHO and its Member States co-operate to promote the use of traditional medicine for health care. The collaboration aims to:
> - Support and integrate traditional medicine into national health systems in combination with national policy and regulation for products, practices and providers to ensure safety and quality.
> - Ensure the use of safe, effective and quality products and practices, based on available evidence.
> - Acknowledge traditional medicine as part of primary health care, to increase access to care and preserve knowledge and resources.
> - Ensure patient safety by upgrading the skills and knowledge of traditional medicine providers.

Other notable reasons for the continued existence and escalating interest in traditional, complementary and alternative medicine include the fact that traditional medical practitioners are usually well-known and highly respected in their communities, and that traditional, complementary and alternative medicine is embedded in the wider belief systems and values of the populations they serve, thereby forming an integral and important part of many people's lives (WHO, 2002). Similarly, allopathic medicine is embedded in the wider belief systems and values of the populations it serves, including the public health care sector and mainstream medical educators and insurers.

The concept of integrative medicine is in part a response to all these factors. Emerging primarily in a modern, Western context, it is an acknowledgement of the importance of incorporating science with the wisdom of ancient systems to provide a medicine that is truly aligned with the values and philosophies of the people and cultures it represents.

Theory and philosophy of integrative medicine

The definition of health

If health is the absence of something, then *what is present* when illness and disease are absent? If your answer to this question is *health*, can you explain what health is? The WHO defines health as "a state of complete physical, mental and social wellbeing and not merely the absence of disease or infirmity". This definition evolved as a response to the long-held biomedical stance that health was the absence of disease. It reflects the growing awareness of the importance of not only biological but also psychosocial factors in determining the health of an individual or community.

Biomedicine has focused on the patient as a passive recipient of medical intervention that largely views the body as a machine. Behavioural medicine has linked health to specific behaviours, for example healthy eating, and seeks to educate people about these and other lifestyle choices. Psychology has emphasised psychological wellbeing. Sociology has challenged us to recognise the impact of physical and psychological environments on health and disease. The bio-psychosocial approach and patient-centred, interdisciplinary, community-orientated health care that is strongly advocated by family medicine have emerged out of this context.

Whilst this evolutionary process reflects an expanded understanding of health, it is still based primarily on the fundamental premise that health is "the absence of disease". People are considered healthy if they are able to avoid disease on multiple levels (physical, emotional, mental and social), and the success of a medical intervention is determined by its capacity to diagnose, treat, prevent, reverse or eliminate the signs and symptoms of disease. This attitude determines the focus of treatment and the necessary stance of research, which is mostly disease-focused in its orientation. Even preventive medicine is exactly that – a bid to prevent disease. Integrative medicine acknowledges the validity of this paradigm *and* emphasises the wellness paradigm.

Q What does a state of complete physical, mental and social wellbeing look like?

How do we know that someone has achieved this state?

What does "complete" mean in the context of health?

How do we recognise someone who is healthy? Do we base it on physical appearance and if so, does physical appearance necessarily indicate good health?

Can someone who has a physical disease or disability be considered healthy?

Can someone who has a healthy body, but is capable of committing ruthless murder be considered healthier than someone with a terminal disease but sound mind and spirit?

Are you healthy? Do you consider yourself to be in "a state of complete physical, mental and social wellbeing?" Consider the reasons for your answer to this question.

The wellness paradigm

John Travis and Don Ardell described the wellness paradigm almost 20 years ago. They defined health as a continuum of illness and wellness, rather than something we either have or don't have (Figure 14.1). On one end of the continuum people might experience high-level wellness, that is "giving good care to your physical self, using your mind constructively, expressing your emotions effectively, being creatively involved with those around you, and being concerned about your physical, psychological and spiritual environments" (Benedict, 2005). On the other end of the continuum people might die a premature death as part of a progressive devolution that went from signs to symptoms to disease to disability. Somewhere in the middle of the spectrum a neutral point of no discernible illness or wellness prevails, and vague signs and symptoms that cannot be labelled as disease are commonplace at this point, for example headache, backache, indigestion and insomnia.

Figure 14.1 The wellness paradigm

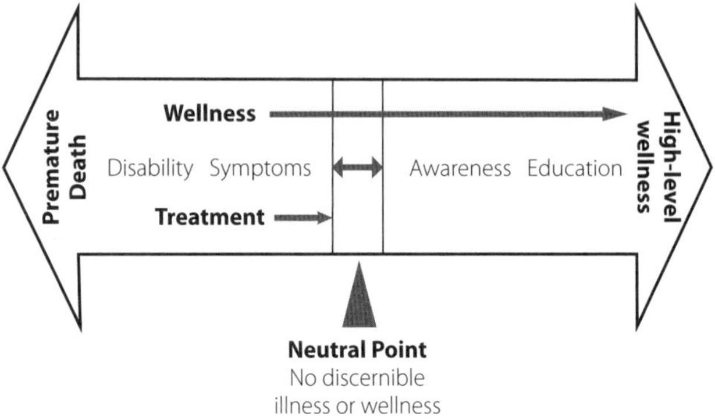

SOURCE: Travis, JW and Ryan, RS 2004.

Travis and Ryan's perspective was that the biomedical treatment paradigm seeks mainly to return people to the neutral point while the wellness paradigm seeks to support them in growing beyond this point even while treating them. Growth is defined as an increase in self-awareness, knowledge and consciousness, that allows for an expanded experience of life. This may sometimes be through and with illness rather than despite it. Most importantly, the model acknowledges that a state of wellness does not have to imply that you are disease-free, strong, successful or young. On the contrary, someone who is well might simultaneously be physically disabled, aged, in pain, and imperfect. The difference lies in the direction the person is headed on the continuum. Are they growing in their awareness, knowledge and consciousness of self? Or are they shrinking, constricting, withdrawing and limiting themselves? Someone with a progressively debilitating and perhaps terminal illness may be optimally well in their capacity to continue to grow and learn from the experience. True health (wholeness) might therefore be defined as the entire spectrum of human experience on the continuum, including *both* the experience of illness *and* the movement towards optimal wellness.

Ardell defines health as a continual striving to live a life that is full, meaningful, zestful and exuberant (2009). "The eventual goal of well-ness is the actualisation of one's true psychophysical/spiritual potential. Wellness is Maslow's notion of self-actualisation carried to its natural extension as growth towards the full integration of mind, body, spirit and environment. This end point is not really an end. It is not perfection.

Better than a continuum in this case is a spiral model, continually cycling through the ebb and flow of life towards higher levels of wellness" (Arloski, 2009).

Healing-orientated medicine

Travis and Ryan's continuum allows for a distinction to be drawn between healing and curing. The treatment paradigm is typically concerned with curing, that is a focus on the alleviation or elimination of symptoms and disease (**disease-orientated medicine**). The wellness paradigm emphasises healing, that is the physical, emotional, mental and spiritual wholeness or wellness, of human beings (**healing-orientated medicine**). Whilst someone may be cured and healed, it is also true that they might be cured of a disease but not healed of it, or healed of a disease and not cured of it.

Allopathic medicine typically intervenes on the left side of the continuum with an emphasis on treatment and cure. It is primarily disease-orientated and focuses on alleviating or eliminating symptoms. Traditional, complementary and alternative medicine is primarily healing-orientated and seeks to intervene along the right side of this continuum. It focuses on engaging the innate healing ability of patients and encouraging them to be more active and aware participants in the maintenance of their own health. Integrative medicine brings the two paradigms together, recognising that treating the disease process effectively is as important as promoting wellness. Most importantly, the two can occur simultaneously.

The classification of traditional, complementary and alternative medicine

The National Centre for Complementary and Alternative Medicine (NCCAM) (http://nccam.nih.gov/health/whatiscam/) groups complementary and alternative medicine into four domains, recognising that there is some overlap between them.

Mind-body medicine

Mind-body medicine uses a variety of techniques designed to enhance the mind's capacity to affect bodily function and symptoms. Some techniques that were considered as complementary and alternative in the past have become mainstream (for example, patient support groups, cognitive-behavioural therapy, mindfulness-based stress reduction). Other mind-body techniques are still considered complementary and alternative, including meditation, visual imagery, hypnosis, relaxation methods, biofeedback and therapies that use creative outlets such as art, music, or dance. A large body of research on psycho-neuro-immunology is beginning to substantiate theories of a mind-body connection.

Biologically-based and botanical therapies

Biologically-based and botanical practices in complementary and alternative medicine use substances found in nature, such as herbs, foods, and vitamins. Some examples of biologically-based therapies include diet and nutritional supplements. Herbal medicine falls into this category, as well as other, as yet scientifically unproven, therapies, for example, the use of shark cartilage in the treatment of cancer. Many medications that are accepted as mainstream allopathic treatments were initially derived from botanical sources, for example digoxin from the foxglove (*Digitalis ianata*) or aspirin from the willow tree.

Manual and body-based therapies

Manual and body-based practices in complementary and alternative medicine are based on manipulation (the application of controlled force to a joint) and other forms of bodywork such as therapeutic massage. Manipulation may be performed as a primary component of treatment (for example chiropractic), or as part of other therapies (for example osteopathy), or whole medical systems (for example naturopathy or Ayurvedic medicine). Therapeutic massage, reflexology and aroma-therapy are typically classified in this category.

Energy medicine

The NCCAM describes two types of energy therapies:
- Bio-field therapies are intended to affect the energy fields that are believed to surround and penetrate the human body. These energy fields purportedly maintain physiological as well as psycho-spiritual balance of human beings, and whilst their existence is still a scientific controversy, there are many practitioners and patients who report significant benefit from the use of these therapies. Some forms of energy therapy manipulate bio-fields by applying pressure and/or manipulating the body. In other forms, practitioners seek to restore balance by transmitting or holding the energy through their

hands, either from a distance or by placing their hands on or near the person. Examples of bio-field therapies include acupuncture, reiki, jin shin jyitsu, cranio-sacral therapy and therapeutic touch.

- Bio-electromagnetic-based therapies involve the unconventional use of electromagnetic fields, such as pulsed fields, magnetic fields, or alternating-current or direct-current fields to influence the human energy field via a wide spectrum of therapeutic devices.

In addition, the following therapies may be considered a part of this last category:

- Vibrational medicine which influences the human energy fields, for example homeopathy, flower essences, light therapy, colour therapy, sound therapy, meridian therapy, radionics and crystal therapy
- Non-linear concepts consistent with distant healing, the healing impact of prayer and the role of intention in healing.

NCCAM refers to whole medical systems which typically incorporates all four of the categories. Whole medical systems are built upon theory and practices that have a complex, comprehensive and holistic understanding and approach to health. Usually, these systems have evolved separate from and long before the advent of conventional medicine, and include all aspects of a person's life. Examples of whole medical systems that have developed in Western culture include homeopathy and naturopathy. Examples of whole medical systems that have developed in non-Western cultures include traditional Chinese medicine, traditional African medicine and Ayurvedic medicine (India) amongst others.

The wisdom of other systems

As we have seen, there are many different systems and therapies that fall under the banner of complementary, alternative and traditional medicine. Each of these systems offers a different perspective and understanding of illness/disease and has a specific set of methodologies, treatments and interventions for promoting health and wellness. Interesting themes that emerge from a study of these systems include:

First do no harm

Most traditional, complementary and alternative approaches use methods and medicinal preparations with minimal risk of side-effects.

The intention is to apply the least possible force or intervention necessary to restore health. Whenever possible, the suppression of symptoms is avoided since this is considered to interfere with the healing process.

Holism

Holism refers to treating the whole person and emphasises a systems approach to health and disease. Systems theory asserts that seemingly separate units join together to create and transcend the individual functions of each unit (for example individual organs) in such a way that a totally new and original entity becomes apparent (a living, breathing human being). The abundance of emergent research in psycho-neuro-immune-endocrinology confirms a view of the human body as a network of interconnected systems, rather than individual systems functioning autonomously and without effect on each other.

The healing power of nature

The belief in the healing power of nature was a basic tenet of the Hippocratic school of medicine. Rejected by allopathic medicine at the turn of the twentieth century, this vitalist approach was adopted by naturopathic physicians as their core academic and clinical principle. Almost all systems of traditional, complementary and alternative medicine acknowledge the presence of an animating *vital force* (vital principle, life force, God, spirit, pepo, energy, chi, qi, and so on) that is responsible for healing. Disturbances in this vital force are considered to play a major role in the development of disease.

The life force is considered to be self-determining, linked to nature, and an aspect of a greater spiritual presence or natural, creative force. Matter, mind, energy and spirit are all considered part of nature and the premise is that good medicine should observe, respect and work within the laws of nature. In ancient healing systems and traditions, the particular emphasis of vitalist principles in a healing context is directly or indirectly aligned with the spiritual beliefs of the culture where the healing tradition originated.

Understanding causality

Allopathic biomedicine tends towards a mechanistic, reductionist perspective that attempts to understand the underlying cause of disease by way of a linear path in which there is a single, underlying initiating cause for any pathology. Identifying and treating "the cause" is a primary therapeutic goal of this pathology-based disease-care approach. The additional assumption is that each disease or illness has the same, or very similar, underlying cause in every individual who exhibits the disease. This results in standardised approaches for treating people with the same disease as a collective group, rather than as unique, complex individuals displaying similar pathology.

Traditional, complementary and alternative medical philosophy takes a broader, wider stance, which asserts that multiple causative factors (genetic, environmental, nutritional, physiological, psychological, spiritual etc.) may come together in a particular individual in a particular way at a particular time to precipitate a particular disease process. This allows for recognition of biochemical individuality and individualised application of therapeutic interventions (including biomedical ones). The causative combination will be unique to each individual even though the ultimate manifestation might be a similar disease process. Treatment will be therefore be individualised in a way that acknowledges the whole person, their vital force and the innate intelligence of the human body.

Intentionality

Many traditional, complementary and alternative medical philosophies do not consider illness or disease to be a negative phenomenon. Instead, the body is believed to have an innate intelligence and the ability to heal itself. This is closely linked to the concept of a vital force or principle that is an aspect of larger natural forces. In this context, health is a state of dynamic balance between internal and external, individual and collective, constructive and destructive forces that impact on the vital energy. Rather than being caused by a morbific agent, such as virus or bacteria, symptoms of disease are the result of the body's intrinsic response or reaction to that morbific agent as it attempts to defend or heal itself (Neuberger, 2006). Symptoms and disease are therefore not an enemy to be destroyed, but a constructive phenomenon that is the best choice the body can make to correct an imbalance, given its circumstances. Imbalance and susceptibility can occur at multiple levels, namely physical, emotional, mental, spiritual or environmental. Asking what the purpose of a disease process is becomes as important as identifying and addressing the imbalance.

The *intention* of the innate intelligence is to make the person aware of the imbalance and garner the support of the whole organism in the healing process. The physician's role is to understand and support the body in its efforts rather than take over or attempt to manipulate the functions of the body; this is unless the self-healing process has become so exhausted or overwhelmed that it cannot rally without external intervention. Suppression of symptoms (for example inflammation with anti-inflammatories or fever with antipyretics) or treatment of infection (for example with antibiotics), without comprehending the underlying imbalance or unique susceptibility, may cause greater distress and disease.

The doctrine of signatures

The doctrine of signatures attempts to draw parallels between the appearance, structure and biological behaviour of natural substances, particularly plants, and the symptomatic disease expressions of the human body and psyche. Natural remedies are usually made from leaves, roots, flowers, minerals, and even insects. Each of these is considered to have some basic quality or essence that sets it apart and makes it unique – its own signature.

Herbalists through the ages have closely studied these signatures and linked them to particular human organ systems and pathology. Symbolism, intuition, biological observation and the study of medicinal properties all serve as guides in the doctrine of signatures, and it is believed that God/ nature/a higher order creative force assigned this signature to these life forms in order to emphasise their specific, curative potential and to guide humans in their quest to find medicinal substances and cures (Richardson-Boedler, 1999).

The idea is that classes of nature can share a pattern of function with human beings and, when they do, their congruence creates a resonance that can be harnessed therapeutically. Symptoms reflect a pattern of disorder and treatment requires a plant that exhibits that same pattern. Introducing the plant into the diseased person allows for reorganisation to occur and results in healing. The congruence between nature and person can be with a physiological ailment or even a mental and emotional one, for example the aspen tree has leaves that tremble or quake in the wind - its flower essence is frequently used to calm the anxious mind (Ballentine, 1999).

This philosophy still forms the foundation for most herbal traditions and homeopathic medicine. It can also be seen in more modern associations, for example the discovery that walnuts, shaped like the human brain, contain omega-oils which have an important influence on neurological function. Strawberries, shaped and coloured like the human heart, have powerful antioxidant properties that may protect against free radical damage to the heart.

Biotypes and body maps

The philosophy of a doctrine of signatures is further evident in the numerous approaches that define different biological types in human beings such as the doshas in Ayurveda, miasms and constitutions in homeopathy, four elements in traditional and complementary medicine and nyepas in Tibetan medicine.

Similarly, there are a large number of systems that consider specific parts of the body to be a map or reflection of the general state of health of various organ systems and the whole body. These biomaps include the iris (iridology), the hands and feet (reflexology) and the tongue (traditional and complementary medicine).

A study of biotypes and maps allows practitioners to determine specific constitutional vulnerabilities or tendencies and individualise treatment approaches. This is not dissimilar from the allopathic preoccupation with the human genome as a means of determining predispositions, susceptibilities and therapeutic guidelines or our typing of patients based on their disease categories.

Birth and death are part of life

Acknowledgement and alignment with the natural cycles of life is a core principle of traditional, complementary and alternative medicine. This includes respect for the different ages and stages of development of human beings, as well as consideration of the different ages and stages of the world that we live in. In traditional African medicine this also includes a belief that good health is a function of one's relationship with deceased ancestors, who possess many powers and continue to interact with the living beyond death (Omonzehele, 2008).

Recognising the needs of each age and stage allows for individualised approaches to treatment of patients. Most importantly, the awareness of life as a series of cycles of birth and death (within one lifetime or even many lifetimes) allows practitioners to include the acceptance of death as a natural process in their approach to health. Dying is not unhealthy, but attempting to preserve life at all costs is.

Spirituality as integral to health

"Humans are spiritual beings. They are inevitably, in some sense, orientated towards the transcendent, whether that is defined as the cosmos, God, or something that is simply greater than

> the individual alone. Caring for a patient in an integrative way requires attention to this spiritual realm".
>
> *(Guinn, 2001).*

Traditional, complementary and alternative therapies and systems almost always include an awareness of mind and spirit in their approach or foundational principles. According to Guinn (2001), two important ways that spirituality may typically be integrated into patient care include:

1. A recognition that it can be an active force employed by patient, practitioner or community in the care of patients, for example prayer, the use of mantras, invocation or exorcism of spirits.
2. Recognition that spiritual care of patients is a critical component of healing, even in situations where physical cure is impossible.

An emphasis on lifestyle and function

Integrative medicine incorporates a functional approach to patients. This approach is systems-orientated and based on the understanding that complex and chronic diseases result from long-term disturbances in the normal physiological function of organ systems in the body. Intervening to restore physiological function and prevent these disturbances is paramount to the prevention of illness and restoration of health. In order to do this, practitioners carefully consider how multiple factors influence the physiological function of the individual patient. These factors include:

- Environmental inputs, for example air, water, toxic exposure, pollution
- Lifestyle choices, for example diet, nutrient intake, exercise habits, sleep patterns
- Mind-body elements, including psychological, spiritual and social factors
- Genetic make-up.

Treatment plans are customised for each patient and focus on interventions that will have the most impact on restoring physiological function as a way of promoting, restoring and maintaining health. This may include combinations of drugs, botanical medicines, nutritional supplements, therapeutic diets, detoxification programmes, as well as counselling on lifestyle, exercise and stress-management techniques.

The therapeutic relationship

Rakel and Jonas (2007) define an optimal healing environment (OHE) as one in which "the social, psychological, spiritual, physical, and behavioural components of health care are orientated toward support and stimulation of our innate healing capacities and the achievement of wholeness". The emphasis on patient-centredness, communication skills and the role of the family physician is critical to this type of healing environment. Integrative medicine is also concerned with the presence and awareness of the doctor, as well as the reciprocal influence that doctors and patients have on each other.

Resonant leadership

Researchers in the field of emotional and social intelligence describe resonant leadership as a quality of emotionally intelligent leaders. This quality allows leaders to tune into feelings and situations - their own and others' - in a way that allows for them to be constructive and powerful forces of influence and change. By contrast, a lack of emotional intelligence can create dissonance and collective distress which results in people feeling off-balance and performing poorly (Goleman *et al.*, 1995). Resonant leadership requires skills in the four domains of emotional intelligence, namely self-awareness, self-management, social awareness and relationship-management. Social intelligence is the mechanism whereby we use emotional intelligence to build resonance (Goleman, 2006).

In a health care setting this implies that a resonant leader (for example a doctor) has the capacity to influence the emotional state and health of the people they interact with. Health professionals might have the capacity to influence not only the outcome of an intervention, but also the longer-term health of their patients simply by paying attention to who they are, how they are being, the health behaviours they exhibit, their level of emotional intelligence and their capacity for emotional empathy. Becoming a resonant health professional requires a range of skills. Reflection, therapy, supervision, journaling and mindfulness practice are all tools in cultivating emotional intelligence.

Mindfulness

Whitesman (2008) asserts that the "mindful practitioner, grounded in self-awareness, is effective in attending to the full range of patients' needs as well as retaining sensitivity to their own well-being". Mindfulness is most simply defined as moment-to-moment, non-judgemental aware-ness, or bringing one's complete attention to the present experience on a moment-to-moment basis (Baer, 2008). Cultivating mindfulness as a way of being is validated by clinical trials that show correlation with parts of the brain associated with interception and emotional regulation in particular (Whitesman, 2008). Mindfulness-based stress reduction (MBSR) has yielded promising results in initial trials and mindfulness-based cognitive therapy (MBCT) resulted in significant reduction in relapse rates of patients with three or more episodes of major depres-sion (Whitesman, 2008). Mindfulness practice is an important tool for the integrative practitioner and their patient.

Self-care

In a famous Harvard address, physician Francis Peabody said that "the secret of caring for the medical patient is in caring for the medical patient" (Shanafelt *et al.*, 2003). Candib rephrased this statement as follows: "The secret of the care of the patient is in caring for oneself while caring for the patient". According to Jonas and Crawford (2007), "being fully present with positive intention for another human is perceived by those we are with and enhances the healing effects of the encounter".

There is a large amount of literature on physician distress and very little on physician wellness. Most studies focus on negative aspects of professional practice such as depression, burnout, substance abuse and divorce (Shanafelt *et al.*, 2003). The concept of physician wellness, ways for doctors to cultivate wellness, and the potential influence of a well physician on patients remain opportunities for further research and investigation. Shanafelt *et al.*, (2003) highlight the following key concepts of effective wellness strategies used by physicians:

1. Relationships: Protect time to spend with family and intimate others. Develop a sense of connection with colleagues. Pursue opportuni-ties to reflect on and share with colleagues about the emotional and existential aspects of being a physician.
2. Religious beliefs/spiritual practice: Nurture the spiritual aspects of self.
3. Work attitudes:
   a. Find meaning in work
   b. Actively choose to expand the scope of medical practice by creating opportunities for diverse experiences and fulfilment of interests that add balance to the routine of regular consultations, for example get involved in medical education or community-building activities, and pursue research interests.

    c.   Set clear limits for practice, for example work part-time, manage schedules effectively and discontinue unfulfilling aspects of practice.
4. Self-care practices: Actively cultivate personal interests and self-awareness in addition to professional and family responsibilities. Seek professional help for personal, physical or psychological illness as needed.
5. Life philosophy: Develop a philosophic approach to life that incorporates a positive outlook, identify and act on values, and stress balance between personal and professional life.

Self-care is vital to physician wellbeing and the health of the health care services as a whole. This understanding has implications for academic, administrative and organisational levels of the health care sector.

Reflection

Regulatory boards and patients, as well as the demands of our own intrinsic professionalism, expect us to keep our knowledge and skills current and to practise the best possible medicine. The capacity to assess, manage, monitor and evaluate our thoughts, feelings, choices, actions and the knowledge that influences them is critical to this process, as is the ability to write concise summaries and articulate focused arguments.

Typically, health professionals are encouraged to engage in reflective practice in response to complex clinical problems or cases that are difficult to diagnose and manage: *reflection-in-action* or *reflection-on-action*. In these situations reflection may improve diagnostic accuracy, minimise errors or prevent errors from happening again in the future and provide learning opportunities for other clinicians.

Integrative medicine requires us to take this process one step further and reflect not only on what we are doing and how we are doing it, but also on who we are and how we are being in our interactions with patients. This is with regard to three important elements:
- Our own and our patients humanity
- Our knowledge and the way we convey and apply it
- The relationship we create with our patients and the choices that are available to them and to us within this relationship.

Exploring our inner nature (what motivates us, what challenges us, why we chose this career path, what influences the personal and professional choices we make on a daily basis) and a commitment to taking care of ourselves is a critical component of patient care. As our connection to ourselves grows, our capacity to sit fully with another suffering human being will be enhanced and our appreciation for our work will deepen. (Rakel and Jonas, 2007).

Integrative medicine and the African context

Integrative medicine is still a new field in South Africa, although South Africa is one of the few countries that have made progress towards integrating traditional and complementary medicine into their legislative framework. At the same time, legislation surrounding the practice and implementation of traditional, complementary and alternative medicine is unclear. There is no clear legal framework regarding the rights of medical practitioners registered with the Health Professions Council of South Africa to practice integrative medicine, particularly with regard to the integration of alternative and complementary practices into their clinical practice.

At the same time, complementary and alternative practices have been legalised and the legislative framework for traditional medicine is under development. There is also evidence that medical professionals are seeking further training in complementary and alternative medical systems - the Allied Health Professions Council of South Africa currently has approximately 4 000 registered practitioners, interns and students of which an estimated 15% are also medical doctors (Gqaleni *et al.*, 2007).

The South African Constitution specifically provides for fundamental human rights with respect to freedom of religion, belief and opinion; language and culture; and equality. It also provides for equal access to health care services and this is understood to refer to all health care services.

In essence, this implies that patients have the right to freedom of choice regarding the health care services they utilise, whether these are the services of a medical doctor or a traditional healer. The government in turn has a responsibility to ensure that people have access to these services in a way that ensures their safety and wellbeing, and this necessitates appropriate legislation and regulation of health professionals. (Mokoena, 2009)

The Allied Health Professions Council of South Africa

The Allied Health Professions Council of South Africa is a statutory health body established in terms of the Allied Health Professions Act 63 of 1982 in order to regulate the allied health professions. At this stage,

recognised allied health professions include:
- Ayurveda
- Chinese medicine and acupuncture
- Chiropractic
- Homoeopathy
- Naturopathy
- Osteopathy
- Phytotherapy and herbalism
- Therapeutic aromatherapy
- Therapeutic massage therapy
- Therapeutic reflexology
- Unani-Tibb.

The Traditional Health Practitioners Act 22 of 2007

For many years traditional medicine was illegal in South Africa. The Witchcraft Suppression Act 3 of 1957, and subsequent amendments to this act, prohibited traditional healers from practising their trade. The Traditional Health Practitioners Act 22 of 2007 finally provided for legal recognition and regulation of traditional medicine in South Africa as demanded by constitutional requirements. Under this Act, which expressly states that it is not applicable to persons who are registered as medical practitioners or dentists, five categories of traditional healers are recognised, including:
- Traditional surgeons
- Traditional birth attendants
- Herbalists
- Diviners
- Apprentices of traditional healing.

The Traditional Health Practitioners Council, which was established under the same Act, aims to promote public health awareness; ensure quality of services; promote and maintain appropriate ethical and professional standards; encourage research, education and training; promote contact between the various fields of training within traditional health practice and set standards for such training; compile and maintain a professional code of conduct; and ensure that traditional health practices comply with universally accepted health care norms and values. Similarly, the Department of Health's draft policy on African traditional medicine (July 2008) recommends that a legal framework be established to regulate and register African traditional medicine and medicinal products; protect African traditional medicine knowledge and intellectual property rights; and protect the rights of persons involved in the practice of African traditional medicine. It has also been recommended that a National Institute of African Traditional Medicines of South Africa and a national pharmacopoeia be established. (Mokoena, 2009)

Education in integrative medicine

Across the globe, increased efforts are being made to facilitate the adoption of integrative medicine curriculae in medical education. The Consortium of Academic Health Centres for Integrative Medicine (CACHIM) comprises 44 highly esteemed academic centres in the USA and Canada that are working together to transform health care through rigorous scientific studies, new models of clinical care and innovative educational programmes that include diverse therapeutic systems. The mission of the consortium is to advance the principles and practices of integrative health care within academic institutions (www. imconsortium.org).

The role of traditional medicine, driven by WHO initiatives, is also being more widely recognised in national and international policy, the media and scientific literature. Content on complementary and alternative medicine and integrative health care is being taught in hundreds of educational programmes across the United States, Canada and Europe (Jones *et al.*, 2009).

In South Africa, various academic institutions offer qualifications in the Allied Health Professions as classified by the Allied Health Professions Council of South Africa, for example chiropractic, homeopathy, Chinese medicine and naturopathy, or brief didactic content on integrative health care as part of other qualifications, for example nursing. More recently, the University of Stellenbosch's Division of Family Medicine and Primary Care has established a postgraduate certificate in integrative medicine for doctors. The South African Society of Integrated Medicine (SASIM) was initiated in 2001 and is an association of registered health practitioners who practice or have an interest in, integrative medicine. The society is committed to furthering the cause of integrative medicine in South Africa.

Integrative medicine in family practice

The South African Constitution asserts the right of all South African citizens to have access to health care services that acknowledge the diversity of our society and its needs. This will require conventional, complementary, alternative and traditional health practitioners to operate alongside each other within the parameters of the law. Several legislative challenges will need to be overcome and the myriad of concerns from across the spectrum of patients and providers will need to be addressed in an equitable and satisfactory manner. The family physician sits at the crossroads of these challenges, concerns and opportunities. Integrative medicine offers a way to bridge the divide.

Incorporating an integrative approach in your practice requires a pioneering spirit, a strong commitment to the quality of ongoing learnership advocated by family medicine, and the willingness to examine and challenge your own belief systems. You will need to learn about the principles and philosophies of integrative medicine and seek out collaborative relationships with colleagues across the spectrum of health disciplines, including those classified as allied health professions. You will also need to cultivate an attitude of curiosity and tolerance towards worldviews other than your own.

As health professionals it is important for us to consider how the worldview that we subscribe to, consciously and unconsciously, enables or disables us and therefore influences what we offer to our patients. It may be true that each of the traditional, complementary and alternative systems, theories and philosophies offered here hold part of the truth that is the whole spectrum of healing. Integrative medicine seeks to define and implement this holistic approach to health and healing.

Bibliography

Abas, M & Broadhead, J (1997) 'Depression and Anxiety among Women in an Urban Setting in Zimbabwe.' *Psychological Medicine*, Vol 27, pp. 59–71.

Abramson, JH (1988) 'Community-Oriented Primary Care – Strategy, Approaches, and Practice: A Review.' *Public Health Reviews*, Vol 16, pp. 35–98.

Alles, V, Mäkelä, M, Persson, I & Seuntjies, I (1998) *Tools and Methods for Quality Improvement in General Practice*. Helsinki: National Research and Development Centre for Welfare and Health.

Arlosky, M. 2009. *Wellness coaching for lasting lifestyle change*. Whole Person Associates, Michigan, USA.

Australian Health Ministers Conference 1994.

Barker, E (1998) 'Ethical Issues in HIV Infections.' *South African Family Practice*, Vol 19, pp. 44–7.

Baum MK, Lai S, Sales S, Page JB, Campa A. (2010) 'Randomized, controlled clinical trial of zinc supplementation to prevent immunological failure in HIV-infected adults.' *Clinical Infectious Diseases,* Vol 50, pp. 1653–1660.

Bauman, Z (1993) *Postmodern Ethics*. Cambridge: Blackwell.

Bauman, A, Fardy, H & Harris, P (2003) 'Getting it right:Why bother with patient centred care?' *Medical Journal of Australia*. Vol 179, pp. 253–256.

Beauchamp, TL & Childress, JF (2001) *Principles of Biomedical Ethics*. New York: Oxford University Press.

Becker, MH (1979) 'Psychological Aspects of Health-related Behaviour', in Freeman, H, Levine, S & Reader, LG (eds), *Handbook of Medical Sociology*. Englewood Cliffs, NJ: Prentice Hall.

Beckman, H & Frankel, R (1984) 'The Effect of Physician Behaviour on the Collection of Data.' *Annals of Internal Medicine*, Vol 101, pp. 692–6.

Benedict, S.L. (2005) 'Wellness Coaching: A Life Coach's Collaborative Approach to Integrative Healthcare.' *Journal of Integrative Medicine*, Vol 4, pp. 24–33.

Bird, K, Hulme, D, Moore, K & Shepherd, A (2003) *Chronic Poverty and Remote Rural Areas*. (CPRC Working Paper No 13) Birmingham and Manchester: Chronic Poverty Research Centre. Accessible at http://www.chronicpoverty.org.

Bodeker, G. & Kronenberg, F. (2002) 'A Public Health Agenda for Traditional, Complementary and Alternative Medicine.' *American Journal of Public Health*, Vol 92, pp. 1582–1591.

Bodenheimer T, Wagner EH, Grumbach K. (2002) 'Improving primary care for patients with chronic illness.' *Journal of the American Medical Association,* Vol 288, pp. 1775-1779.

Boyle, D, Dwinnell, B & Platt, F (2005) 'Invite, Listen and Summarize: A Patient-Centered Communication Technique.' *Academic Medicine,* Vol 80, pp. 29–32.

Bradshaw D, Norman R, Schneider M. A clarion call for action based on refined DALY estimates for South Africa. S Afr Med J. 2007 Jun;97(6):438, 440

Bresick, G & Harvey, C (1997) 'Caring for the Carer: Managing the Family of the Stroke Patient.' *South African Medical Journal*, Vol 15, No 3, pp. 305–12.

Bryant, J (1969) *Health and the Developing World.* Ithaca and London: Cornell University Press.

Cabana, MD & Jee, SH (2004) 'Does Continuity of Care Improve Patient Outcomes?' *Journal of Family Practice,* Vol 53, pp. 974–80.

Campbell TL, McDaniel SH, Cole-Kelly K et al. (2002) 'Family Interviewing: A Review of the Literature.' *Primary Care Family Medicine* Vol 34, pp. 312–318.

Cantillon, P & Jones, R (1999) 'Does Continuing Medical Education in General Practice Make a Difference?' *British Medical Journal*, Vol 318, pp. 1276–9.

Chalmers, J. (2002) 'The criminalisation of HIV transmission.' *Sexually Transmitted Infections*, Vol 78, pp. 448–451.

Chou, R, Fu R, Carrino, JA. & Deyo R. (2009) Imaging strategies for low-back pain: systematic review and meta-analysis. *Lancet* Vol 373, pp. 463–471.

Chou, R, Qaseem, A, Snow, V, Casey, D, Cross TJ, Shekelle, P, Owens, DK, for the Clinical Efficacy Assessment Subcommittee of the American College of Physicians American Pain Society Low Back Pain Guidelines Panel. (2007) 'Diagnosis and treatment of low back pain: a joint clinical practice guideline from the American College of Physicians and the American Pain Society' *Annals of Internal Medicine*, Vol 147, pp. 478–491.

Christie, RJ & Hoffmaster, CB (1986) *Ethical Issues in Family Medicine.* New York: Oxford University Press.

Claassen, JN (1998) 'The benefits of CAGE as a Screening Tool for Alcoholism in a Closed Rural South African Community.' *South African Medical Journal*, Vol 89, No 9, pp. 976–9.

Cole-Kelly, K & Seaburn, DB (2005) Chapter 4: 'A Family Orientated Approach to Individual Patients', in McDaniel, SH, Campbell, TL,

Hepworth, J & Lorenze, A, *Family-Oriented Primary Care*. New York: Springer.

Coombs, M (2004) *Power and Conflict between Doctors and Nurses: Breaking Through the Inner Circle in Clinical Care*. London: Routledge, p 12.

Coovadia H, Jewkes R, Barron P, Sanders D, Mcintyre D. (2009) 'The health and health system of South Africa: historical roots of current public health challenges.' *Lancet*. Vol 374, pp. 957–959.

Couper I (2006) Growing our own: The university and the rural health workforce challenge [inaugural address: Chair of Rural Health]. Johannesburg: Witwatersrand University www.wits.ac.za/files/res3833c5ec34124a6eb1d4e0f03fdb2b5b.doc

Couper ID, Hugo JFM, Conradie H, Mfenyana K (2007) 'Influences on the choice of health professionals to practise in rural areas.' *South African Medical Journal*. Vol 97, pp. 1082–1086.

Couper ID. (2007) 'Further reflections on chronic illness care.' *SA Family Practice*. Vol 49, pp. 4–10.

Couper, ID & Hugo, J. (2005) 'Management of District Hospitals – Exploring Success.' *Rural and Remote Health*, Vol 5, p 433. Available online http://rrh.deakin.edu.au

Couper, I.D. & Mash, B. 2008, 'Obtaining consensus on core clinical skills for family medicine training.' *South African Family Practice*, Vol 50, pp. 41.

Crouch, MA & Roberts, L (eds) (1987) *The Family in Medical Practice: A Family Systems Primer*. New York: Springer-Verlag.

Day, C & Gray A. (2008). 'Health and Related Indicators.' In Barron P, Roma-Reardon J (Eds). *South African Health Review 2008*. Durban: Health Systems Trust.

Day, C & Hedber, G C. (2004). 'Health Indicators.' In Ijumba P, Day C, Ntuli A (Eds). *South African Health Review 2003/04* Durban: Health Systems Trust

De Jong, J (1987) *A Descent into African Psychiatry*. Amsterdam: Foris.

Department of Health. (2009) *Guidelines for the Prevention of Malaria in South Africa*. Pretoria: Department of Health.

Deyo, RA. & Weinstein, JN. (2001) Low Back pain. *New England Journal of Medicine*. Vol 344, pp. 263–370.

Doherty, WJ & Baird, MA (1986) 'Developmental Levels of Physician Involvement with Families.' *Family Medicine*, Vol 18, pp. 153–6.

Donnelly WJ. (2005) 'Patient-centered medical care requires a patient-centered medical record.' *Academic Medicine*. Vol 80, pp. 33–38.

Ellis, C (1994) 'Patient-centered care.' *SA Family Practice*, Vol 15, No 11, pp. 648–56.

Elwyn, G, Edwards, A & Kinnersley, P (1999) 'Shared Decision-Making in Primary Care: The Neglected Second Half of the Consultation.' *British Journal of General Practice,* Vol 49, pp. 477–482.

Engel, GL (1980) 'The Clinical Application of the Biopsychosocial Model.' American Journal of Psychiatry, Vol 137, No 5, pp. 535–44.

Epping-Jordan J, Begoa, R, Rania, K & Eduardo, S (2001) 'The Challenge of Chronic Conditions: WHO Responds.' *British Medical Journal*, Vol 323, pp. 947–48.

Epstein RM, Mauksch L, Jaén CR. (2008) 'Have you really addressed your patient's concerns?' *Family Practice Management.* Vol 15, p 35.

Evans, M (1997) 'Critical Appraisal.' *Canadian Family Physician*, Vol 43, p 449.

Fawzi, WW, Msamanga, GI, Spiegelman, D, Wei, R, Kapiga, S, Villamor, E, Mwakagile, D, Mugusi, F,

Hertzmark, E & Essex, M. (2004) 'A randomized trial of multivitamin supplements and HIV disease progression and mortality,' *New England Journal of Medicine*, Vol. 351, , pp. 23–32.

Fehrsen, GS & Henbest, RJ (1993) 'In Search of Excellence. Expanding the Patient-centered Clinical Method: A Three-Stage Assessment.' *Family Practice,* Vol 10, pp. 49–54.

Fowler, HW & Fowler, FG (eds) (1964) *The Concise Dictionary of Current English*. London: Oxford University Press.

Frankel, S (1992) 'Overview', in Frankel, S (ed), *The Community Health Worker: Effective Programmes for Developing Countries*, pp. 1–61. Oxford: Oxford University Press.

Fredlund, VG (2003) 'Total Hip Replacement for Mseleni Joint Disease Undertaken in a Rural Hospital: Five-year Follow-up.' *South African Family Practice*, Vol 45, pp. 10–14.

Gibbons RJ, Chatterjee K, Daley J, *et al.* (1999) 'ACC/AHA/ACP Guidelines for the Management of Patients with Chronic Stable Angina.' *Journal of the American College of Cardiology.* Vol 33, pp. 2092

Gill, JM, Mainous, AG, Diamond, JJ & Lenhard, MJ (2003) 'Impact of Provider Continuity on Quality of Care for Persons with Diabetes Mellitus.' *Ann Fam Med*, Vol 1, pp. 162–70.

Gillon, R (1994) 'Medical Ethics: Four Principles plus Attention to Scope.' *British Medical Journal*, Vol 309, pp. 184–8.

Goleman, D. 2006. *Social intelligence.* Hutchinson, London, p. 84.

Goleman, D., Boyiatzis, R. & McKee, A. 1995. *The New Leaders, Transforming the art of leadership into the science of results.* Time Warner Books, London.

Gqaleni, N. Moodley I, Kruger H, Ntuli A, McLeod H. 2007. Traditional and Complementary Medicine, in S.

Harrison, R. Bhana & A. Ntuli (eds), *South African Health Review 2007*. Durban: Health Systems Trust, Chapter 12, pp. 175–188.

Green, J & Britten, N (1998) 'Qualitative Research and Evidence Based Medicine.' *British Medical Journal*, Vol 316, pp. 1230–1232.

Greenhalgh, P (1996) 'Is my practice evidence based?' *British Medical Journal*, Vol 313, pp. 957–8.

Grimley, EJ (1995) 'Evidence Based and Evidence Biased Medicine.' *Age and Ageing*, Vol 24, pp. 461–3.

Grol, R & Lawrence, M (1995) *Quality Improvement by Peer Review (Oxford General Practice Series*, No 32). Oxford: Oxford University Press.

Grosskurth, H, Mosha, F, *et al* (1995) 'Impact of Improved Treatment of Sexually Transmitted Diseases on HIV Infection in Rural Tanzania: Randomised Controlled Trial', *Lancet*, Vol 346, pp. 530–6.

Guinn D. An integrative ethics: A health care ethics of the everyday. Second Opinion. 2001;7:55–72 http://www.parkridgecenter.org/Page534.html

Guyatt, G, *et al.* (1992) 'Evidence Based Medicine. A New Approach to Teaching the Practice of Medicine.' *Journal of American Medical Association*, Vol 268, pp. 2420–5.

Hammond-Tooke, D (1989) *Rituals and Medicines*. Johannesburg: Donker.

Harley, B (1999) *HIV/AIDS Primary Care: Clinical Guidelines for the Cape Metropolitan Area*. (Second edn). Cape Town: South Peninsula Municipality.

Hartman, E. (1978) 'Using eco-maps and genograms in family therapy.' *Social casework*, Vol 464, pp. 76.

Hausler, H (2000) Tuberculosis and HIV/AIDS, Clinical Guidelines, October 2000, National Dept of Health. Accessible at http://www.doh.gov.za/aids/docs/tuberculosis.html

Haynes, RB, Montague, P, Oliver, T, McKibbon, KA, Brouwers, MC & Kanani, R (1999) 'Interventions to Help Patients to Follow Prescriptions for Medications.' *The Cochrane Library*, Issue 2 (2000). Oxford: Update Software.

Health Professions Council of South Africa (1999) *New Curriculum for Medicine and Dentistry*. Pretoria: Health Professions Council.

Health Professions Council of South Africa (HPCSA) (2003) Minutes of Medical and Dental Professions Board Meeting, September 2003. Pretoria: Health Professions Council of South Africa

Health Systems Trust (1997) *Rational Drug Prescribing Training Course*. Durban: Health Systems Trust.

Health Systems Trust (1997) *South African Health Review.* Durban: Health Systems Trust.

Helman CG. *Culture, health and illness.* Oxford University Press, New York: 2001

Helman, RJ (1981) 'An Approach to Prescribing in Family Practice.' *South African Family Practice*, January, pp. 8–12.

Henbest RJ., Fehrsen S. (1992) 'Patient-centredness: is it applicable outside the West? Its measurement and effect on outcomes.' Family Practice. Vol 9, pp. 311.

Institute for Alternative Futures (IAF). Patient-Centered Care 2015 Scenarios. The Picker Institute, report 2004. http://www.altfutures.com/pubs/Picker%20Final%20Report%20May%2014%202004.pdf

Institute of Medicine (2005) *Quality Through Collaboration: The Future of Rural Health.* Committee on the Future of Rural Health Care, Board on Health Care Services. Washington DC: The National Academies Press.

International Fund for Agricultural Development (IFAD) (2001) *Rural Poverty Report 2001: The Challenge of Ending Rural Poverty.* Oxford: Oxford University Press. Accessible at http://www.ifad.org/poverty/index.htm

International Headache Society Classification Subcommittee. (2004) The International Classification of Headache Disorders. 2nd edition. Cephalalgia Vol 24 (Suppl 1), pp. 1–160.

Jackson R, Ameratunga S, Broad J, Connor J et al (2006). 'The GATE frame: Critical Appraisal with pictures.' *ACP Journal Club* Vol 144, pp. A8-11

Jacobson, L, Edwards, AG, *et al.* (1997) 'Evidence Based Medicine and General Practice.' *British Journal of General Practice*, Vol 47, pp. 449-52.

Jacques, P, Reid, S, Chabikulu, O & Fehrsen, S (1998) *Developing Appropriate Skills for Rural Doctors – Phase 1: Procedural Skills of Rural Doctors in South Africa.* Durban: Health Systems Trust.

Jones, D, Templet, A, Sierpina, V & Kreitzer, M.J (2009) 'Functional Medicine: Theory, Education, and Practice.' *Explore*, Vol 5, pp. 177-179.

Jongbloed, L (1994) 'Adaptation to a Stroke: The Experience of One Couple.' *American Journal of Occupational Therapy*, Vol 11, pp. 1006-13.

Joyner K, & Mash B. (2010) Chapter 5: How to provide comprehensive, appropriate care for survivors of intimate partner violence in Joyner K (Ed) Aspects of Forensic Medicine – An Introduction for Healthcare Professionals. Cape Town: Juta.

Kale, R (1995) 'Traditional Healers in South Africa: A Parallel Health Care System.' *British Medical Journal*, Vol 310, pp. 1182–5.

Kantor, JE (1989) *Medical Ethics for Physicians-in-Training*. New York and London: Plenum Medical Book Company.

Kark, S & Kark, E (1999) *Promoting Community Health: From Pholeta to Jerusalem*. Johannesburg: Witwatersrand University Press.

Kark, SL (1942) 'A Health Service among Rural Bantu.' *South African Medical Journal*, Vol 16, pp. 197–8.

Kark, SL & Cassell, JC (1952) 'The Pholela Health Centre.' *South African Medical Journal*, Vol 26, pp. 101–4, 132–6.

Kerse, N, Buetow, S, Mainous, AG, Young, G, Coster, G & Arroll, B (2004) 'The Doctor-Patient Relationship and Compliance with Medication: A Primary Care Investigation.' *Ann Fam Med*, Vol 2, pp. 455–61.

Kibel, MA & Wagstaff, LA (1991) *Child Health for All: A Manual for Southern Africa*. Cape Town: Oxford University Press.

Kim, J & Watts, C (2005) 'Gaining a Foothold: Tackling Poverty, Gender Inequality, and HIV in Africa.' *British Medical Journal*, Vol 331, pp. 769–72.

Kinkade S. Evaluation and treatment of low back pain. Am Fam Physician 2007; 75:1181–8, 1190–2.

Kinmonth, A (1995) 'Understanding Meaning in Research and Practice.' *Family Practice*, Vol 12, pp. 1–2.

Kontoyannis A, Conway K. Surgery. Edinburgh: Mosby-Elsevier, 2008.

Kringos, DS, Boerma, WG, Hutchinson, A, van der Zee, J & Groenewegen, PP. (2010) 'The breadth of primary care: a systematic literature review of its core dimensions.' *BMC health services research*, Vol. 10, pp. 65.

Kroene, K & Mandelsdorff, A (1989). 'Common Symptoms in Ambulatory Care: Incidence, Evaluation, Therapy, and Outcome.' *American Journal of Medicine*, Vol 86, No 3, pp. 262–6.

Kurtz, S, Silverman, J, Benson, J & Draper, J (2003) 'Marrying Content and Process in Clinical Method Teaching: Enhancing the Calgary–Cambridge Guides.' *Academic Medicine*, Vol 78, pp. 802–809.

Lang, F, Marvel K, Sanders D, et al. (2002) 'Interviewing when family members are present.' *American Family Physician*, Vol 65, pp. 1351–1354

Larson, EH & Hart, LG (2001) 'The Rural Physician', in Geyman, JP, Norris, TE & Hart, LG (eds), *Textbook of Rural Medicine*. New York: McGraw-Hill, pp. 27–40.

Larson, J, Risor, O & Putnam, S (1997) 'P-R-A-C-T-C-A-L: A Step-by-Step Model for Conducting the Consultation in General Practice.' *Family Practice*, Vol 14, pp. 295–301.

Lehmann U, Dieleman M, Martineau T (2008) Staffing remote rural areas in middle- and low-income countries: A literature review of attraction and retention. *BMC Health ServicesResearch* Vol 8, pp. 1–10.

Levenstein, S (1994) 'Patient-Centered Care – Do we Really Believe in it?' *South African Family Practice*, Vol 15, pp. 301–306.

Levenstein, SL (1988) 'Compliance – What's it all about?' *South African Family Practice*, pp. 305–311.

Lewin, SA, Skea, ZC, Entwistle, V, Zwatenstein, M & Dick, J (2001) 'Interventions for providers to promote a patient-centered approach in clinical consultations.' *The Cochrane Database of Systematic Reviews* 2001, Issue 4, Art No: CD003267. DOI:10.1002/14651858. CD003267.

Little, P, Everitt, H, Williamson, I, Warner, G, Moore, M, Gould, C, Ferrier, K, & Payne, S (2001) 'Preferences of patients for patient centred approach to consultation in primary care: observational study.' *British Medcical Journal*, Vol. 322, pp. 468.

Longo, DR & Daugird, AJ (1994) 'The Quality of Ambulatory-Based Primary Care: A Framework and Recommendations.' *International Journal for Quality in Health Care*, Vol 6, pp. 133–146.

Lundahl B, Burke B. (2009) 'The Effectiveness and Applicability of Motivational Interviewing: A Practice-Friendly Review of Four Meta-Analyses.' *Journal of Clinical Psychology*, Vol 65, pp. 1232–1245

Macauley, D (1994) 'READER: An Acronym to Aid Critical Reading by General Practitioners.' *British Journal of General Practice*, Vol 44, pp. 83–5.

MacNaughton, J (1995) 'Anecdotes and Empiricism.' *British Journal of General Practice*, Vol 45, pp. 571–572.

Maguire, P & Pitceathly, C (2002) 'Clinical Review: Key Communication Skills and How to Acquire Them.' *British Medical Journal*, Vol 325, September, pp. 697–700.

Mander, M., Ntuli, L., Diederichs, N. & Mavundla, K. 2007. Economics of the Traditional Medicine Trade in South Africa, in S. Harrison, R. Bhana & A. Ntuli (eds), South African Health Review 2007. Durban: Health Systems Trust, Chapter 13, pp. 189–200.

Mash R, Mash B, & de Villiers, P. (2010)''Why don't you just use a condom?': Understanding the motivational tensions in the minds of South African women.' *African Journal of Primary Health Care & Family Medicine*,Vol 2, Art. #79, 4 pages. DOI: 10.4102/phcfm.v2i1.79

Mash, B & Allen, S (2004) 'Managing Chronic Conditions in a South African Primary Care Context: Exploring the Applicability of Brief Motivational Interviewing', *South African Family Practice*, Vol 46, pp. 21–6.

Mash, B & Levitt, NS (1999) 'Quality Improvement in the Care of People with Diabetes in Khayelitsha, Cape Town.' *South African Family Practice*, Vol 20, pp. 123–5.

Mash, B & Mahomed, H (2000) 'Participatory Development of a Minimum Dataset for the Khayelitsha District.' *South African Medical Journal*, Vol 90, pp. 1024–30.

Mash, B, Couper, I & Hugo, J (2006) 'Building consensus on clinical procedural skills for South African family medicine training using the Delphi technique.' *South African Family Practice,* Vol 48, pp. 14.

Mash, B, Downing, R, Moosa, S & De Maeseneer, J (2008) 'Exploring the key principles of family medicine in sub-Saharan Africa: International Delphi consensus process.' *South African Family Practice,* Vol 50, pp 60.

Mash, RB & Reid, S (2010) 'Statement of consensus on Family Medicine in Africa.' *African Journal of Primary Health Care & Family Medicine,* Vol 2, pp. 4.

Matthes, C (2005) Chapter 9: 'Reducing Sexual Risk Behaviours: Theory and Research, Successes and Challenges', in Abdool Karim SS & Abdool Karim Q (eds), *HIV/AIDS in South Africa*. Cape Town: Cambridge University Press.

May PA, Marais A-S. Gossage JP, Viljoen DL. (2005) 'Epidemiological analysis of a third wave of data about children with fetal alcohol spectrum disorders and controls in the Western Cape Province, South Africa.' *Alcohol Clinical Experience and Research.* Vol 29, p 43A.

Mayosi B, Flisher AJ, Lalloo UG, Sitas, F, Tollman, SM, Bradshaw D. (2009) 'The burden of non-communicable diseases in South Africa.' *Lancet.* Vol 374, pp. 934–947.

McCaffery, K, Forrest, S, Waller, J, Desai, M, Szarewski, A & Wardle (2003) 'Attitudes Towards HPV Testing: A Qualitative Study of Beliefs Among Indian, Pakistani, African and White British Women in the UK.' *British Journal of Cancer*, Vol 88, pp. 42–46.

McDaniel, SH, Campbell, TL, Hepworth, J & Lorenze, A (2002) *Family-Oriented Primary Care*. New York: Springer.

McIntyre, J & Gray, G (2000) 'Preventing Mother-to-Child Transmission of HIV: African Solutions for an African Crisis.' *Southern African Journal of HIV Medicine*, Vol 1, pp. 30–1.

McKeown, T (1979) *The Role of Medicine* (second edn). Oxford: Oxford University Press.

McPherson, A (2005) 'Adolescents in Primary Care.' *British Medical Journal*, Vol 330, pp. 465–467.

McWhinney, I (1972) 'Beyond Diagnosis: An Approach to the Integration of Behavioural Science and Clinical Medicine'. *The New England Journal of Medicine*, Vol 287, pp. 384–387.

McWhinney, I (1981) *An Introduction to Family Medicine*. New York: Oxford University Press.

McWhinney, I (1997) *A Textbook of Family Medicine* (second edn). New York: Oxford University Press.

McWhinney, I.R. 1997, *A textbook of family medicine*, Oxford University Press, USA.

McWhinney, IR (1989) *A Textbook of Family Medicine*. New York: Oxford University Press.

McWilliam, CL (1993) 'Health Promotion: Strategies for Family Physicians'. *Canadian Family Physician*, Vol 39, pp. 1079–85.

Mkhize, N (2004) 'Psychology: An African Perspective', in Hook, D (ed) *Critical Psychology*. Cape Town: UCT Press, pp. 24–52.

Mokoena, JD (2009) 'Integrative healthcare and legislation', in van Wyk, N.C. (ed), *Integrative healthcare: A guide to meet the needs of Africa*, Juta and Co. Ltd., pp. 64–71.

Morgan, S, Bassett, K, Wright, J, Evans, R, Barer, M, Caetano, P & Black, C (2005) '"Breakthrough" Drugs and Growth in Expenditure on Prescription Drugs in Canada'. *British Medical Journal*, Vol 331, pp. 815–6.

Morrell, D (ed) (1988) *Epidemiology in General Practice*. Oxford: Oxford University Press.

Morris, M & Kretzschmar, M (1997) 'Concurrent partnerships and the spread of HIV'. *AIDS*, Vol 11, pp. 641.

Muir Gray, JA (2000) *Evidence Based Healthcare. How to Make Health Policy and Management Decisions*. New York: Churchill Livingstone.

Mushlin, A, Kouides, R, Shapiro, D (1998) 'Estimating the Accuracy of Screening Mammography: A Meta-Analysis'. *American Journal of Preventive Medicine*, Vol 14, Issue 2, pp. 143–153.

Muula AS (2007) How do we define 'rurality' in the teaching on medical demography? Rural and Remote Health, Vol 7, pp. 653 (online). Available from: http://www.rrh.org.au

Naidoo, S (1997) 'Local Government in the Move to a District Health System', in Barron, P (ed), *South African Health Review*, pp. 53–58. Durban: Health Systems Trust.

Neighbour, R (1987) *The Inner Consultation: How to Develop an Effective and Intuitive Consulting Style*. Lancaster: MTP.

Norris, TE & Rosenblatt, RA (2003) *Training Rural Physicians – The 'Pipeline' Concept of Sequential Rural Training Experiences.*

Presentation at 6th Wonca World Rural Health Conference, Santiago de Compostela, Spain, September 2003.

Nutting, PA (1987) *Community-Oriented Primary Care: From Principles to Practice*. (HRS-A-PE 86-1). Washington DC: US Department of Health and Human Sciences.

Omonzehele, P F (2008) 'African Concepts of Health, Disease and Treatment.' *Explore*, Vol 4, pp. 120-126.

Pizzorno, J E Jr. & Snider, P (2006) 'Naturopathic Medicine', in M.S. Micozzi (ed), *Fundamentals of complementary and integrative medicine*. 3rd Edition, Saunders Elsevier, Missouri, pp. 221-255.

Pritchard, P & Pritchard, J (1994) *Developing Teamwork in Primary Health Care: A Practical Workbook*. New York: Oxford University Press.

Rakel, D. & Jonas, W. 2007. 'Creating Optimal Healing Environments', in Rakel, D. (ed), *Integrative medicine,* 2nd Edition, Saunders Elsevier, Philadelphia, pp. 15-21.

Rakel, D. & Weil, A. 2007. 'Philosophy of Integrative Medicine', in Rakel, D. (ed), *Integrative medicine*, 2nd Edition, Saunders Elsevier, Philadelphia, pp. 3-13.

Reid S, Wessely S (2002) "Frequent attenders with medically unexplained symptoms: service use and costs in secondary care.' *The British Journal of Psychiatry*, Vol 180, pp. 248-253.

Reid S, Mash R, Downing R, & Moosa S (2011) 'Perspectives on key principles of generalist medical practice in public service in Sub-Saharan Africa: a qualitative study.' *BMC Family Practice*, Vol 12, pp. 67, doi:10.1186/1471-2296-12-67

Reid, S (2004) *Monitoring the Effect of the New Rural Allowance for Health Professionals*. Durban: Health Systems Trust. Accessible at http://www.hst.org.za/

Rhyne, R, Bogue, R, Kukula, G & Fulmer, H (eds) (1998) *Community-Oriented Primary Care: Health Care for the 21st Century*. Washington DC: American Public Health Association.

Robertson, DW (1996) 'Ethical Theory, Ethnography and Differences between Doctors and Nurses in Approaches to Patient Care.' *Journal of Medical Ethics*, Vol 22, pp. 292-9.

Rogers, CR (1967) *On Becoming a Person: A Therapist's View of Psychotherapy*. London: Constable.

Rolland, JS & Walsh, F. (2005) 'Systemic Training for Healthcare Professionals: The Chicago Center for Family Health Approach.' *Family Process*, Vol 44, pp. 283-301.

Rollnick S, Butler C, Kinnersley P, Gregory J, Mash B. (2010) 'Motivational interviewing.' *British Medical Journal*, Vol 340, p c1900

Rollnick, SR, Mason, P & Butler, C (1999) *Health Behaviour Change: A Guide for Practitioners*. Edinburgh: Churchill Livingstone.

Rosenberg, W & Donald, A (1995) 'Evidence Based Medicine: An Approach to Clinical Problem Solving.' *British Medical Journal*, Vol 310, pp. 1122–6.

Rosenblatt, RA (2001) 'The Health of Rural People and the Communities and Environments in which They Live', in Geyman, JP, Norris, TE & Hart, LG (eds) *Textbook of Rural Medicine*. New York: McGraw-Hill, p 3–14.

Rubak, S, Sanbaek A, Lauritzen T, Christensen B. (2005) 'Motivational interviewing: a systematic review and meta-analysis.' *British Journal of General Practice*. Vol. 55, pp. 305–312.

Rundall, TG, Shortell, SM, Wang, MC, Casalino, L, Bodenheimer, T, Gillies, RR, *et al.* (2002) 'As Good as it Gets? Chronic Care Management in Nine Leading US Physician Organisations.' *British Medical Journal*, Vol 325, pp. 958–61.

Rural Doctors Association of Australia (RDAA), Australian Local Government Association, Country Women's Association of Australia, Health Consumers of Rural & Remote Australia and the National Farmers Federation of Australia (2004) Good Health to Rural Communities: A Collaborative Policy Document. Accessible at http://www.rdaa.com.au/uploaded_documents/ Good_Health to Rural Communities final.pdf

Russell, MAH, Wilson, C, Taylor, C & Baker, D (1974) 'Effect of General Practitioners' Advice Against Smoking.' *British Medical Journal*, Vol 3, pp. 231–234.

Sackett, DL, Richardson, WS, Rosenberg, W & Haynes, RB (2000) *Evidence-Based Medicine. How to Practice and Teach EBM*. Edinburgh: Churchill Livingstone.

Scheffler, RM, Mahoney, CB, Fulton, BD, Dal Poz, MR & Preker, AS (2009) 'Estimates of health care professional shortages in sub-Saharan Africa by 2015.' *Health Affairs,* Vol 28, pp. w849.

Schlemmer, A (2005) 'Exploring the Effects of a Language Barrier between the Patients and Staff at Hottentots Holland Hospital.' M Fam Med Thesis, Stellenbosch University.

Shai-Mahoko, SN (1996) 'Indigenous Healers in the North West Province: A Survey of Their Clinical Activities in the Rural Areas.' *Curationis*, Vol 19, pp. 31–4.

Shanafelt, TD, Sloan, J A & Habermann, T M (2003) 'The Well-Being of Physicians.' *American Journal of Medicine*, Vol 114, pp. 513–519.

Siegfried N, Muller M, Deeks JJ, Volmink J. (2009) 'Male circumcision for prevention of heterosexual acquisition of HIV in men.' *Cochrane Database Systematic Review*. Apr 15, CD003362. Review.

Siegler, M (1979) 'Clinical Ethics and Clinical Medicine.' *Archives of Internal Medicine*, Vol 139, pp. 914–15.

Silverman, J, Kurtz, S & Draper, J (1998) *Skills for Communicating with Patients*. Abingdon, Oxon, UK: Radcliffe Medical Press.

Skelton, JR, Kai, J & Loudon, RF (2001) 'Cross-cultural Communication in Medicine: Questions for Educators.' *Medical Education*, Vol 35, pp. 257–61.

Smilkstein, G (1978) 'The Family APGAR: A Proposal for a Family Function Test and Use by Physicians.' *Journal of Family Practice*, Vol 6, p 1234.

Smith, JD (2004) *Australia's Rural and Remote Health: A Social Justice Perspective*. Croydon, Vic: Tertiary Press.

Sparks, BLW (1998) 'Micro-ethics of the Consultation.' *Continuing Medical Education*, Vol 16, pp. 846–7.

Speed, C. (2004) ABC of Rheumatology. Low Back Pain. *British Medical Journal,* Vol 328, pp. 1119–1121.

Starfield, B (1994) 'Primary Care Tomorrow: Is Primary Care Essential?' *Lancet*, Vol 344, pp. 1129–1133.

Statistics South Africa (2003) Census 2001. Census in Brief. Pretoria: Statistics South Africa. Accessible at http://www.statssa.gov.za/

Stewart H, Elder A, Gosling R. *Michael Balint: Object Relations Pure and Applied*. London: Routledge, 1996.

Stewart, M, Brown, JB, Weston, WW, McWhinney, IR, McWilliam, CL & Freeman, TR (1995) *Patient-Centred Medicine. Transforming the Clinical Method*. Thousand Oaks, CA: Sage Publications.

Stott, NC & Davis, RH (1979) 'The Exceptional Potential in each Primary Care Consultation.' *Journal of the Royal College of General Practitioners*, Vol 29, pp. 201–205.

Swap CJ & Nagurney JT (2005) 'Value and limitations of chest pain history in the evaluation of patients with suspected acute coronary syndromes.' *Journal of the American American Association*, Vol 294, pp. 2623.

Swartz, L & Dick, J (2002) 'Managing Chronic Disease in Less Developed Countries.' *British Medical Journal*, Vol 325, pp. 914–915.

Thrower, SM, Bruce, WF. & Welton, RF (1982) 'The Family Circle Method for Integrating Family Systems Concepts in Family Medicine.' *Journal of Family Practice*, Vol 15, p 451.

Tollman, SM (1991) 'Community Oriented Primary Care: Origins, Evolution, Applications.' *Social Science Medicine*, Vol 32, No 6, pp. 633–42.

Travis JW & Ryan, R S (2004) *Wellness Workbook*, 3rd Edition, Celestial Arts, Berkeley.

Truter I. (2008) 'A therapeutic approach to coughing.' *Professional Nursing Today*, Vol 12, pp. 37–42.

Tuckett, D, Boulton, M & Olson, C (1985) *Meeting Between Experts: An Approach to Sharing Ideas in Medical Consultation*s. London: Tavistock.

US Preventive Services Task Force (2010) *Guide to Clinical Preventive Services: An Assessment of the Effectiveness of 169 Interventions.* Baltimore: Williams and Wilkins.

Van Rensburg, HCJ (2004) 'The Health Professions and Human Resources for Health – Status, Trends and Core Issues', in Van Rensburg, HCJ (ed) *Health and Health Care in South Africa*. Pretoria: Van Schaik.

Visagie, C & Sapa (2009) *Traditional Healers and Medical Schemes.* Health24 articles, June 2009. Retrieved: July 22, 2011, from: http://www.health24.com/natural/General/17-2898,51174.asp

Wagner EH, Austin BT, Davis C, Hindmarsh M, Schaefer J, Bonomi A. (2001) 'Improving chronic illness care: translating evidence into action.' *Health Affairs.* Vol 20, pp. 64–78.

Wagner, EH & Groves, T (2002) 'Care for Chronic Diseases: The Efficacy of Coordinated and Patient-Centred Care is Established, but Now is the Time to Test its Effectiveness.' *British Medical Journal*, Vol 325, pp. 913–14.

Walensky, RP, (2005) 143LB: '2 Million Years of Life Saved: The Survival Benefit of AIDS Therapy in the United States.' 11th Conference on Retroviruses and Opportunistic Infections (CROI), 8–11 February 2004, San Francisco.

Wallace, EZ (1997) 'Doing the Right Things Right: Is Evidence Based Medicine the Answer?' *Annals of Internal Medicine*, Vol 127, pp. 91–4.

Weed, L (1969) *Medical Records, Medical Education and Patient Care.* Cleveland: Case Western Reserve University.

Whitesman. S. 2008. *The Mind-Body Approach to Medicine Recognises the Consciousness of both Patient and Doctor.* CME, vol. 26, no. 1, pp. 12–16.

WHO (1978) 'Primary Health Care.' *Health for All Series*, No 1. Geneva: WHO.

WHO (1986) *Ottawa Charter for Health Promotion. International Conference on Health Promotion.* Ottawa: World Health Organization.

WHO (2002) *Innovative Care for Chronic Conditions: Building Blocks for Action.* Global Report. World Health Organization.

WHO (2003) *Adherence to Long-Term Therapies: Evidence for Action.* WHO accessed at http://www.who.int/chronic_conditions/adherencereport/en/

WHO (2004) *Integrated Management of Adolescent and Adult Illness. Module: General Principles of Good Chronic Care.* World Health Organization. Accessible at http//www.who.int/3by5/publications/documents/en/generalprinciples082005.pdf

WHO 2007

WHO, UNAIDS. Progress in male circumcision scale-up: country implementation and research update. June 2010 | WHO, UNAIDS http://www.who.int/hiv/pub/malecircumcision/mc_country_progress/en/index.html

WHO/UNICEF (1948) Preamble to the Constitution of the World Health Organization as adopted by the International Health Conference, New York, 19–22 June, 1946; signed on 22 July 1946 by the representatives of 61 States (Official Records of the World Health Organization, No 2, p 100) and entered into force on 7 April 1948.

Wileman L, May C and Chew-Graham CA. Medically unexplained symptoms and the problem of power in the primary care consultation: a qualitative study. Family Practice 2002; 19: 178–182.

Wilkins, R (ed) (1991) *The Doctor's Quotation Book: A Medical Miscellany.* London: Robert Hale Ltd.

Wilkinson, D & Strasser, R (2004) 'Context', in Wilkinson, D, Hays, R, Strasser R & Worley, P (eds) *The Handbook of Rural Medicine in Australia.* Melbourne: Oxford University Press.

Williams, JR (2005) World Medical Association Medical Ethics Manual.

Williams, RL, Flocke, SA, Sysanski, SJ, Mettee, TM & Martin, KB (1995) 'A Practical Tool for Community Oriented Primary Care: Community Diagnosis using a Personal Computer.' *Family Medicine*, Vol 27, pp. 39–43.

Wilson NW, Couper ID, De vries E, Reid S, Fish T & Marais BJ (2009) 'A critical review of interventions to redress the inequitable distribution of healthcare professionals to rural and remote areas.' Rural and Remote Health 9: 1060. (Online) Available from: http://www.rrh.org.au

Winkler, ER (1993) From Kantianism to Contextualism. The Rise and Fall of the Paradigm Theory in Bioethics, in Applied Ethics: A Reader, pp. 343–65. Oxford and Cambridge: Blackwell.

Wonca Working Party on Rural Practice, Health for All Rural People Planning Committee (2003) Creating Unity for Action: An Action

Plan for Rural Health. Monash University School of Rural Health, Traralgon, Victoria.

Wood, B (1993) 'Interpreters in Medical Consultations – a Literature Review.' South African Family Practice, Vol 14, pp. 347–53.

World Health Organisation 2008, World Health Report – Primary Health Care: Now more than ever. World Health Organisation, Geneva.

WORLD HEALTH ORGANIZATION (2010) Increasing access to health workers in remote and rural areas through improved retention: Global Policy Recommendations WHO, Geneva. Available at http://www.who.int/hrh/en/

Zola, K (1973) 'Pathways to the Doctor – from Person to Patient.' Social Science and Medicine, Vol 7, pp. 677.

Index

Page numbers in italics refer to figures and tables.